www.bma.o

ADVANCES IN
SURGICAL PATHOLOGY

GASTRIC CANCER

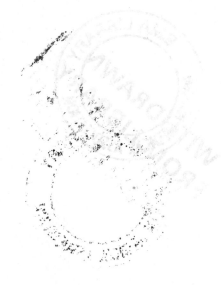

ADVANCES IN SURGICAL PATHOLOGY

GASTRIC CANCER

Dongfeng Tan, MD
Professor
Department of Pathology and Laboratory
  Medicine
University of Texas MD Anderson Cancer Center
Houston, Texas

Gregory Y. Lauwers, MD
Professor
Department of Pathology
Harvard Medical School
Director, Division of Surgical Pathology
Director, Gastrointestinal Pathology Service
Department of Pathology
Massachusetts General Hospital
Boston, Massachusetts

SERIES EDITORS

Philip T. Cagle, MD
Professor of Pathology and Laboratory Medicine
Weill Medical College of Cornell University
New York, New York
Director, Pulmonary Pathology
The Methodist Hospital
Houston, Texas

Timothy Craig Allen, MD, JD
Professor and Chairman
Department of Pathology
The University of Texas Health Sciences
  Center at Tyler
Tyler, Texas

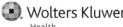
Wolters Kluwer | Lippincott Williams & Wilkins
Health
Philadelphia • Baltimore • New York • London
Buenos Aires • Hong Kong • Sydney • Tokyo

Senior Executive Editor: Jonathan W. Pine, Jr.
Product Manager: Marian A. Bellus
Vendor Manager: Alicia Jackson
Senior Marketing Manager: Angela Panetta
Senior Manufacturing Manager: Benjamin Rivera
Senior Designer: Stephen Druding
Production Service: SPi Technologies

© 2011 LIPPINCOTT WILLIAMS & WILKINS, a WOLTERS KLUWER business
Two Commerce Square
2001 Market Street
Philadelphia, PA 19103 USA
LWW.com

Printed in the People's Republic of China

Library of Congress Cataloging-in-Publication Data

Advances in surgical pathology. Gastric cancer / [edited by] Dongfeng Tan, Gregory Lauwers.
    p. ; cm.
Other title: Gastric cancer
Includes bibliographical references and index.
ISBN 978-1-60831-617-5 (alk. paper)
1. Stomach—Cancer. I. Tan, Dongfeng. II. Lauwers, Gregory. III. Title: Gastric cancer.
[DNLM: 1. Stomach Neoplasms—pathology. WI 320]

RC280.S8A38 2010
616.99'433—dc22

2010033882

Care has been taken to confirm the accuracy of the information presented and to describe generally accepted practices. However, the authors, editors, and publisher are not responsible for errors or omissions or for any consequences from application of the information in this book and make no warranty, expressed or implied, with respect to the currency, completeness, or accuracy of the contents of the publication. Application of the information in a particular situation remains the professional responsibility of the practitioner.

The authors, editors, and publisher have exerted every effort to ensure that drug selection and dosage set forth in this text are in accordance with current recommendations and practice at the time of publication. However, in view of ongoing research, changes in government regulations, and the constant flow of information relating to drug therapy and drug reactions, the reader is urged to check the package insert for each drug for any change in indications and dosage and for added warnings and precautions. This is particularly important when the recommended agent is a new or infrequently employed drug.

Some drugs and medical devices presented in the publication have Food and Drug Administration (FDA) clearance for limited use in restricted research settings. It is the responsibility of the health care provider to ascertain the FDA status of each drug or device planned for use in their clinical practice.

To purchase additional copies of this book, call our customer service department at (800) 638-3030 or fax orders to (301) 223-2320. International customers should call (301) 223-2300.

Visit Lippincott Williams & Wilkins on the Internet: at LWW.com. Lippincott Williams & Wilkins customer service representatives are available from 8:30 am to 6 pm, EST.

10 9 8 7 6 5 4 3 2 1

This book is dedicated to my wife Hong (Helen) Zou, my daughters Connie and Christina, my mother Shubao Tang, and my late father Jiaqi Tan.

Dongfeng Tan, MD, FCAP

This book is dedicated first to my parents, Renée and Maurice Lauwers, for teaching me the value of hard work and for their incredible love and support. Also, I would like to acknowledge the hard work and dedication of all the contributors and also of my assistant, Laura Nakatsuka, who puts up with me and tries to keep me focused. Most of all, I dedicate this book to my wife, Cindy, and my children, Damian, Sean, and Timothy, who always encourage and support me, and bring completeness to my life.

Gregory Y. Lauwers, MD

Series Overview

Expectations for the pathologist practicing today exceed those for pathologists in practice only a few years ago. In addition to the rapid growth of knowledge and new technologies in the field of pathology, recent years have seen the emergence of many trends that significantly impact the traditional practice of pathology including the sub specialized multidisciplinary approach to patient care, personalized therapeutics including targeted molecular therapies and imaging techniques such as endoscopic microscopy, molecular radiology and imaging multimodality theranostics that compete with conventional light microscopy. In order to remain a viable member of the patient care team, the pathologist must keep up with growing knowledge in traditional subjects as well as in new areas of expertise such as molecular testing. Additionally, the pathologist is subject to an increasing number of credentialing requirements and, for those now completing training, Self-Assessment Modules for Maintenance of Certification which require the pathologist to be examined on the recent advances in pathology in order to sustain their qualifications to practice.

Each volume in the new series "Advances in Surgical Pathology" focuses on a specific subject in pathology that has undergone recent advancement in terms of knowledge, technical procedures, application and/or integration as part of current trends in pathology and medicine. Each book includes an accompanying Solution site with a fully searchable online version of the text and image bank. This series of books not only updates the pathologist on recently acquired knowledge but emphasizes the new uses of that knowledge within the context of the changing landscape of pathology practice in the 21st century. Rather than information in a vacuum, the pathologist is educated on how to apply the new knowledge as part of a sub specialized multidisciplinary team and for purposes of personalized patient therapy.

Each volume in the series will be divided into the following Sections: (1) Overview— updates the pathologist on the general topic, including epidemiology, bringing the pathologist generally up-to-date on a topic as a basis for the more specialized sections that follow. (2) Histopathology—reviews histopathology and specific recent changes that warrant more description and more illustration, for example, recently described entities and recent revisions in classifications. This will also emphasize histopathology figures to illustrate recently described entities and to demonstrate the basis for classification changes so that the pathologist is able to understand and recognize these changes. (3) Imaging—reviews the impact of imaging techniques on histopathologic diagnosis and on the practice of pathology. An example of the former is the use of increasingly sensitive high resolution CT scan in the diagnosis of interstitial lung diseases. An example of the latter is the use of multimodality theranostics rather than traditional histopathology for the diagnosis and treatment of lung cancer. Figures linking the radiologic images to the histopathology will be emphasized. (4) Molecular Pathology—a review and update on specific molecular pathology as it applies to specific diseases for the practicing pathologist in regards to molecular diagnostics and molecular therapeutics. An example of the former is the identification of a specific fusion gene to diagnose synovial sarcoma. An example of the latter is the identification of specific EGFR mutations in pulmonary adenocarcinoma and its relationship to treatment with EGFR antagonists. (5) For those volumes dealing with cancers (Lung Cancer, Breast Cancer, Prostate Cancer, Colon Cancer, etc.), additional Sections will include Preneoplastic and Preinvasive Lesions, which will emphasize histopathologic figures and Staging, particularly emphasizing the new staging systems and to illustrate specific problems in staging.

These books will assist the pathologist in daily practice in the modern setting and provide a basis for interacting with other physicians in patient care. They will also provide the timely updates in knowledge that are necessary for daily practice, for current credentialing and for Maintenance of Certification. As such, this series is invaluable to pathologists in practice at all levels of experience who need to keep up with advances for their daily performance and their periodic credentialing and to pathologists-in-training who will apply this knowledge to their boards and their future practice. In the latter case, this series will serve as a useful library for pathology training programs.

Contributors

Shinichi Ban, MD, PhD

Chief
Department of Pathology
Saiseikai Kawaguchi General Hospital
Kawaguchi, Japan

Annie On On Chan, MD

Gastroenterology and Hepatology Centre
The Hong Kong Sanatorium & Hospital
Hong Kong

Wei Feng, MD

Instructor
Department of Pathology and Laboratory
    Medicine
University of Texas Medical School at Houston
Houston, Texas
Pathologist, Pathology Lab
North Cypress Medical Center
Cypress, Texas

Masashi Fukayama, MD, PhD

Professor, Chairman
Departments of Pathology and Diagnostic
    Pathology
Graduate School of Medicine
The University of Tokyo
Chief
Department of Diagnostic Pathology
Tokyo University Hospital
Tokyo, Japan

Robert M. Genta, MD, DTM&H

Clinical Professor of Pathology and Medicine
    (Gastroenterology)
Department of Pathology and Medicine
University of Texas Southwestern Medical Center
Dallas, Texas
Chief, Academic Affairs
Caris Life Sciences
Irving, Texas

Mahmoud Goodarzi, MD

Attending Pathologist
Caris Diagnostics, a division of Caris Life Sciences
Newton, Massachusetts

Abha Goyal, MD, PhD

GI Pathology Fellow
Department of Pathology
University of Pennsylvania
Philadelphia, Pennsylvania

David Y. Graham, MD

Professor of Medicine and Molecular Virology and
    Microbiology
Department of Medicine
Baylor College of Medicine
Michael E. DeBakey VA Medical Center
Houston, Texas

Hye Seung Han, MD, PhD

Associate Professor
Department of Pathology
Konkuk University School of Medicine
Konkuk University Medical Center
Seoul, Korea

Rumi Hino, MD

Department of Pathology
Graduate School of Medicine
University of Tokyo
Tokyo, Japan

Zhiwei Huang, PhD

Assistant Professor
Division of Bioengineering
Faculty of Engineering
National University of Singapore
Singapore, Republic of Singapore

Woo Ho Kim, MD, PhD

Professor
Department of Pathology
Seoul National University College of Medicine
Seoul National University Hospital
Seoul, Korea

Shawn Kinsey, MD

Gastrointestinal Pathologist
Department of Pathology
Caris Life Sciences
Irwing, Texas

Hiroto Kita, MD, PhD

Professor, Director
Department of Gastroenterology
International Medical Center
Saitama Medical University
Hidaka, Saitama, Japan

Richard H. Lash, MD

Chief Medical Officer
Department of Pathology
Caris Life Sciences
Irwing, Texas

Gregory Y. Lauwers, MD

Professor
Department of Pathology
Harvard Medical School
Director, Division of Surgical Pathology
Director, Gastrointestinal Pathology Service
Department of Pathology
Massachusetts General Hospital
Boston, Massachusetts

John J. Liang, MD, PhD

Assistant Professor
Department of Pathology
Penn State University Medical Center
Hershey, Pennsylvania

Mikhail Lisovsky, MD, PhD

Assistant Professor
Department of Pathology
Dartmouth Medical School
Hanover, New Hampshire
Staff Pathologist
Department of Pathology
Dartmouth Hitchcock Medical Center
Lebanon, New Hampshire

Koji Nagata, MD, PhD

Assistant Professor
Department of Pathology
Saitama Medical University
Staff, Department of Pathology
International Medical Center
Hidaka, Saitama, Japan

Min En Nga, MBBS, FRCPath, FRCPA

Assistant Professor
Department of Pathology
National University of Singapore
Consultant Pathologist
Department of Pathology
National University Hospital
Singapore, Republic of Singapore

Donato Nitti, MD

Full Professor
Department of Oncological and Surgical Sciences
University of Padova
Chief, Department of Surgery
University Hospital of Padova
Padova, Italy

Do Youn Park, MD, PhD

Associate Professor
Department of Pathology
Pusan National University School of Medicine
Associate Pathologist
Department of Pathology
Pusan National University Hospital
Busan, Republic of Korea

Madhavi Patnana, MD

Assistant Professor
Department of Diagnostic Radiology
University of Texas MD Anderson Cancer Center
Houston, Texas

William Payne, MD

Attending Pathologist
Fort Worth Pathology
Fort Worth, Texas

Asif Rashid, MBBS, PhD

Professor
Department of Pathology
University of Texas MD Anderson Cancer Center
Houston, Texas

Guido Rindi, MD, PhD

Full Professor of Pathology
Institute of Anatomic Pathology
Università Cattolica del Sacro Cuore (UCSC)
Head, Histopathology and Cytodiagnostic Service
Department of Microbiological, Molecular and
    Morphological Diagnostics and Haematology
Policlinico Gemelli
Roma, Italy

Massimo Rugge, MD, FACG

Department of Diagnostic Sciences & Special
    Therapies
Pathology Unit
University of Padova, Italy
Professor of Medicine (non-tenure)
Department of Gastroenterology VA Medical Center
Baylor College of Medicine
Houston, Texas
Department of Pathology
Padova Teaching Hospital
Padova, Italy

Antonia R. Sepulveda, MD, PhD

Professor
Department of Pathology and Laboratory
    Medicine
University of Pennsylvania
Director
Surgical Pathology Fellowship
Hospital of the University of Pennsylvania
Philadelphia, Pennsylvania

Michio Shimizu, MD, PhD

Professor
Department of Pathology
Saitama Medical University
Chief
Department of Pathology
International Medical Center
Hidaka, Saitama, Japan

Aya Shinozaki, MD

Department of Pathology
Graduate School of Medicine
University of Tokyo
Tokyo, Japan

Enrico Solcia, MD

Professor Pathological Anatomy
Department of Pathology and Genetics
University of Pavia
Consultant
Department of Pathology
IRCCS Fondazione Policlinico San Matteo
Pavia, Italy

Amitabh Srivastava, MD

Assistant Professor
Department of Pathology
Dartmouth Medical School
Staff Pathologist
Department of Pathology
Dartmouth Hitchcock Medical Center
Lebanon, New Hampshire

Sanford A. Stass, MD

Professor and Chairman
Department of Pathology
University of Maryland School of Medicine
Director
Pathology Laboratories
University of Maryland Medical Center
Baltimore, Maryland

Dongfeng Tan, MD

Professor
Department of Pathology and Laboratory
    Medicine
University of Texas MD Anderson Cancer
    Center
Houston, Texas

Ming Teh, MD, FRCPath

Head/Associate Professor
Department of Pathology
Yong Loo Lin School of Medicine
National University of Singapore
Chief/Senior Consultant
Department of Pathology
National University Hospital
Singapore, Republic of Singapore

**Thomas Paulraj Thamboo, MBChB,
FRCPath, FRCPA**

Assistant Professor
Department of Pathology
National University of Singapore
Consultant
Department of Pathology
National University Hospital
Singapore, Republic of Singapore

Raghunandan Vikram, MD

Assistant Professor
Department of Radiology
MD Anderson Cancer Center
Houston, Texas

Shengle Zhang, MD, PhD

Associate Professor
Department of Pathology
SUNY Upstate Medical University
Attending Pathologist
Director of Anatomic Molecular Pathology
    Laboratories
Department of Pathology
SUNY Upstate Medical University
    Hospital
Syracuse, New York

X. Frank Zhao, MD, PhD

Associate Professor
Department of Pathology
University of Maryland
College Park, Maryland

Preface

The past decade has seen rapid growth of knowledge and new technologies in the field of pathology of gastric cancer. The emerging information have significantly affected the traditional practice of pathology, including the subspecialized multidisciplinary approach to patient care and personalized treatments such as targeted molecular therapy, which is based on molecular diagnostics and advanced imaging. To remain viable members of the cancer patient care team, pathologists must keep up with the growing knowledge not only about traditional subject areas such as differential diagnosis of varied gastric neoplasms and tumor classifications but also the emerging areas of molecular diagnostics and personalized medicine.

This book, *Advances in Surgical Pathology: Gastric Cancer,* provides a concise, updated review of the pathologic characteristics of gastric cancer, with an emphasis on exploring practical issues and recent developments. Gastric cancer is a disease whose management requires a multidisciplinary approach in which pathology plays a key role. Individual chapters have been written by international experts in the fields of pathology, gastrointestinal medical oncology, cancer epidemiology, and gastrointestinal radiology, and they address the fundamental issues surrounding gastric cancer, including its epidemiology, basic diagnostic features, differential diagnoses, pitfalls and complications, and treatments.

The book consists of 6 sections and 22 chapters. Although the chapters follow a sequence from pathogenesis to therapy, each chapter stands alone in its treatment of the subject matter. Section I updates the reader about the general topic and provides a basis for the more specialized sections that follow. Cancer stem cells and the interaction between genetics and environmental factors in gastric cancer carcinogenesis are emphasized. Section II is devoted to the histopathology of gastric cancer. It reviews specific recent changes that warrant more description and more illustration than are given in the overview. In particular, figures are used to illustrate recently described entities and demonstrate the basis for classification changes so that the pathologist is able to understand and recognize these changes. Section III discusses the significance of updated imaging techniques on histopathologic diagnosis and on the practice of pathology. Endoscopic evaluation and histology correlation are emphasized. Section IV reviews and updates data on molecular pathology of gastric cancer, molecular diagnostics, and molecular cancer prognosis assessment as well as personalized medicine and targeted therapy in management of gastric cancer. Emphasis is placed on critical molecules as special treatment targets, particularly genes/DNA, RNA, proteins/antibodies, and nanoparticles. Section V reviews the gastric cancer staging systems and impact of radiological imaging on gastric cancer staging. Specific challenges and problems in staging are discussed. Section VI discusses preneoplastic and preinvasive lesions of gastric cancer. Pathological features, differential diagnosis, patient screening, and cancer prevention are emphasized.

The book is intended to assist the pathologist in daily practice and provide a basis for interacting with other physicians in patient care with the ultimate goal that pathologist take a central role not only in the diagnosis of patients but their clinical management as well. It provides timely updates in knowledge that are necessary for the modern setting and for continued medical education. As such, the book is invaluable to pathologists in practice at all levels of experience and to pathologists-in-training who can apply this knowledge to their boards and their future practice. We are delighted that we were able to recruit the many outstanding contributors who have presented their areas of expertise in the book. In many cases, this has required more time and effort than they initially antici- pated, and we are grateful for their dedicated commitment. We have been also gratefully assisted and encouraged by the professionals of the publisher, such as Jonathan Pine, a senior executive editor at LWW, Marian Bellus, the book project manager and Anoop Kumar at SPi, among many others.

Dongfeng Tan, MD
Gregory Y Lauwers, MD

Contents

SECTION IV. Molecular Pathology

SECTION V. Staging

SECTION VI. Preneoplastic and Preinvasive Lesions

ADVANCES IN
SURGICAL PATHOLOGY

GASTRIC
CANCER

Introduction

Introduction to the Normal Histology and Physiology of the Stomach

1

▶ William Payne

▶ Dongfeng Tan

INTRODUCTION

Understanding the normal anatomy and physiology of the stomach is vitally important in diagnosing disease. Without an accurate understanding of the normal structure and function of the stomach, both at the microscopic and macroscopic levels, it can be difficult to reliably recognize a pathologic condition. This chapter outlines the basic normal gastric anatomy, histology, and physiology.

EMBRYOLOGY

The stomach develops from the caudal aspect of the foregut. Starting around the fourth week after conception, the dorsal border grows faster than the ventral border, creating the lesser and greater curvatures. As the stomach grows, it rotates 90 degrees clockwise, with the ventral border rotating to become the lesser curvature and the dorsal border becoming the greater curvature. In addition, the cranial end moves to the left and the caudal end to the right. The endoderm of the primordial gut forms most of the mucosa of the digestive system. The splanchnic mesenchyme develops into most of the muscle, connective tissue, and associated surrounding soft tissue.[1]

ANATOMY

The stomach lies anterior to the pancreas and extends from just below the diaphragm to its junction with the duodenum. The stomach is surrounded by a rich vascular and neural network, which controls both the secretory action of the stomach and its muscular contractions. The stomach is divided into four main anatomic regions: the cardia, fundus, body (corpus), and antrum. The cardia receives the food from the esophagus, is located just distal to the esophagus, and extends past the esophagus by a few centimeters. The fundus is formed by the left superior aspect of the stomach, which lies under the left diaphragm, and is limited inferiorly by a horizontal line drawn to the left of the incisura cardiaca. The body (corpus) is the largest anatomic region of the stomach, is located between the fundus and antrum, and is bound inferiorly by a line passing from the incisura angularis (on the lesser curvature) to the greater curvature. Distal to the body lies the pyloric antrum, which extends distally to the sulcus intermedius, after which the stomach becomes the pyloric canal. When the stomach is in a nondistended state, prominent rugae (folds) are present on the mucosal surface and are most prominent in the gastric body. As the stomach dilates, these rugae become less apparent.[2]

The stomach is richly vascularized; blood is supplied primarily along the lesser curvature by the left and right gastric arteries and along the greater curvature by the right and left gastroepiploic arteries. In addition, blood is supplied to parts of the fundus and body along the greater curvature by the short gastric arteries. The gastric arteries have many arterial anastomoses, which help to ensure an adequate blood supply and make the stomach more resilient to vascular damage than other parts of the gastrointestinal (GI) system.[2,3] While the venous drainage is much more variable than the arterial supply, the stomach drains venous blood through veins named similarly to the corresponding arteries. The venous system drains into the hepatic portal vein, which in turn drains into the liver.[2]

The lymphatic drainage pattern of the stomach is important, especially in gastric cancers. Lymphatics are present in the lamina propria and the submucosa. They drain through the muscle into the deeper layers of the stomach.[4] While the patterns of drainage do vary somewhat, the drainage patterns tend to follow the course of the arteries and veins. The gastric lymphatics drain in four main drainage patterns, approximately as follows: the proximal aspect of the body and fundus, along the great curvature, drains into the left gastroepiploic and splenic nodes, while the inferior half of the body and the pyloris along the greater curvature drain to the right gastroepiploic nodes and the subpyloric nodes. The body, fundus, and cardia along the lesser curvature drain to the left gastric nodes. The pylorus along the lesser curvature drains to the right gastric, hepatic, suprapyloric, and right superior pancreatic nodes. The lymphatic system from the different gastric areas then drains into the celiac nodes.[3,5,6]

HISTOLOGY AND PHYSIOLOGY

The stomach is made of several distinct functional layers: the mucosa, the submucosa, the muscularis propria, and the serosa. The mucosa comprises three layers: the epithelium; the underlying lamina propria, which is separated from the epithelium by a basement membrane and consists of loose connective tissue, including fibroblasts, histiocytes, and varying amounts of lymphoid cells; and the muscularis mucosae, which consists of thin layers of smooth muscle. The submucosa lies underneath the mucosa and contains blood vessels and nerves, including Meissner plexus. The muscularis propria consists of large bundles of smooth muscle that are arranged in perpendicular patterns to assist peristalsis. The stomach is unique compared to other GI organs in that it has three (vs. two) layers of smooth muscle. The innermost layer is the inner oblique layer, which is unique to the stomach, next is the middle circular layer, and last is the outer longitudinal layer. Auerbach plexus (myenteric plexus) is located between the inner circular and the outer longitudinal layers. Surrounding the stomach is a serosal layer.[7,8]

Roughly corresponding to, but not strictly adhering to, the anatomic regions of the stomach, the type of mucosa varies depending on its location. The cardiac mucosa is located in the proximal stomach, adjacent to the gastroesophageal junction. The border between the esophageal and gastric junction, while irregular, has a rather sharp histologic transition. Distal to the cardiac mucosa, fundic-type mucosa lines both the fundus and the body (corpus). At the most distal end of the stomach is the pyloric-type mucosa (sometimes referred to as antral-type mucosa).[7,8] This mucosa extends proximally in a triangular pattern, with the tip of the triangle extending further along the lesser curvature than the greater curvature.[9] The transition from the pyloric to the fundic mucosa can occur histologically over a 1- to 2-cm region and is less well defined than other histologic transitions, with features of both pyloric and fundic mucosa present.[6]

Lymphoid Elements

Small primary follicles can occasionally be seen within the normal stomach. However, secondary follicles (with germinal centers) should not be present in the normal stomach. Other lymphoid elements such as the occasional lymphocyte, plasma cell, and mast cell can also be present in the normal stomach.[6]

Neural Control

The autonomic nervous system helps to control the movement of the stomach. Auerbach plexus primarily controls gastric motility and is located between the inner circular and outer longitudinal layers of the muscularis propria. Meissner plexus (submucosal plexus) primarily controls regional blood flow and gastric secretions. While the enteric system can act independently of external neural stimulus, it is innervated by the autonomic nervous system, which can stimulate or inhibit it.[10]

Foveolae (Gastric Pits)

Mucous-secreting cells line the surface of the stomach and extend into invaginations of the gastric mucosa called gastric pits. The gastric glands lie beneath the gastric pits and open into them. While the entire surface of the stomach is lined with foveolar epithelium, its appearance (depth of gastric pits, thickness of foveolae) varies depending on the location.[7]

Fundic Mucosa

The majority of the stomach is lined with fundic mucosa, and the fundic glands perform the majority of the secretory work of the stomach. Both the fundus and the body are lined with fundic-type mucosa. The surface epithelium is made up of gastric pits, which extend into the upper one fourth of the epithelium (the fundic mucosa has the shortest gastric pits of the gastric mucosa) and contain mucous-secreting cells that serve many functions, including acting as a protective barrier and providing lubrication. Beneath this layer lie the gastric glands, which contain parietal (oxyntic), peptic (chief or zymogenic), mucous neck, neuroendocrine, and stem cells in varying proportions. These gastric glands appear as relatively straight, tubular glands that empty into the gastric pits above them and are subdivided into the isthmus, neck, and base regions, as the glands progress deeper into the mucosa (Fig. 1-1). Within the isthmus region, there are mucous neck cells and a few neuroendocrine cells, especially enterochromaffin and enterochromaffin-like cells. In the neck region, there are mucous neck, stem, parietal, and neuroendocrine cells. The base region contains primarily chief cells, occasional parietal cells, and some neuroendocrine cells.[7,8] The cells within the fundic mucosa have varying lifespan, with the surface mucous cells only lasting 3 days and the mucous neck cells lasting 1 week. The other cell types typically have a longer lifespan, with the parietal, chief, and enteroendocrine cells lasting several years.[5]

Pyloric Mucosa

In contrast to the fundic mucosa, the gastric pits in the pyloric mucosa are deeper, occupying approximately the upper third to the upper half of the mucosa,[8] and the foveolae are spread

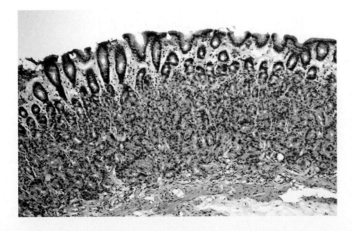

FIGURE 1-1 Gastric fundic (body) mucosa. Note the shallow gastric pits and the more linear gastric glands.

FIGURE 1-2 Gastric pyloric (antral) mucosa. The gastric pits are relatively shallow and the antral glands are heavily branched and coiled (in comparison with the gastric body).

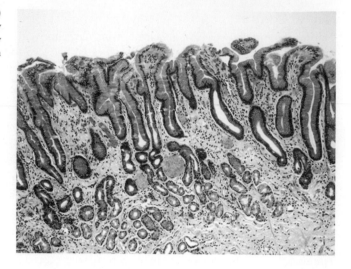

further apart than in the cardiac mucosa. The gastric pits are lined with mucous-secreting cells. The pyloric glands are heavily branched and coiled, in contrast to the relatively straight, tubular glands in the fundus (Fig. 1-2). While the pyloric glands contain cells types similar to those found in the fundic mucosa, their proportions are vastly different, with the pyloric glands beneath the pits lined predominantly with mucous cells and only the occasional peptic cells and rare parietal cells. In addition to neutral mucin,[5] these cells secrete a small amount of pepsinogen. Varying types of neuroendocrine cells are present in the pylorus, including "G" cells, which secrete gastrin, and other neuroendocrine cells, such as "D" cells, which secrete somatostatin.[10]

Cardiac Mucosa

The cardiac glands resemble the pyloric glands, with only minor differences, and contain the same basic cell types as the pyloric mucosa.[5] Mucous-secreting cells predominate, but some parietal and chief cells are also present. The depth of the cardiac gastric pits is variable, but the pits are generally deeper than the pyloric gastric pits and can be up to 50% of the depth of the cardiac epithelium (Fig. 1-3). The cardiac glands range in shape from simple tubular to compound, branched tubular glands but, in general, are less compact than the pyloric glands, with more lamina propria.[2] In normal gastric cardiac mucosa, the glands also occasionally have cystic dilation. While there is some debate as to the extent of the cardiac mucosa in the normal stomach

FIGURE 1-3 Gastric cardiac mucosa taken adjacent to the gastroesophageal junction. Note the variable depth of the gastric pits and the similarity to antral mucosa.

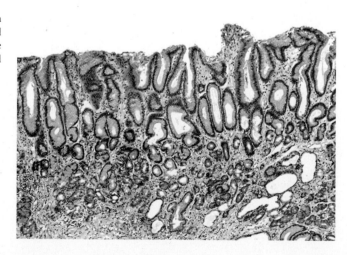

(and whether or not it even exists), studies have suggested that cardiac mucosa is found in the normal stomach, but in small and variable amounts.[6,11]

MUCOSAL CELL TYPES AND THEIR FUNCTIONS

Mucous-Secreting Cells

On the surface of the epithelium, the mucous-secreting cells secrete a protective layer of mucin, which is thick and adheres to the surface epithelium. These cells are high columnar cells and contain abundant mucin. Bicarbonate ions are secreted and trapped within this mucous layer, helping to neutralize gastric acid and protecting the underlying epithelium.[12] Additionally, the mucous serves a lubricating function.

Mucous Neck Cells

The mucous neck cells are present within the gastric glands, predominantly in the neck and isthmus, and bear some resemblance to the superficial mucous-secreting cells. They contain fewer cytoplasmic mucin granules and are more cuboidal than the surface mucous cells. The mucous neck cells are derived from stem cells and help to replace the mucosa.[5]

Parietal Cells

The parietal (oxyntic) cells are pyramidal in shape and have an eosinophilic cytoplasm (because of the abundant mitochondria), with a centrally located nucleus, and they secrete gastric acid and intrinsic factor[7](Fig. 1-4). The gastric acid is produced by a hydrogen/potassium transmembrane ATPase, causing the secretion of HCl. Intrinsic factor is needed for vitamin B_{12} absorption in the ileum. In chronic autoimmune gastritis, which can destroy the parietal cells, reduced levels of HCl and intrinsic factor can cause achlorhydria and pernicious anemia.[10]

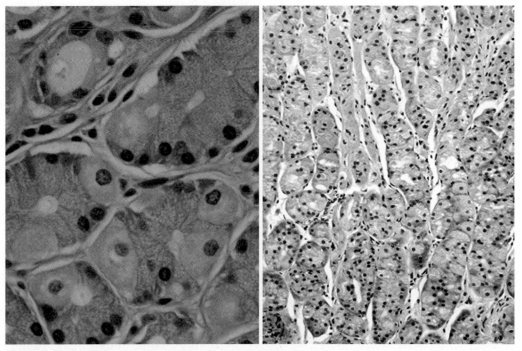

FIGURE 1-4 Fundic glands. The parietal cells are more pink and pyramidal in shape, compared with the basophilic chief cells (**left**). The linearity of the glands is evident, with more basophilic chief cells located at the base and more parietal cells at the surface (**right**).

Chief Cells

The chief (peptic or zymogenic) cells have a more basophilic granular cytoplasm (because of the abundant rough endoplasmic reticulum) and basally located nuclei (Fig. 1-4). These cells make up the majority of the cells at the base of the fundic glands. Pepsinogen is manufactured within these cells and then stored in secretory granules. Upon stimulation of the chief cells, pepsinogen is released into the gastric lumen. When it is exposed to an acidic pH (and pepsin), the pepsinogen is converted into pepsin. Pepsin is active in a highly acidic environment and loses most of its activity as the pH rises.[10] Chief cells also secrete rennin and gastric lipase.[7]

Enteroendocrine Cells

The enteroendocrine cells are typically found at the base of the gastric glands, but their location can vary.[8] They are pleomorphic cells with irregular nuclei and a granular cytoplasm but are not always readily apparent on routinely analyzed (hematoxylin-and-eosin stained) tissue sections. By immunohistochemistry, however, the enteroendocrine cells are immunopositive for endocrine markers, such as chromogranin, synaptophysin, and CD57. These immunohistochemical markers are commonly used in histologic diagnosis and differentiation diagnosis of neuroendocrine neoplasms (Fig. 1-5).

While there are over 13 different enteroendocrine cell types throughout the GI system, the ones found in the stomach include the "A" (secrete glucagon), "D" (secrete somatostatin), enterochromaffin "EC" (secrete serotonin), enterochromaffin-like "ECL" (secrete histamine), "G" (secrete gastrin), "GL" (secrete glicentin), and "VIP" (secrete vasoactive intestinal peptide) cells. These cells release their secretions (hormones) into the lamina propria, where they either act in the immediate area (paracrine) or travel to act on the vascular system (endocrine).

Physiologically, gastrin is one of the most important gastric hormones, which is primarily produced by G cells in the pyloric glands (Fig. 1-6). It is released in response to physical and chemical stimuli. It travels to the enterochromaffin cells within the body of the stomach, which release histamine into the deep glands of the gastric body, causing release of gastric acid by the parietal cells. Gastrin also acts directly on the parietal cells to induce the release of gastric acid.[5] Gastrin also causes pepsinogen secretion by the chief cells[10] and increases gastric motility. Somatostatin and an acidic environment inhibit gastrin. Gastrin is the main hormone that increases the activity of the stomach, although many other hormones, including cholecystokinin, secretin, and gastric inhibitory peptide, reduce either the gastric motility or the secretion of gastric acid.

FIGURE 1-5 Scattered enteroendocrine cells, highlighted by chromogranin immunostain, among the oxyntic glands.

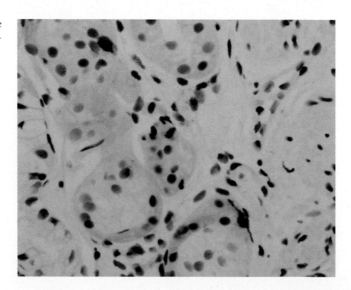

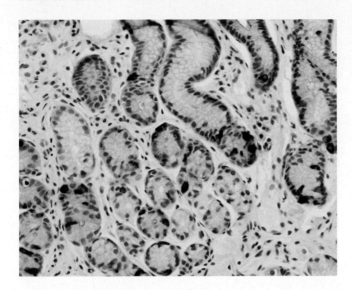

FIGURE 1-6 "G" cells, gastrin-producing cells in the pyloric/antral mucosa, are highlighted by immunostaining of gastrin.

Stem Cells

The stem cells are thought to be located in the middle portion of the gastric glands and to migrate up or down the glands as they mature. A wide variety of stem cells has been reported to exist within the GI system. Stem cells and cancer have become a hot topic in recent years.[13–16]

To detect a possible "stemness" signature, a group of French investigators applied a data integration algorithm from several DNA microarray datasets generated by the Stem Cell Genome Anatomy Project (SCGAP) Consortium to several mouse and human tissues to generate a cross-organism compendium that they submitted to a single-layer artificial neural network trained to attribute differentiation labels to the cells, which ranged from totipotent stem cells to differentiated ones.[13] The authors showed that the inherent architecture of the system allowed the study of the biology behind the different stages of stem cell differentiation, and the artificial neural network isolated a 63-gene "stemness" signature. Currently, all data and source code of the Stem Cell characterization by Artificial Neural Networks (SCANN) project are available on the SourceForge Web site (http://scann.sourceforge.net).

A study using in vivo cell lineage tracing indicated that Lgr5 was expressed in the stomach and suggested that Lgr5 (+ve) cells were stomach stem cells.[14] In particular, in neonates, Lgr5 was expressed in both the prospective corpus and pyloric glands. In contrast, in the adult, Lgr5 was predominantly restricted to the mature pyloric glands. In an in vitro cell culture system, single Lgr5 (+ve) cells efficiently generated long-lived organoids resembling mature pyloric epithelium. Lineage tracing revealed that the Lgr5 (+ve) cells were self-renewing, multipotent stem cells responsible for the long-term renewal of the gastric epithelium.

Studies with *Helicobacter felis*–infected mice have shown that bone marrow–derived cells can repopulate the gastric epithelium and progress to cancer.[15] A recent study further demonstrated that bone marrow–derived mesenchymal stem cells (MSCs) expressing cytokeratin 19 (K19) contribute to the development and differentiation of gastric epithelium.[13] In that study, MSC cultures were established from whole bone marrow, and expression of K19 was detected in a minority (1 of 13) of clones by real-time polymerase chain reaction analysis and immunostaining. Transfection of a K19-green fluorescent protein (GFP) vector and isolation of GFP-expressing colonies generated high K19-expressing MSC clones (K19GFPMSCs). Incubation of MSCs with gastric tissue extract markedly induced the mRNA expression of gastric phenotypic markers, and this effect was observed to a greater extent in K19GFPMSCs than in parental MSCs or mock transfectants. Both K19GFPMSCs and GFP-labeled control MSCs gave rise to gastric epithelial cells after injection into the murine stomach. It is of interest to note that after blastocyst injections,

K19GFPMSCs gave rise to GFP-positive gastric epithelial cells in all 13 pups, whereas only 3 of 10 offspring showed GFP-positive gastric epithelial cells after injection of GFP-labeled control MSCs. Although K19 expression could not be detected in murine whole bone marrow, *H. felis* infection increased the number of K19-expressing MSCs in the circulation. Therefore, the K19-positive MSC fraction that is induced by chronic *H. felis* infection appears to be the important subset in this process.

Cancer stem cells (CSCs) are a unique subpopulation that possesses the capacity to repopulate tumors, drive malignant progression, and mediate chemoresistance.[16] Stem cell markers, such as CD44 and nestin, are used in CSCs studies.

References

1. Moore KL, Persaud TVN, Torchia MG. *Before we are born: essentials of embryology and birth defects.* 7th ed. Philadelphia, PA: Saunders/Elsevier; 2008:x, 353.
2. Standring S, Gray H. *Gray's anatomy: the anatomical basis of clinical practice.* 40th ed. Edinburgh, UK: Churchill Livingstone/Elsevier; 2008:xxiv, 1551.
3. Netter FH. *Atlas of human anatomy.* 4th ed. Philadelphia, PA: Saunders/Elsevier; 2006: 47,548.
4. Listrom MB, Fenoglio-Preiser CM. Lymphatic distribution of the stomach in normal, inflammatory, hyperplastic, and neoplastic tissue. *Gastroenterology.* 1987;93(3):506–514.
5. Fenoglio-Preiser CM. *Gastrointestinal pathology: an atlas and text.* 3rd ed. Philadelphia, PA: Wolters Kluwers/Lippincott Williams & Wilkins; 2008:xiii, 1296.
6. Mills SE. *Histology for pathologists.* 3rd ed. Philadelphia, PA: Lippincott Williams & Wilkins; 2007:xi, 1272.
7. Gartner LP, Hiatt JL. *Color textbook of histology.* 3rd ed. Philadelphia, PA: Saunders/Elsevier; 2007:xi, 573.
8. Young B. *Wheater's functional histology: a text and colour atlas.* 5th ed. Edinburgh: Churchill Livingstone/ Elsevier; 2006:x, 437.
9. Stave R, Brandtzaeg P, Nygaard K, et al. The transitional body-antrum zone in resected human stomachs. Anatomical outline and parietal-cell and gastrin-cell characteristics in peptic ulcer disease. *Scand J Gastroenterol.* 1978;13(6):685–691.
10. Guyton AC, Hall JE. *Textbook of medical physiology.* 10th ed. Philadelphia, PA: Saunders; 2000: xxxii, 1064.
11. Derdoy JJ, Bergwerk A, Cohen H, et al. The gastric cardia: to be or not to be? *Am J Surg Pathol.* 2003;27(4):499–504.
12. Allen A, Flemstrom G. Gastroduodenal mucus bicarbonate barrier: protection against acid and pepsin. *Am J Physiol Cell Physiol.* 2005;288(1):C1–C19.
13. Bidaut G, Stoeckert CJ Jr. Large scale transcriptome data integration across multiple tissues to decipher stem cell signatures. *Methods Enzymol.* 2009;467:229–245.
14. Barker N, Huch M, Kujala P, et al. Lgr5(+ve) stem cells drive self-renewal in the stomach and build long-lived gastric units in vitro. *Cell Stem Cell.* 2010;6(1):25–36.
15. Okumura T, Wang SS, Takaishi S, et al. Identification of a bone marrow-derived mesenchymal progenitor cell subset that can contribute to the gastric epithelium. *Lab Invest.* 2009;89(12):1410–1422. [Epub Oct 19, 2009]
16. Dhingra S, Feng W, Zhou D, et al. Expression of stem cell markers in human gastric adenocarcinoma and non-neoplastic gastric mucosa: a study of 209 cases. *Mod Pathol.* 2010;23(1):142–143.

Epidemiology of Gastric Carcinoma

2

▶ Woo Ho Kim

DEMOGRAPHIC FEATURES

Gastric carcinoma is a malignancy that arises from the gastric mucosa, and its incidence and mortality rates have fallen dramatically over the past 70 years.[1] However, despite these dramatic declines, stomach cancer is the fourth most prevalent cancer and the second most common cause of cancer death worldwide.[2] Approximately 880,000 people were diagnosed with gastric cancer, and approximately 700,000 succumbed to the disease annually worldwide.[3]

Sixty percent of gastric cancer cases occur in developing countries. Incidence rates are highest in Eastern Asia, the Andean region of South America, and Eastern Europe, whereas incidence rates are lowest in North America and Northern Europe. The majority of countries in Africa and Southeast Asia have low incidence rates. There is a >20-fold difference in the incidence rates between regions with high incidence rates, such as Korea or Japan, and those with low incidence rates, such as North America. Furthermore, the mortality rates follow the same trends as the incidence rates (Fig. 2 1).[4]

To compare the gastric cancer incidence rates in different nations or regions, age-standardized incidence rates (ASRs) and cumulative incidence rates (CRs) until the age of 64 or 74 are commonly used. Between 1998 and 2002, the Yamagata and Miyagi prefectures in Japan had the highest incidence rates in the world (Table 2-1),[4] with an ASR for men of 70 to 80/100,000 and an ASR for women of around 30/100,000. In addition, the CRs up to 74 years of age for men were 9.4% to 9.7% and for women 3.3% to 3.5%. The areas with the second highest incidence rates were also in Japan and Korea. The populations that show the lowest gastric cancer incidences are whites in the United States, Indians, and Kuwaitis. Gastric cancer incidence rates in the low-incidence regions are approximately 1/10 to 1/14 that of the high-incidence regions, with ASRs of 2 to 7/100,000 for men and 1 to 4/100,000 for women.

The reported decline in the incidence of gastric carcinoma since 1968 is dramatic in low-incidence countries (Table 2-2). However, declines in high-incidence countries, such as Japan and Chile, have been negligible, which has increased the gap between incidence rates in low- and high-incidence countries.

In the 1930s, gastric cancer was the most common cause of cancer death in the United States and Europe. The decline in gastric carcinoma in the United States since World War II is demonstrated by the following age-adjusted mortality rates for white males: 16.3 per 100,000 between 1950 and 1969 and 7.33 per 100,000 between 1970 and 1994. In fact, in the 50 years following 1950, the incidence of gastric cancer decreased by 60% in Western Europe and North America. A comparison of gastric cancer risk in 34 European countries over the period between 1975 and 2004 revealed that gastric cancer mortality rates decreased continuously in all European nations. From 1990–1994 to 2000–2004, gastric cancer mortality rates in European nations declined from 14.1 to 9.9/100,000 in men and from 6.4 to 4.5/100,000 in women, and this steady fall in gastric cancer mortality rates has persisted in recent years. During the period 2000 to 2004, the highest mortality rate among European nations was in Belarus (29.3/100,000 in men;

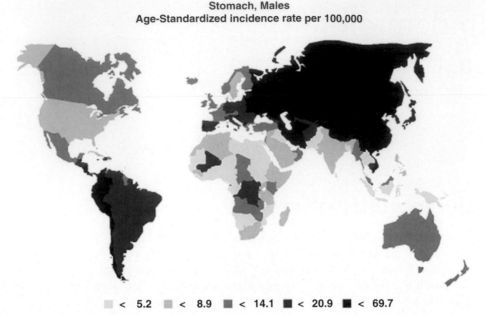

Stomach, Males
Age-Standardized incidence rate per 100,000

■ < 5.2 ■ < 8.9 ■ < 14.1 ■ < 20.9 ■ < 69.7

FIGURE 2-1 Age-standardized incidence rate per 100,000 of gastric cancer in male (estimate at the year of 2002). (*Source*: Ferlay J, Bray F, Pisani P, et al. GLOBOCAN 2002: Cancer incidence, mortatity and prevalence wordwide. Lyon: IARC Press; 2004.)

11.5/100,000 in women). The lowest incidence areas were Switzerland, France, and the Nordic countries (5–6/100,000 in men). England and Wales had a temporal decline in noncardia gastric cancer incidence, which fell from 8.5 to 4.1/100,000 in men and from 3.8 to 1.9/100,000 in women between 1971 and 1998. A further decrease of at least 24% in the incidence of noncardia

Table 2-1	Geographic variation of age-adjusted gastric carcinoma incidence rates per 100,000 in men	
Area		**Incidence**
High incidence		
Japan, Yamagata Prefecture		91.4
Japan, Miyagi Prefecture		83.2
Korea, Busan		72.5
Intermediate incidence		
China, Shanghai		46.5
Belarus		46.8
Low incidence		
United States, Utah		4.7
India, Bombay		6.5
Non-Kuwaitis in Kuwait		2.4

Source: Ferlay J, Bray F, Pisani P, et al. *GLOBOCAN 2002: Cancer incidence, mortality and prevalence worldwide*. Lyon: IARC Press; 2004.

Table 2-2	Temporal trends in gastric carcinoma incidence rates (age-standardized rate) in men	
	1968–1972	**1993–1997**
Japan, Osaka	91.9	60.7
Estonia	53.6	32.3
Singapore	43.7	25.7
Finland	34.8	12.6
Jews in Israel	20.0	11.8
Denmark	19.9	8.2
Sweden	19.7	8.6
United Kingdom, South Thames	19.2	11.4
Canada, Quebec	14.5	10.4
Canada, Alberta	13.6	8.4

gastric cancer is anticipated during the next decade in Western countries, without additional preventive effort.[5]

Although the reasons underlying the different mortality rates have not been established, improved diet, increased food variety, and reduced prevalence of *Helicobacter pylori* infection are possible reasons. Improved diagnosis and treatment are also likely factors underlying the observed reduction in mortality rates.[6] On the other hand, increases in the prevalence of obesity may explain the observed increases in the incidences of gastric cardia cancer in certain Western countries, because the risk of gastric cardia cancer increases with body mass index.[7]

Gastric cancer is rarely encountered in people younger than 30 years of age, but thereafter, its incidence increases steadily with age, which is a characteristic feature of most carcinomas in both men and women. The gastric cancer incidence rate among men is about twice that among women for individuals older than 50 years of age. On the other hand, the male-to-female ratio is less than two for individuals younger than 50 years of age. The predominance of gastric cancer in men is seen in high-incidence areas as well as in low-incidence areas, suggesting, but not yet proving, that hormonal factors may be involved in gastric carcinoma.[8]

The incidence of gastric carcinoma increases steeply after 50 years of age in all populations, and an exceptionally high incidence of 673/100,000 has been reported in Miyagi, Japan, for individuals aged 80. The incidence rate for individuals aged 80 in low-risk area such as Los Angeles is 103/100,000. The incidence rate is high even in young individuals living in high-risk countries. The incidence at age 25 is 4.1/100,000 in the Korean population and only 0.3/100,000 in Caucasian residents of Los Angeles (Table 2-3).

EPIDEMIOLOGY AND HISTOLOGICAL SUBTYPES OF GASTRIC CANCER

The most commonly used gastric carcinoma classifications are the World Health Organization (WHO) and Lauren classifications. The Lauren classification describes two main histological types, the intestinal type, which consists of a gland-forming tumor, and the diffuse type, which consists of discohesive individual cells supported by a dense stroma.[9] The intestinal type is more frequently observed in older patients and follows multifocal atrophic gastritis or intestinal metaplasia, whereas the diffuse type carcinoma occurs commonly in young patients, is not

Table 2-3	Age-standardized incidence of stomach cancer per 100,000 people	
Sex	Race	Incidence
Male	Caucasian	7.07
	African American	11.74
	Korean American	30.24
	Native Korean	66.5–72.5
Female	Caucasian	3.37
	African American	5.95
	Korean American	15.25
	Native Korean	19.5–30.4

accompanied by intestinal metaplasia, and can be hereditary. Furthermore, the intestinal-type carcinoma predominates in high-risk areas, whereas the diffuse type is more common in low-risk areas.[10] In addition, men are more likely to have the intestinal-type carcinoma.[11]

Clinicopathological factors suggest that the environment contributes more to the development of intestinal-type carcinoma than to diffuse-type carcinoma, and conversely, the genetic contribution to the diffuse-type carcinoma may be greater than that to intestinal-type carcinoma.[12] The intestinal-type carcinoma is more likely to show vascular spread and hepatic metastasis, and the diffuse type is less likely to have hepatic metastasis and is more prone to transperitoneal spread.

The Surveillance Epidemiology and End Results (SEER) registry of the National Cancer Institute shows that the incidence of diffuse-type gastric carcinoma increased between 1973 and 1990, whereas that of intestinal-type carcinoma decreased.[13] In Japan, a similar trend was noted in gastric antral carcinoma relative to gastric carcinoma in the middle third of the stomach, that is, there was a larger proportion of diffuse carcinoma in the more proximal stomach. Differences between the intestinal versus the diffuse types of gastric carcinoma are summarized in Table 2-4.[14]

The intestinal-type adenocarcinomas arise in the setting of chronic inflammation. Genetic changes can be detected in intestinal metaplasia, a precancerous lesion that shows p16 methylation[15] or reduced E-cadherin expression in the gastric mucosa of *H. pylori*–infected individuals.[16]

Table 2-4	Epidemiology and clinicopathological characteristics of gastric carcinoma	
	Intestinal-type Carcinoma	Diffuse-type Carcinoma
Epidemiology	Common in high-risk countries	Incidence similar in most countries
Predilection site	Antrum	Corpus
Gross pathology	Fungating	Linitis plastica
Histology	Gland forming	Single cell
Distant metastasis	Hepatic	Transperitoneal
Sex, age	Men, over 60	Women, young age (<60 y)
Prognosis	Better survival	Poor survival

Intestinal metaplasia is an irreversible lesion, which suggests a permanent change in the genetic and epigenetic features of the gastric stem or progenitor cells. Furthermore, biological detection of genomic instability in intestinal metaplasia has been suggested as a surrogate marker for gastric carcinoma risk and a predictor of its malignant potential.[17]

EPIDEMIOLOGY AND ANATOMIC LOCATION OF GASTRIC CANCER

Gastric cancer was the most common malignancy in the world until the end of the first half of the 20th century, after which its incidence and mortality rates have dramatically decreased, especially in Western countries. On the other hand, the incidence of gastric cardia cancer has increased by five- to sixfold in developed countries over the past 30 years.[18] Gastric cardia cancer now accounts for approximately half of all gastric carcinomas among men in the United States and the United Kingdom.[19] A similar increase in incidence has been observed for esophageal adenocarcinoma, in which obesity, gastroesophageal reflux disease, and Barrett esophagus are the major etiologic factors. Gastric cardia cancers share the epidemiologic features of adenocarcinomas of the distal esophagus and those of the gastroesophageal junction. Many genetic and nongenetic findings suggest that noncardia and cardia gastric adenocarcinomas are distinct biological entities, and the epidemiologic differences between the two are summarized in Table 2-5. Furthermore, for unknown reasons, H. pylori infection is inversely associated with the risk of gastric cardia cancer,[20] but it is a strong risk factor for noncardia gastric cancer. In addition, men are diagnosed with gastric cardia cancer five times more often than women, and Caucasians are diagnosed with gastric cardia cancer twice as often as African Americans.[21] In addition, the incidence rates of proximal gastric cancers are higher among professional classes.

Table 2-5	Epidemiologic difference between cardia and noncardia gastric cancer	
	Cardia Cancer	Noncardia Cancer
Incidence	Increasing	Decreasing
Geographic location		
Western countries	+	−
East Asia	−	+
Developing countries	−	+
Age	++	++
Male	++	+
Caucasian	+	−
Low socioeconomic status	+	−
H. pylori infection	−	+
Diet		
Preserved food	+	+
Fruits and vegetables	−	−
Obesity	+	−
Smoking	+	+
Gastroesophageal reflux disease	+	−

EPIDEMIOLOGICAL RISK FACTORS

Gastric cancer is a multifactorial disease and shows marked geographic variations, time trends, and migration effects, which suggests that environmental and lifestyle factors contribute significantly to its etiology. The higher incidence of gastric carcinoma in Korean Americans than in Caucasians and African Americans probably reflects early life experience and persisting cultural habits, although differences in stomach cancer screening rates probably explain some of the differences in the stomach cancer incidences of Caucasians, African Americans, Korean Americans, and native Koreans. In native Koreans, early cancer accounts for almost half of all stomach cancers. In contrast, early cancer is rare in Caucasians and Korean Americans in the United States.

H. pylori INFECTION

H. pylori infection represents one of the most significant environmental risk factors. *H. pylori* increases the risk of gastric cancer approximately 2.8- to 6.0-fold, according to prospective cohort studies (details in Chapter 3). *H. pylori* increases the risk of both the intestinal- and the diffuse-type cancers, and this increased risk is higher for women than men. Many in vivo and in vitro studies have demonstrated the etiologic role of *H. pylori* in gastric cancer, and the details of the role of *H. pylori* in gastric carcinogenesis is described in a separate chapter. However, it is improbable that *H. pylori* infection alone is responsible for the development of gastric cancer, and evidence supports the notion that consumption of certain foods affects the risk of gastric cancer development. *H. pylori* gastritis facilitates the growth of bacteria that catalyze the production of carcinogenic *N*-nitroso compounds.[22]

FOODS

It has been shown that salt-preserved foods and dietary nitrite in preserved meats are potentially carcinogenic. In a study performed in Japan between 1995 and 1998, a high salt consumption was not found to increase the risk of gastric cancer per se. However, salted foods, such as pickled vegetables, salted fish, and salted fish roe, were found to increase the risk of gastric cancer significantly. Therefore, dietary sodium and salted foods have been suggested to have different effects on the development of gastric cancer.[23] In animal models, the ingestion of salt is known to cause gastritis and to enhance the effects of gastric carcinogens,[24] and several case-control studies have shown that high intake of salt or salt-preserved foods is associated with gastric cancer risk, but evidence from prospective studies is inconsistent.[25] *N*-nitroso compounds are carcinogenic in animal models and are produced in the stomach from dietary nitrite, but case-control studies have shown only a slight or insignificant increase in the risk of gastric cancer among cases with high vs. low nitrite intake.[26]

On the other hand, prospective studies have reported that fruit and vegetable consumption significantly reduces gastric cancer risk.[27] In a prospective study performed in Europe, a Mediterranean diet, which includes large amounts of fruits, vegetables, legumes, fish, and cereal, was found to be associated with a lower risk of gastric cancer.[28] Furthermore, animal studies have shown that polyphenols in green tea have antitumor and anti-inflammatory effects. In preclinical studies, polyphenols have been shown to have antioxidant activities and can inhibit nitrosation, both of which have been implicated as etiologic factors in gastric cancer.[29] In addition, green tea has been shown to affect the methylation status of genes.[30] Although various case-control studies have shown a reduced risk of gastric cancer in relation to green tea consumption, recent prospective cohort studies found that green tea had no protective effect.[31]

The worldwide decline in gastric cancer incidence may be partly due to the widespread use of refrigerators, which reduces the consumption of preserved foods and increases the intake of fresh fruits and vegetables. In a case-control study performed in a Portuguese population with a high rate of *H. pylori* infection, high fruit and dairy product consumption and low consumption of alcoholic beverages were associated with a reduced incidence of gastric cancer that was not modulated by *H. pylori* infection. This association was similar for cardia and noncardia gastric cancer, but the association was weaker for cancers with the diffuse-type histology.[32] Cereal fiber intake has also been reported to reduce the risk of adenocarcinoma, particularly of the diffuse type,[33] and in several epidemiologic studies, a monotonous diet was found to be a risk factor. In addition, dietary deficiencies of vitamins, such as vitamins A, B, C, and E, calcium, folic acid, and potassium are also known to increase the risk of adenocarcinoma, which concurs with the finding regarding the protective effects of fruits and vegetables. Similar protective effects have been described for ascorbic acid, carotenoids, folates, and tocopherols, which all act as antioxidants.[34]

SMOKING

Smoking is another well-known risk factor of gastric carcinoma. In the most recently published meta-analysis, which included 42 articles featuring cohort, case-cohort, and nested case-control studies up to 2007, the relative risk of gastric cancer among current smokers was 1.62 for men (95% CI: 1.50–1.75) and 1.20 for women (95% CI: 1.01–1.43), as compared with those who never smoked.[35] Relative risk increased from 1.3 for those with the lowest consumption of cigarettes to 1.7 for those smoking approximately 30 cigarettes per day, by trend estimation analysis. Smoking was significantly associated with both cardia (RR = 1.87) and noncardia (RR = 1.60) gastric cancer, and several other meta-analyses support the etiologic role of tobacco smoking in gastric carcinoma.[36] In a Korean study, the risk of gastric cancer among smokers was found to be two to three times that of nonsmokers, and in a Danish study, the concentration of *N*-nitroso compounds in gastric juice was higher in smokers than in nonsmokers. These studies demonstrated that tobacco smoking is an important behavioral factor and one that has been consistently linked with gastric carcinoma.

OTHER ENVIRONMENTAL RISK FACTORS

Some types of industrial exposure are known to increase the risk of gastric cancer. Workers who have been exposed to asbestos or iron for several decades have a two to three times higher risk.[37] Exposure to ionizing radiation >250 rad is also a risk factor, and Hiroshima atomic bomb survivors have a slightly higher risk of developing gastric cancer.

Changing patterns of cancer incidence after immigration provide valuable information regarding the weight of environmental and genetic influences. First-generation immigrants from high-risk countries to low-risk countries continue to have the higher rates of gastric cancer incidence of their original countries, whereas their children and grandchildren show lower rates approaching those of the host countries. The above results support the concept that environmental exposure during early life generates cancer precursors that persist into adulthood and are not easily reversed in a favorable environment.

The risks of stomach cancer between Korean American men and women sharply declined compared with their native counterparts. Korean American men have a four times higher rate of stomach cancer than Caucasian men and a three times higher rate than African American men (SEER 1997–2000) (Table 2-4). Korean American women have a seven times higher stomach cancer rate than Caucasian women and a three times higher rate than African American women.

PRECANCEROUS LESIONS AND EPIDEMIOLOGY

Gastric carcinogenesis is considered a multistep process involving generalized and specific genetic alterations that drive the progressive transformation of cells. In one study, an average of 4.18 genomic alterations are necessary for the transformation to the cancerous state.[38] Chronic gastritis, especially that induced by *H. pylori*, is common in regions of high incidence. Intestinal metaplasia is characterized by the appearance of small intestinal-type goblet cells in the gastric mucosa, and intestinal metaplasia has been proven to be a preneoplastic lesion in several population and animal studies. Chronic gastritis induced by *H. pylori* is the major underlying cause of intestinal metaplasia. Autoimmune gastritis induced by antiparietal cell antibodies is also a precancerous lesion with a threefold higher risk of cancer development.[39] Furthermore, the remnant stomach after gastrectomy is known to have an increased risk of gastric cancer, and the Billroth II method, which involves the anastomosis of the gastric mucosa to the jejunum, is associated with a higher risk of gastric cancer than the Billroth I method, which involves the anastomosis of the stomach to the duodenum. The underlying mechanism of the increased risk posed by a remnant stomach is probably associated with the regurgitation of bile and pancreatic fluids into the stomach.

Recently, genetic polymorphisms of many genes have been shown to be etiologically associated with gastric cancer. A detailed discussion on this topic is included in the chapter entitled "Molecular Epidemiology of Gastric Cancer." Familial clustering of gastric cancer has been shown to be about two to three times higher in the offspring of gastric cancer patients. However, this does not directly support a genetic predisposition to gastric cancer, because family members invariably share a common diet and environment, for example, one twin study failed to find a higher concordance rate in identical twins than in dizygotic twins.

PREVENTION

Because gastric cancer is associated with a poor prognosis, the main strategy for improving clinical outcomes places a focus on primary prevention. However, the reduction in gastric cancer mortality rates during the past 70 years has been largely the result of unplanned efforts. The widespread introduction of refrigerators may have reduced the consumption of chemically preserved foods and increased the consumption of fresh fruits and vegetables.[40] The decline in the prevalence of *H. pylori* infection is probably due as much to improvements in sanitary and housing conditions as it is to the use of eradication therapy. In addition, reduced tobacco smoking, at least by men, has also contributed to this decline in the gastric cancer incidence.[36] Therefore, modifiable risk factors, such as high levels of salt and nitrites in the diet, low fruit and vegetable intake, cigarette smoking, and *H. pylori* infection, are targets for prevention.

Several intermediate-sized intervention trials have indicated that in some patients, *H. pylori* eradication therapy leads to the regression of and prevents the progression of precancerous lesions.[41] Furthermore, eradication therapy reduces gastric cancer incidence in patients without any precancerous lesions at baseline and is effective before the development of atrophic gastritis. A few recent interventional studies in Japan have demonstrated a significant prophylactic effect of eradication therapy on the development of gastric cancer. However, gastric cancer may still develop despite successful eradication therapy, and a study in an animal model confirmed that the use of eradication therapy at an early point after infection increased its effectiveness in preventing gastric cancer development.[42]

One ongoing intervention study in China is investigating a comprehensive approach to gastric cancer prevention that includes *H. pylori* eradication, nutritional supplements, and aggressive screening by double-contrast radiographic or endoscopic examination. During the first 4 years after intervention, the relative risk of overall mortality for this intervention in a high-risk group was 0.51 (95% CI: 0.35–0.74),[43] which suggests that targeting high-risk populations for aggressive screening and prevention may be an effective strategy for reducing gastric cancer mortality.

PROGNOSIS AND EPIDEMIOLOGY

Although survival rates are increasing rapidly, the prognosis for gastric cancer remains poor and mortality rates remain high. Gastric cancer is the second only to lung cancer as the leading cause of cancer-related death worldwide. In general, countries with higher incidence rates of gastric cancer show better survival rates than countries with lower incidence rates.[44] This association is partly due to the relationship between survival rates and tumor location in the stomach. Tumors located in the gastric pyloric antrum have a much better prognosis than those in the gastric cardia, and in particular, patients with gastric pyloric antrum tumors have better 5-year survival rates and lower intraoperative mortality rates.[45] In addition, the availability of early detection screening in Japan and Korea substantially increased the proportion of early-stage cancers detected, and in areas with an active mass screening program, gastric cancer mortality rates have been reduced by half from those in the early 1970s. When gastric cancer is limited to the mucosa, the 5-year survival rate approaches 95%; however, few early-stage gastric cancers are discovered in the United States, which explains the 5-year survival rate of <20%. In European countries, the 5-year survival rates for gastric cancer are similar to those in the United States (between 10% and 20%).[46] Host-related factors might also affect prognosis. In a U.S. study, gastric cancer patients of Asian descent were found to have better prognoses than non-Asian patients.[47] The above findings strongly suggest that host-related factors affect prognosis.

Because of the high risk of gastric cancer in Japan and Korea, both nations have been operating national surveillance programs. Annual or biannual screening using a double-contrast barium technique or endoscopy is recommended for persons over the age of 40. In Korea and Japan, about half of all gastric tumors are detected at an early stage in asymptomatic individuals, and the mortality rate from gastric cancer has been halved as compared with the early 1970s.

EPIDEMIOLOGY AND CHEMOPREVENTION

High intake of antioxidants, such as vitamin C, vitamin E, and beta-carotene, may reduce the risk of gastric cancer. High serum levels of beta-carotene, lycopene, and vitamin C were found to be significantly associated with a lower risk of gastric cancer in a Chinese cohort.[48] In a randomized trial conducted in Lin Xian Province, China, individuals supplemented with a combination of selenium, beta-carotene, and alpha-tocopherol were found to have a lower risk of both cardia and noncardia gastric cancers.[49] However, a randomized trial in Finland found no association between alpha-tocopherol or beta-carotene supplementation and the prevalence of gastric cancer in elderly men with atrophic gastritis,[50] and the prospective Cancer Prevention Study II cohort conducted in the United States concluded that vitamin supplementation did not significantly reduce the risk of stomach cancer mortality.[51] Therefore, it appears that dietary supplementation has a preventive effect in populations with a high incidence of gastric cancer and/or a low intake of nutritional supplements.

Cyclooxygenase-2 (COX-2) plays a role in cell proliferation, apoptosis, and angiogenesis and, therefore, may be involved in gastrointestinal carcinogenesis.[52] It is known that COX-2 levels are elevated during the progression from atrophic gastritis to intestinal metaplasia and adenocarcinoma of the stomach and that exposure to cigarette smoke, excessively acidic conditions, or *H. pylori* infection induces COX-2 expression. Aspirin and other nonsteroidal anti-inflammatory drugs (NSAIDs) are believed to inhibit cancer cell growth primarily by inhibiting COX-2, and increasing evidence indicates that COX-2 inhibitors may help prevent gastrointestinal malignancies. The association between NSAID usage and the development of gastric cancer has been studied less extensively than its association with colorectal cancer. However, a recent meta-analysis showed that NSAID use is associated with a reduction in the risk of noncardia gastric cancer.[53] Thus, COX-2 inhibitors may provide a chemopreventive strategy against gastric carcinogenesis.

References

1. Parkin DM, Pisani P, Ferlay J. Estimates of the worldwide incidence of eighteen major cancers in 1985. *Int J Cancer*. 1993;54:594–606.
2. Parkin DM. International variation. *Oncogene*. 2004;23:6329–6340.
3. Stewart BW, Kleihues P, eds. *World Cancer Report*. Lyon: IARC Press; 2003.

4. Ferlay J, Bray F, Pisani P, et al. *GLOBOCAN 2002: Cancer incidence, mortality and prevalence worldwide.* Lyon: IARC Press; 2004.

5. de Vries AC, Meijer GA, Looman CW, et al. Epidemiological trends of pre-malignant gastric lesions: a long-term nationwide study in the Netherlands. *Gut.* 2007;56:1665–1670.

6. La Vecchia C, Bosetti C, Lucchini F, et al. Cancer mortality in Europe, 2000–2004, and an overview of trends since 1975. *Ann Oncol.* 2010;21:1323–1360.

7. Merry AH, Schouten LJ, Goldbohm RA, et al. Body mass index, height and risk of adenocarcinoma of the oesophagus and gastric cardia: a prospective cohort study. *Gut.* 2007;56:1503–1511.

8. Chandanos E, Lagergren J. Oestrogen and the enigmatic male predominance of gastric cancer. *Eur J Cancer.* 2008;44:2397–2403.

9. Lauren P. The two histological main types of gastric carcinoma: diffuse and so-called intestinal-type carcinoma. An attempt at a histo-clinical classification. *Acta Pathol Microbiol Scand.* 1965;64:31–49.

10. Hamilton SR, Aaltonen LA, eds. *WHO classification of tumours. Pathology and genetics of tumors of digestive system.* Lyon: IARC Press; 2000.

11. Derakhshan MH, Liptrot S, Paul J, et al. Oesophageal and gastric intestinal-type adenocarcinomas show the same male predominance due to a 17 year delayed development in females. *Gut.* 2009;58:16–23.

12. Milne AN, Carneiro F, O'Morain C, et al. Nature meets nurture: molecular genetics of gastric cancer. *Hum Genet.* 2009;126:615–628.

13. Henson DE, Dittus C, Younes M, et al. Differential trends in the intestinal and diffuse types of gastric carcinoma in the United States, 1973–2000: increase in the signet ring cell type. *Arch Pathol Lab Med.* 2004;128:765–770.

14. Fenoglio-Preiser CM, Noffsinger AE, Stemmermann GN, et al., eds. *The neoplastic stomach in Gastrointestinal pathology: an atlas and text.* Lippincott Williams & Wilkins, Philadelphia, 2008.

15. Dong CX, Deng DJ, Pan KF, et al. Promoter methylation of p16 associated with *Helicobacter pylori* infection in precancerous gastric lesions: a population-based study. *Int J Cancer.* 2009;124:434–439.

16. Terres AM, Pajares JM, O'Toole D, et al. *H. pylori* infection is associated with downregulation of E-cadherin, a molecule involved in epithelial cell adhesion and proliferation control. *J Clin Pathol.* 1998;51:410–412.

17. Zaky AH, Watari J, Tanabe H, et al. Clinicopathologic implications of genetic instability in intestinal-type gastric cancer and intestinal metaplasia as a precancerous lesion: proof of field cancerization in the stomach. *Am J Clin Pathol.* 2008;129:613–621.

18. Pera M, Cameron AJ, Trastek VF, et al. Increasing incidence of adenocarcinoma of the esophagus and esophagogastric junction. *Gastroenterology.* 1993;104:510–513.

19. Brown LM, Devesa SS. Epidemiologic trends in esophageal and gastric cancer in the United States. *Surg Oncol Clin N Am.* 2002;11:235–256.

20. Kamangar F, Dawsey SM, Blaser MJ, et al. Opposing risks of gastric cardia and noncardia gastric adenocarcinomas associated with *Helicobacter pylori* seropositivity. *J Natl Cancer Inst.* 2006;98:1445–1452.

21. El-Serag HB, Mason AC, Petersen N, et al. Epidemiological differences between adenocarcinoma of the oesophagus and adenocarcinoma of the gastric cardia in the USA. *Gut.* 2002;50:368–372.

22. Sanduleanu S, Jonkers D, De Bruine A, et al. Non-*Helicobacter pylori* bacterial flora during acid-suppressive therapy: differential findings in gastric juice and gastric mucosa. *Aliment Pharmacol Ther.* 2001;15:379–388.

23. Takachi R, Inoue M, Shimazu T, et al. Consumption of sodium and salted foods in relation to cancer and cardiovascular disease: the Japan Public Health Center-based Prospective Study. *Am J Clin Nutr.* 2009;91:456–464.

24. Takahashi M, Hasegawa R. Enhancing effects of dietary salt on both initiation and promotion stages of rat gastric carcinogenesis. *Princess Takamatsu Symp.* 1985;16:169–182.

25. Kato I, Tominaga S, Matsumoto K. A prospective study of stomach cancer among a rural Japanese population: a 6-year survey. *Jpn J Cancer Res.* 1992;83:568–575.

26. Hansson LE, Nyren O, Bergstrom R, et al. Nutrients and gastric cancer risk: a population-based case-control study in Sweden. *Int J Cancer.* 1994;57:638–644.

27. McCullough ML, Robertson AS, Jacobs EJ, et al. A prospective study of diet and stomach cancer mortality in United States men and women. *Cancer Epidemiol Biomarkers Prev.* 2001;10:1201–1205.

28. Buckland G, Agudo A, Lujan L, et al. Adherence to a Mediterranean diet and risk of gastric adenocarcinoma within the European Prospective Investigation into Cancer and Nutrition (EPIC) cohort study. *Am J Clin Nutr.* 2009.

29. Wang ZY, Cheng SJ, Zhou ZC, et al. Antimutagenic activity of green tea polyphenols. *Mutat Res.* 1989;223:273–285.

30. Yuasa Y, Nagasaki H, Akiyama Y, et al. DNA methylation status is inversely correlated with green tea intake and physical activity in gastric cancer patients. *Int J Cancer.* 2009;124:2677–2682.

31. Tsubono Y, Nishino Y, Komatsu S, et al. Green tea and the risk of gastric cancer in Japan. *N Engl J Med.* 2001;344:632–636.

32. Bastos J, Lunet N, Peleteiro B, et al. Dietary patterns and gastric cancer in a portuguese urban population. *Int J Cancer.* 2009;127:433–441.

33. M AM, Pera G, Agudo A, et al. Cereal fiber intake may reduce risk of gastric adenocarcinomas: the EPIC-EURGAST study. *Int J Cancer.* 2007;121:1618–1623.

34. Jenab M, Riboli E, Ferrari P, et al. Plasma and dietary carotenoid, retinol and tocopherol levels and the risk of gastric adenocarcinomas in the European prospective investigation into cancer and nutrition. *Br J Cancer.* 2006;95:406–415.

35. Ladeiras-Lopes R, Pereira AK, Nogueira A, et al. Smoking and gastric cancer: systematic review and meta-analysis of cohort studies. *Cancer Causes Control.* 2008;19:689–701.

36. Tredaniel J, Boffetta P, Buiatti E, et al. Tobacco smoking and gastric cancer: review and meta-analysis. *Int J Cancer.* 1997;72:565–573.

37. Raj A, Mayberry JF, Podas T. Occupation and gastric cancer. *Postgrad Med J.* 2003;79:252–258.

38. Nishimura T. Total number of genome alterations in sporadic gastrointestinal cancer inferred from pooled analyses in the literature. *Tumour Biol.* 2008;29:343–350.

39. Brinton LA, Gridley G, Hrubec Z, et al. Cancer risk following pernicious anaemia. *Br J Cancer.* 1989;59:810–813.

40. La Vecchia C, Negri E, D'Avanzo B, et al. Electric refrigerator use and gastric cancer risk. *Br J Cancer.* 1990;62:136–137.

41. Wong BC, Lam SK, Wong WM, et al. *Helicobacter pylori* eradication to prevent gastric cancer in a high-risk region of China: a randomized controlled trial. *JAMA.* 2004;291:187–194.

42. Kabir S. Effect of *Helicobacter pylori* eradication on incidence of gastric cancer in human and animal models: underlying biochemical and molecular events. *Helicobacter.* 2009;14:159–171.

43. Guo HQ, Guan P, Shi HL, et al. Prospective cohort study of comprehensive prevention to gastric cancer. *World J Gastroenterol.* 2003;9:432–436.

44. Verdecchia A, Corazziari I, Gatta G, et al. Explaining gastric cancer survival differences among European countries. *Int J Cancer.* 2004;109:737–741.

45. DeMeester SR. Adenocarcinoma of the esophagus and cardia: a review of the disease and its treatment. *Ann Surg Oncol.* 2006;13:12–30.

46. Faivre J, Forman D, Esteve J, et al. Survival of patients with oesophageal and gastric cancers in Europe. *Eur J Cancer.* 1998;34:2167–2175.

47. Theuer CP, Kurosaki T, Ziogas A, et al. Asian patients with gastric carcinoma in the United States exhibit unique clinical features and superior overall and cancer specific survival rates. *Cancer.* 2000;89: 1883–1892.

48. Yuan JM, Ross RK, Gao YT, et al. Prediagnostic levels of serum micronutrients in relation to risk of gastric cancer in Shanghai, China. *Cancer Epidemiol Biomarkers Prev.* 2004;13:1772–1780.

49. Blot WJ, Li JY, Taylor PR, et al. Nutrition intervention trials in Linxian, China: supplementation with specific vitamin/mineral combinations, cancer incidence, and disease-specific mortality in the general population. *J Natl Cancer Inst.* 1993;85:1483–1492.

50. Varis K, Taylor PR, Sipponen P, et al. Gastric cancer and premalignant lesions in atrophic gastritis: a controlled trial on the effect of supplementation with alpha-tocopherol and beta-carotene. The Helsinki Gastritis Study Group. *Scand J Gastroenterol.* 1998;33:294–300.

51. Jacobs EJ, Connell CJ, McCullough ML, et al. Vitamin C, vitamin E, and multivitamin supplement use and stomach cancer mortality in the Cancer Prevention Study II cohort. *Cancer Epidemiol Biomarkers Prev.* 2002;11:35–41.

52. Sawaoka H, Tsuji S, Tsujii M, et al. Cyclooxygenase inhibitors suppress angiogenesis and reduce tumor growth in vivo. *Lab Invest.* 1999;79:1469–1477.

53. Wang WH, Huang JQ, Zheng GF, et al. Non-steroidal anti-inflammatory drug use and the risk of gastric cancer: a systematic review and meta-analysis. *J Natl Cancer Inst.* 2003;95:1784–1791.

3

Helicobacter pylori and Gastric Neoplasms

▶ Antonia R. Sepulveda

▶ Abha Goyal

INTRODUCTION

Helicobacter pylori, a Gram-negative bacterium, is the most important human pathogen of the Helicobacter genus. Studies by Warren and Marshal[1] were the first to implicate *H. pylori* as the causative agent of chronic gastritis and ulcers. This discovery led to the Nobel Prize for Medicine and Physiology in 2005. *H. pylori* infection results in chronic injury of the stomach and chronic gastritis, which significantly increases the risk of gastric adenocarcinoma and mucosa-associated lymphoid tissue (MALT) lymphoma, generally described in the current World Health Organization (WHO) classification as extranodal marginal zone B-cell lymphoma.[2–4]

In this chapter, we review the evidence supporting a role for *H. pylori* in gastric carcinogenesis, the stepwise pathologic changes of the gastric mucosa (gastritis, gastric atrophy, intestinal metaplasia, and dysplasia/adenoma) that underlie gastric cancer, the role of *Helicobacter* virulence factors in gastric cancer risk, the molecular mechanisms underlying *H. pylori*–associated gastric cancer, human genetic susceptibility factors including proinflammatory gene polymorphisms, and the potential contribution of bone marrow–derived stem cells in gastric carcinogenesis. We also review the evidence supporting a role for *H. pylori* in gastric lymphomagenesis, the mechanisms that may underlie *H. pylori*–associated MALT lymphoma, the molecular features of gastric MALT lymphomas, and the role of *H. pylori* eradication in the treatment of these low-grade lymphomas.

H. pylori AND GASTRIC CANCER

Evidence for a Role of *H. pylori* in Gastric Carcinogenesis

Gastric cancers are heterogeneous neoplasms that include several adenocarcinoma subtypes characterized by unique genetic and molecular features. This heterogeneity is likely a result of alternative underlying mechanisms of neoplastic development and progression. Since the early 1990s, much has been learned regarding the molecular basis and biological behavior of gastric adenocarcinoma and precursor lesions. The scientific breakthroughs that have led to and continue to propel our understanding of gastric carcinogenesis include the following: (a) the demonstration that *H. pylori* gastritis is associated with an increased risk of gastric cancer development, (b) the identification of a genetic basis for some familial forms of gastric cancer, and (c) the availability of robust molecular approaches that expand the traditional morphology-based characterization of gastric cancer subtypes.

The association of *H. pylori* infection and gastric adenocarcinomas led to the classification of *H. pylori* as a human carcinogen by a WHO panel in 1994,[2] nearly a decade after the first report by Warren and Marshal[1] implicating *H. pylori* as the bacteria that causes chronic gastritis. *H. pylori* infection appears to play a role predominantly during the initiating steps of gastric cancer, although the environment established by the ongoing inflammatory response to the infection may contribute to neoplastic progression.

Gastric cancers result from the action of several causal mechanisms and their interactions. The factors known to play a role in gastric cancer development include host genetic suscepti- bility factors, environmental exogenous factors that have carcinogenic activity such as dietary components and smoking, and the cellular injury that is caused by chronic gastritis (reviewed in Ref. [5]).

The evidence supporting a role for *H. pylori* in gastric carcinogenesis includes the following: (a) epidemiological studies reporting a close association between *H. pylori* and gastric cancer in several populations around the world, (b) characteristic histopathologic changes that mark the steps of gastric mucosal injury associated with gastric cancer risk (the Correa cascade), (c) animal models of *H. pylori* and gastric cancer, and (d) data showing that *H. pylori* eradication may reduce the risk of gastric cancer development.

H. pylori was initially classified as a human carcinogen based on the strong epidemiologi- cal association of *H. pylori* gastritis and gastric cancer.[2,3] This association was explained by the fact that the majority of gastric cancers arise in a background of chronic gastritis, which is most commonly caused by *H. pylori* infection of the stomach.[6,7] Overall, the risk of gastric cancer in patients with *H. pylori* gastritis is sixfold higher than that of people without *H. pylori* gastritis,[8] and this risk increases for patients with more extensive degrees of gastric atrophy and intestinal metaplasia. Even for *H. pylori*–infected patients with nonatrophic gastritis, their gastric cancer risk is approximately twofold higher than that of healthy non–*H. pylori*–infected individuals. In addition, prospective studies demonstrated gastric cancer development in 2.9% of *H. pylori*– infected patients over a period of 7.8 years, but this incidence was higher in patients with extensive atrophic gastritis and intestinal metaplasia, reaching an incidence rate of 8.4% during a 10-year surveillance.[9,10] Underscoring the importance of *H. pylori* in gastric carcinogenesis, the gastric cancer risk attributable to *H. pylori* infection has been estimated to be 75%.[7]

In addition, several animal models, including Mongolian gerbils and mice, develop gastritis as well as other *H. pylori*–associated gastric diseases, including intestinal metaplasia, dysplasia, and gastric cancer, following *Helicobacter* infection.[11,12]

Furthermore, *H. pylori* eradication reduced the incidence of gastric cancer in patients with- out atrophy and intestinal metaplasia at study baseline,[13] and eradication of *H. pylori* infection in patients with early gastric cancer resulted in a decreased frequency of new cancers,[14] supporting the notion that eradication may contribute to preventing progression from gastritis to gastric cancer.

Histologic Changes in the Progression of Chronic *H. pylori* Gastritis to Cancer

The chronicity associated with *H. pylori* gastritis is critical to the carcinogenic potential of the infection. *H. pylori* infection is generally acquired during childhood and persists throughout life unless the patient undergoes eradication treatment.[15] Gastric cancer generally develops several decades after acquisition of the infection and is associated with the progression of mucosal dam- age during chronic gastritis.

Histologically, the progression of *H. pylori*–associated chronic gastritis to gastric cancer is characterized by a stepwise acquisition of mucosal changes, starting with chronic gastritis, the progressive damage of gastric glands resulting in mucosal atrophy, the replacement of normal gastric glands by intestinal metaplasia, and the development of dysplasia and carcinoma in some patients (Figs. 3-1 and 3-2). Gastritis is the first and longest lasting response to *H. pylori* infec- tion of the stomach and is mediated by the activation of both humoral and cellular inflamma- tory responses within the gastric mucosa involving dendritic cells, macrophages, mast cells, the recruitment and expansion of T and B lymphocytes, plasma cells, and neutrophils.[16] Despite the continued host inflammatory response, *H. pylori* is able to evade the host immune mechanisms and persist, causing chronic gastritis.

The pathologic changes of the gastric mucosa in which *H. pylori*–associated gastric cancer generally occurs may be described as atrophic gastritis, where, in a background of active chronic

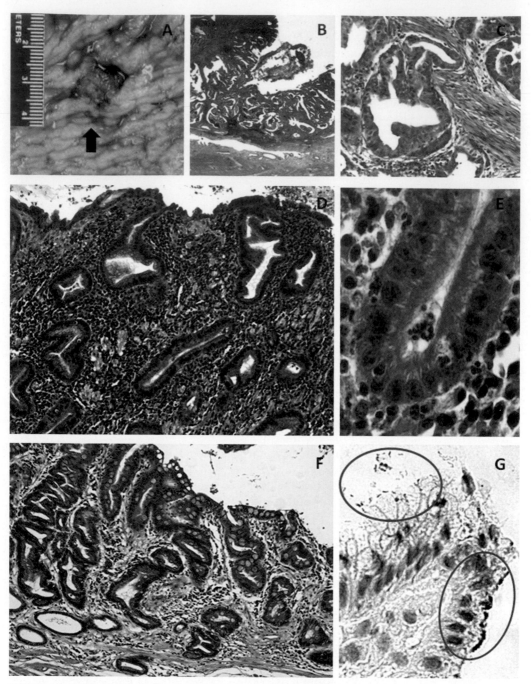

FIGURE 3-1 Classic findings in *H. pylori*–associated gastric carcinogenesis. A: Gross photograph of ulcerated adeno-carcinoma in gastric antrum (*arrow*). **B:** Histology of ulcerated adenocarcinoma. **C:** Invasive moderately differentiated adenocarcinoma (intestinal type). **D:** Background mucosa reveals marked inflammation of the lamina propria (chronic gastritis). **E:** High-power view of gastric epithelium with associated neutrophils (active gastritis). **F:** Foci of intestinal metaplasia in the gastric mucosa affected by chronic gastritis. **G:** High-power view of *H. pylori* immunohistochemical analysis. *H. pylori* bacteria are present in the surface mucus (*left-upper oval shape*) and are attached to the apical aspect of gastric surface epithelial cells (*right-lower oval shape*), original magnification 400×. Hematoxylin and eosin stains original magnification 100× (**B,C,F**) and 200× (**E**).

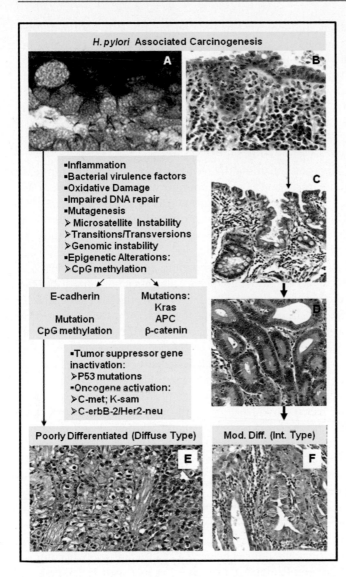

FIGURE 3-2 *H. pylori*–associated gastric carcinogenesis: alternative pathways and associated molecular patterns. **A:** *H. pylori* bacteria closely associate with the gastric epithelium (thiazine stain, 400×). **B:** Gastric mucosa with chronic active gastritis in response to *H. pylori* infection. **C:** Intestinal metaplasia stage of gastric carcinogenesis, progressing to dysplasia/adenoma (**D**) an invasive moderately differentiated (Mod. Diff.) adenocarcinoma of intestinal type (Int. Type) (**F**). **E:** Some cases of gastric cancer arising in association with *H. pylori* chronic gastritis do not progress through the stages of intestinal metaplasia and dysplasia, but rather abruptly present as poorly differentiated (diffuse type) adenocarcinomas. Hematoxylin and eosin stains original magnification 200× (**B–F**).

inflammation, there is a progressive loss of the normal glandular structures of the gastric mucosa (gastric atrophy) and the replacement of the normal glandular epithelium by intestinal metaplasia. This stepwise series of histopathologic changes are named the Correa cascade. Given the association of gastric glandular atrophy and intestinal metaplasia and an increased risk of gastric cancer, these changes, in particular intestinal metaplasia, are accepted as a marker of gastric cancer risk and may be interpreted as preneoplastic epithelial changes in gastric carcinogenesis. Progression to gastric cancer is higher in patients with more extensive forms of atrophic gastritis with intestinal metaplasia involving large areas of the stomach, including the gastric body and fundus. This pattern of gastritis has been described as pangastritis or multifocal atrophic gastritis.[6,17] Extensive gastritis involving the gastric body and fundus results in hypochlorhydria, allowing for bacterial overgrowth and increased carcinogenic activity in the stomach through the conversion of nitrites to carcinogenic *N*-nitroso compounds. *H. pylori*–associated pangastritis is frequently seen in the relatives of gastric cancer patients, which may contribute to gastric cancer clustering in some families.[18]

Stomach cancers are classified according to the WHO classification on the basis of their grade of differentiation, which is categorized as well, moderately, and poorly differentiated adenocarcinomas.[19] The Lauren classification reported in 1965 has been widely used in studies of gastric adenocarcinomas, separating gastric cancer into the intestinal and diffuse types, on the basis of the morphologic features of the tumor. The cancers that arise in the inflammatory background of *H. pylori*–associated chronic gastritis are most commonly intestinal-type adeno-carcinomas, which are predominantly well to moderately differentiated (Figs. 3-1 and 3-2), but diffuse-type tumors, which are poorly differentiated and may include a variable component with signet ring cell features, also occur in association with *H. pylori*[9,20] (Fig. 3-2).

Inflammatory Cascades in *H. pylori* Chronic Gastritis

H. pylori infection of the stomach elicits a host inflammatory response that includes both humoral and cellular responses and involves both innate and acquired immune responses.[16] Once *H. pylori* colonizes and infects the stomach, the disease persists as chronic gastritis, unless treatment is applied to eradicate the infection.[15] Because of the long-term chronic inflammatory status of the gastric mucosa, *H. pylori* must be able to evade the immune system, and this evasion is thought to be the main contributor to gastric cancer development. The mechanisms that lead to *H. pylori* immune evasion and chronic gastritis are being unraveled. The immune response to *H. pylori* is induced when the bacterial products contact the gastric epithelial cells lining the stomach and the macrophages and dendritic cells in the lamina propria, which are reached after the epithelial cells and intercellular junctions are damaged by *H. pylori* virulence factors such as the vacuolating cyto-toxin (VacA). This cellular damage permits the bacteria and bacterial products to move through the interrupted epithelial cell layer to the subepithelial lamina propria (reviewed in Ref. [16]). The steps involved in the host immune response to *H. pylori* can be described as follows: (a) *H. pylori* bacteria adhere to the apical aspect of epithelial cells that are primarily located on the mucosal surface and eventually move into the gastric foveolae, where the organisms may come into contact with gastric stem cells. The epithelial cells respond to *H. pylori* through cell-signaling events to produce cytokines, which are released into the lamina propria to activate macrophages, dendritic cells, and other inflammatory cells; (b) Some *H. pylori* bacteria are able to enter the lamina propria after the surface epithelial layer is damaged, allowing *H. pylori* to directly interact with innate and acquired immune response cells; (c) Macrophages, dendritic cells, and T-cell mediators released by the epithelial cells activate T lymphocytes with a predominant Th1 response, regulatory T lymphocytes (T-reg), B lymphocytes, which mature into mucosal plasma cells, and neutrophils, which actively phagocytize *H. pylori*. In addition, dendritic cells release IL23 and activate the pro-duction of IL17, which is associated with a Th17 response against *H. pylori*. Recent data indicate that *H. pylori* directs Treg-skewed dendritic cell–induced helper T-cell differentiation, in contrast to the Th17-skewed response seen with proinflammatory bacteria. The increased Treg induction in *H. pylori*–infected hosts forces an imbalance of the Th17/Treg axis, which may lead to ineffec-tive bacterial eradication and the persistence of *H. pylori* as a chronic infection.[21]

Stem Cells and *H. pylori*–associated Gastric Carcinogenesis

Studies of *H. pylori* infection in mouse models have suggested a potential role for bone marrow–derived stem cells in chronic gastritis and *H. pylori*–associated neoplastic progression.[22] The authors hypothesize that *H. pylori*–associated inflammation and glandular atrophy creates an abnormal microenvironment in the gastric mucosa that favors the engraftment of bone marrow–derived stem cells onto the inflamed gastric epithelium. The engrafted bone marrow–derived stem cells would not follow a normal differentiation pathway and would undergo uncontrolled replication, progressive loss of differentiation, and neoplastic behavior.[22] However, the potential role of bone marrow–derived stem cells in human disease remains unclear.

H. pylori Strains and Virulence Factors in Gastric Carcinogenesis

H. pylori is characterized by a unique set of virulence factors that play significant roles in its patho-genesis and influence the course of *H. pylori*–associated diseases.[23] The best known and most significant *H. pylori* virulence factors are VacA and the cytotoxin-associated antigen A (CagA) proteins.[24] Other bacterial factors that are important for *H. pylori*–related carcinogenesis include the *BabA* gene, which plays a role in bacterial adhesion to gastric epithelial cell blood group antigens. The combined presence of BabA, CagA and VacAs1 in *H. pylori* strains has been reported to be associated with duodenal ulcers and gastric adenocarcinomas in Western populations.

VacA is an 88 kDa protein that is secreted by *H. pylori* and causes the vacuolization and apoptosis of epithelial cells. VacA has been shown to have immunomodulatory effects, affecting B-lymphocyte antigen presentation, regulation of the T cell–mediated cytokine response, inhibition of T-lymphocyte activation and proliferation, and inhibition of T lymphocyte–induced B-cell proliferation (reviewed in Ref. [5]). The immunomodulatory actions of the VacA toxin on T and B lymphocytes may contribute to the ability of *H. pylori* to establish persistent chronic gastritis.

The CagA protein is a 125 to 145 kDa protein encoded by the *cagA* gene, which is one of the genes that constitute the Cag pathogenicity island.[24] This segment of the *H. pylori* genome encodes a type IV bacterial secretion system.[24] Recent studies have elucidated the role of CagA in *H. pylori* pathogenesis. These studies include the characterization of the functional domains of the CagA protein, the demonstration that some structural forms are more virulent and that variants of this protein are produced by different *H. pylori* strains (reviewed in Ref. [24]). In addition, the mechanisms by which CagA affects epithelial cells and may contribute to gastric cancer development are becoming better understood.[24] *H. pylori* strains carrying a *cagA* gene have been shown to have a stronger association with gastric cancer.[23,25] *H. pylori* strains that produce the CagA protein are associated with an increased risk of gastric carcinoma, at least in part, because these strains cause greater inflammatory mucosal damage. CagA-positive strains have been shown to induce higher levels of interleukin-8 (IL-8) than CagA-negative strains, resulting in higher levels of inflammation in the gastric mucosa.[26]

Some structural variants of CagA have a stronger association with gastric cancer. The CagA type C strains are associated with more severe degrees of atrophic gastritis and gastric cancer. *H. pylori* strains with unique phosphorylation patterns of the CagA phosphorylation site in the amino acid motif EPIYA are more common in Eastern Asia than in Western countries, which may contribute to the increased incidence of gastric cancer in Eastern Asia.[24] CagA is injected from the bacterium into gastric epithelial cells through the type IV secretion system and then interacts with several intracellular signaling molecules in both tyrosine phosphorylation-dependent and -independent manners. Once in the cell, CagA is phosphorylated on tyrosine residues in the EPIYA sites by the epithelial cell Src protein and other signaling molecules. Once phosphorylated, CagA binds the Src homology 2 domain–containing tyrosine phosphatase (SHP2) and deregulates its phosphatase activity.[24] CagA-related intracellular signaling is likely to have many other roles that may influence gastric carcinogenesis. For example, recent studies show that methylation of the O6-methylguanine DNA methyltransferase (*MGMT*) DNA repair gene was significantly associated with the CagA-positive *H. pylori* strains that are associated with chronic gastritis, suggesting a role for CagA-positive *H. pylori*–mediated effects in epigenetic regulation.[27] Additional support for a contributing role of CagA in gastric carcinogenesis includes the findings that mice carrying a transgenic *cagA* gene had gastric epithelial hyperplasia, and some mice developed gastric polyps and adenocarcinomas of the stomach and small intestine.[28]

Host Genetics and Susceptibility to *H. pylori*–associated Gastric Cancer

Overall, a positive family history of gastric cancer may increase the risk for gastric carcinoma by about threefold. Furthermore, patients with a family history of gastric cancer and infection with a CagA-positive *H. pylori* strain were reported to have a greater than eightfold higher risk of gastric carcinoma than others without these risk factors.[29] The inflammatory response to *H. pylori* is modulated by host genetics, influencing the risk of gastric cancer development. Among the best understood genetic changes are proinflammatory gene polymorphisms in the IL-1β and IL-1RN (receptor antagonist) genes, which have been shown to increase the risk of hypochlorhydria, gastric atrophy, gastric cancer, and cancer precursors in the presence of *H. pylori*.[30]

Molecular Pathways of *H. pylori*–associated Gastric Carcinogenesis

Both *H. pylori* bacteria and bacterial factors released in the gastric mucosa environment, as well as inflammatory mediators and oxygen radicals released by activated or injured epithelial and inflammatory cells alter the normal regulation of molecular signaling, epigenetic events, and gene transcription. *H. pylori* also increases mutagenesis, and all of these cellular alterations result in changes in cell behavior, such as altered apoptosis, increased cell proliferation, and progression to neoplasia.[5,24,31]

Mutagenesis and epigenetic and gene expression changes in *H. pylori*–associated carcinogenesis.

Mutagenesis, epigenetic changes, and a complex pattern of changes in gene expression and molecular pathways are key events in gastric carcinogenesis, occurring from the early stages of *H. pylori* gastritis to the subsequent formation of preneoplastic and neoplastic mucosal lesions.[5]

Characterization of mutations in gastric carcinogenesis has identified microsatellite instability (MSI-)type mutations, point mutations, and genomic instability, including loss of heterozygosity (LOH) and gene amplifications, in the stepwise formation of lesions of gastric carcinogenesis (intestinal metaplasia, dysplasia/adenoma, and adenocarcinoma).

Mutagenesis in *H. pylori*–associated gastritis occurs by several mechanisms. Increased DNA damage during *H. pylori* infection may be caused by oxidative damage from the action of reactive oxygen species (ROS) and reactive nitrogen species (RNS; reviewed in Ref. [5]). Recent studies show that epithelial expression of activation-induced cytidine deaminase (AID) in inflammatory conditions, such as *H. pylori* gastritis, may induce C/G to T/A transitions by its cytidine deaminase activity.[32] Because of an overall deficiency of some DNA repair functions during *H. pylori* gastritis, the mutations in the genome persist. Further increasing the risk of mutation, the mucosal atrophy and hypochlorhydria that are associated with long-lasting chronic gastritis may enhance the action of environmental carcinogens in the stomach.

Mutations associated with oxidative damage include point mutations in genes such as the tumor suppressor *P53* and other genes involved in gastric carcinogenesis. ROS are generated by inflammatory cells as well as by gastric epithelial cells after activation by *H. pylori*. In addition, *H. pylori* gastritis is associated with increased levels of inducible nitric oxide synthase (iNOS), nitric oxide (NO), and cyclooxygenase (COX-2), which lead to increased mutagenesis through oxidative stress. Furthermore, the limited availability of oxygen radical scavengers, such as glutathione and glutathione S-transferase, during *H. pylori* gastritis may contribute to the relatively higher levels of oxygen radicals in the mucosa of chronically infected patients. Gastric mucosa with *H. pylori* gastritis and intestinal metaplasia and gastric atrophy preneoplastic lesions contain increased levels of DNA 8-hydroxydeoxyguanosine (8OHdG), which can be used as a marker for oxidative DNA damage. Interestingly, the levels of 8OHdG in the gastric mucosa significantly decrease after eradication of *H. pylori* infection.

The deficiency of DNA repair that allows for the accumulation of mutations during *H. pylori* gastritis and throughout the carcinogenesis process involves alterations in DNA mismatch repair as well as other proteins that primarily repair DNA lesions induced by oxidative and nitrosative stress, including MGMT and polymorphic glycosylase (OGG1). The DNA mismatch repair proteins are required for the repair of DNA replication–associated sequence errors. Fully functional DNA mismatch repair requires active MutS (hMSH2, hMSH3, and hMSH6) and MutL proteins (hMLH1, hPMS1, hPMS2, and hMLH3). A deficiency in DNA mismatch repair leads to frameshift mutations, which can alter the coding region of genes as well as repetitive regions known as short tandem repeats or microsatellite regions, resulting in MSI. Because of the close relationship between MSI and DNA mismatch repair deficiency, MSI is used as a test of DNA mismatch repair deficiency in tissues.[33] Specifically, high levels of MSI, defined as MSI-H, detected in >30% of the microsatellite marker loci tested, correlate well with loss of DNA mismatch repair function in tissues.[33] Several studies have reported a role for DNA mismatch repair deficiency in mutation accumulation during *H. pylori* infection.[31,34,35] MSI can be detected in intestinal metaplasia from patients with gastric cancer, indicating that MSI can occur in preneoplastic mucosa (reviewed in

Ref. [5]). MSI was reported in 13% of chronic gastritis cases, 20% of intestinal metaplasias, 25% of dysplasias, and 38% of gastric cancers, indicating a stepwise acquisition of MSI in gastric carcinogenesis. Identical MSI patterns were observed in some cases at the gastritis stage several years before the diagnosis of adenocarcinoma. Supporting the role of *H. pylori* in MSI and underlying DNA mismatch repair deficiency in the various steps of gastric carcinogenesis, several studies have reported that patients with MSI-positive tumors showed a significantly higher frequency of active *H. pylori* infection.[5] In an *in vitro* coculture system, gastric cell lines exposed to *H. pylori* expressed reduced levels of the DNA mismatch repair proteins hMLH1 and hMSH2,[34] and these changes were associated with increased mutagenesis of a reporter vector, including MSI-type frame-shift mutations as well as point mutations.[31]

MSI was reported in 17% to 35% of gastric adenomas and in 17% to 59% of gastric carcinomas (reviewed in Ref. [5]). High levels of MSI in gastric adenomas and cancers were shown to be caused by loss of expression of *hMLH1*, which is associated with hypermethylation of its promoter. Gastric cancers with MSI-H may carry frame-shift mutations that may affect the function of cancer-related genes, such as *BAX, IGFRII, TGFβRII, hMSH3*, and *hMSH6*. In MSI-H adenomas, frame-shift mutations in *TGFβRII* were detected in 38% to 88% of the cases, *BAX* mutations were detected in 13%, *hMSH3* mutations in 13%, and *E2F-4* mutations in 50% of the cases (reviewed in Ref. [5]).

Point mutations and genomic imbalances such as LOH at multiple gene loci have been characterized in intestinal metaplasia, adenomas, and gastric carcinomas (reviewed in Ref. [5]). Mutations in the *P53* and *APC* genes can be detected in some cases of intestinal metaplasia and gastric dysplasia. Similar to other cancers, *P53* mutations in exons 5 through 8, resulting in G:C to A:T transitions, are detected in gastric neoplasia. *APC* mutations, including stop codon and frame-shift mutations, were reported in 46% of informative cases of gastric adenomas and 5q allelic loss in 33% of informative cases of gastric adenomas and in 45% of carcinomas. *K-ras* mutations in codon 12 are rare in gastric carcinogenesis and were reported in 14% of cases with atrophic gastritis and in <10% of adenomas, dysplasias, and carcinomas (reviewed in Ref. [5]).

Several other DNA repair proteins are involved in the correction of mutations induced by the oxidative stress associated with *H. pylori* infection such as repair of 8-OIIdG by polymorphic glycosylase (OGG1). A gene polymorphism that may affect the function of OGG1 was reported frequently in patients with intestinal metaplasia and gastric cancer, suggesting that deficient OGG1 function may contribute to increased mutagenesis during gastric carcinogenesis.[36] MGMT can remove O6-alkyl-guanine-DNA adducts. In the absence of functional MGMT, these adducts are not removed and mispair with T during DNA replication, resulting in G-to A mutations. *MGMT*-promoter methylation has been reported in various stages of gastric carcinogenesis, suggesting a role for this DNA repair protein in gastric cancer development. The role of MGMT is supported by recent studies showing that *H. pylori* gastritis is associated with hypermethylation of the *MGMT* gene and reduced levels of MGMT proteins in the gastric epithelium, particularly in patients infected with CagA-positive *H. pylori* strains. *MGMT*-promoter methylation was partially reversible after eradication of *H. pylori* infection. These data indicate that MGMT-dependent DNA repair is disrupted during *H. pylori* gastritis, increasing mutagenesis in *H. pylori*–infected gastric mucosa.[27]

Gene regulation through epigenetic modification, such as CpG methylation, appears to be an important mechanism in early gastric carcinogenesis, affecting genes such as *hMLH1, p14, p15, p16, E-cadherin, RUNX3*, thromobospondin-1 (*THBS1*), tissue inhibitor of metalloproteinase 3 (*TIMP-3*), *COX-2*, and *MGMT*.[5,27] The mechanisms that regulate CpG methylation and reduce gene expression during *H. pylori*–associated gastritis and subsequent mucosal lesions are still poorly understood. A study by Chen et al. showed that proinflammatory IL-1β polymorphisms were associated with CpG-island methylation of target genes such as the *E-cadherin*.[37] Interestingly, CpG methylation in gastric mucosa has been shown to be partially reversible after eradication of *H. pylori* infection.[27]

The patterns of gene expression that characterize the stepwise lesions of gastric carcinogenesis have been reported, leading to the identification of specific expression profiles that characterize gastritis, intestinal metaplasia, and subtypes of gastric adenocarcinoma, such as different gastric cancer prognostic groups.[5,38,39]

MicroRNAs (miRNAs) are small noncoding RNAs that regulate gene expression at a post-transcriptional level. The role of miRNAs in *H. pylori*–associated disease is under active investigation.[40] Recent studies addressing miRNA alterations in gastric carcinogenesis have shown that most gastric cancers overexpress miR-21, and increased expression of miR-21 was detected in *H. pylori*–infected gastric mucosa, as compared with noninfected tissue, while *miR-218-2* was downregulated.[41]

H. pylori AND EXTRANODAL MARGINAL ZONE B-CELL LYMPHOMA OF MALT LYMPHOMA

Extranodal marginal zone B-cell lymphomas develop from lymphoid tissue with a composition similar to native MALT, which is typically present in the gut and is most prominent in the Peyer patches in the terminal ileum. Most of the gastric marginal zone B-cell lymphomas arise in the background of MALT that is acquired as a result of *H. pylori* infection of the stomach.[4,42]

Evidence for a Role of *H. pylori* in the Development of MALT Lymphoma

Epidemiological, histopathologic, and experimental studies have provided evidence linking *H. pylori* infection and MALT lymphoma. Importantly, *H. pylori* eradication alone may be sufficient to cure early-stage MALT lymphoma.[43]

The first studies implicating *H. pylori* in the pathogenesis of gastric MALT lymphoma were published in the early 1990s, reporting that *H. pylori* infection was present in 92% of the stomachs with MALT lymphomas,[4] and other studies subsequently confirmed that gastric MALT lymphoma is more frequent in geographic regions with a higher incidence of *H. pylori* gastritis. Furthermore, the stomach represents the primary organ affected by *H. pylori* infection and is also the most common site for primary gastrointestinal lymphomas, accounting for >75% of cases.[44] Recent studies have reported that 70% to 95% of MALT lymphoma cases are *H. pylori* positive.[45] The etiology of gastric MALT lymphomas that are not associated with *H. pylori* infection is poorly understood. It is possible that in some of the *H. pylori*–negative cases there is low bacterial load such that *H. pylori* infection is not detected. Alternatively, they may be associated with infection caused by other *Helicobacter* species, such as *Helicobacter heilmannii*, which also responds to antibiotic therapy.[46] The disparity in the literature regarding the proportion of *H. pylori*–positive MALT lymphomas may relate to the diverse patient demographic characteristics in the various studies, differences in study approaches, such as the number of biopsies examined, the different grades and stages of lymphoma included in the studies, and the approaches used to determine *H. pylori* status. *H. pylori* may be detected in biopsies of gastric mucosa using routinely stained hematoxylin and eosin sections, with the aid of special stains (thiazine, Warthin-Starry, genta stains) or by immunohistochemical analysis. Evidence of *H. pylori* infection can also be determined by the urea breath test, rapid urease test, bacterial isolation from tissue cultures of stomach biopsy samples, polymerase chain reaction (PCR) using DNA extracted from gastric mucosa samples, fecal antigen testing, and anti–*H. pylori* serology. It has been suggested that serologic testing should be performed if the biopsy results are negative owing to its high sensitivity.[47]

Animal models have provided support for the association between *H. pylori* and MALT lymphoma. BALB/c mice infected with *Helicobacter felis* developed lymphoid follicles and lymphoepithelial lesions that were morphologically similar to those seen in gastric MALT lymphoma in humans.[48] The role of *H. pylori* gastric infection in the development of gastric MALT lymphoma has been further supported by the fact that eradication of *H. pylori* with antibiotic-based therapies results in the regression of MALT lymphomas in as many as 60% to 80% of cases, and *H. pylori* eradication therapy with antibiotics is currently accepted as the first-line treatment for stage I gastric MALT lymphomas.[43,49]

Pathogenic Mechanisms of *H. pylori*–associated MALT Lymphoma

H. pylori infection induces a host immunologic response that results in the expansion of the gastric mucosa by lymphoid tissue, ranging from an increased number of mononuclear cells to lymphoid aggregates and prominent lymphoid follicles. Usually the host response to *H. pylori* only results in chronic active gastritis, with variable grades of activity, from mild to severe.[6] However, in some cases, the B-cell lymphoid population progresses to a neoplastic pathway that manifests as MALT lymphoma (Figs. 3-3 and 3-4). In vitro studies have demonstrated that the B-cell lymphoid proliferation that ensues in response to *H. pylori* infection of the stomach is dependent on T cells that are activated by *H. pylori* antigens.[50] B lymphocytes interact with T cells through CD40 and CD40 ligands, such that persistent *H. pylori* infection results in the emergence of a clonal B-cell population.[51,52]

CagA is an important virulence factor of *H. pylori* and has been causally associated with MALT lymphoma; however, its role in MALT lymphoma is poorly understood. Transgenic mice expressing *H. pylori* CagA proteins developed myeloid leukemias and B-cell lymphomas,[28] supporting a role for CagA-associated mechanisms in MALT lymphoma. These studies show that tyrosine phosphorylation of the CagA protein results in an interaction with the SHP-2 oncoprotein, leading to its deregulation and promoting lymphoma development.[28] In addition, CagA-positive *H. pylori* strains are significantly associated with chromosomal translocation t(11;18)(q21;q21) in

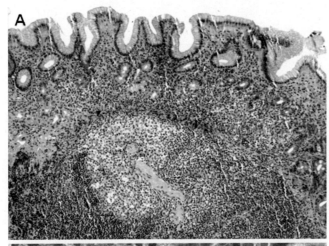

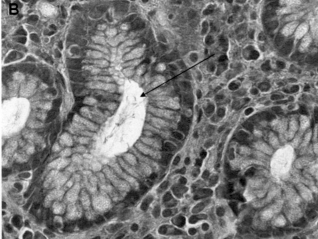

FIGURE 3-3 *H. pylori* gastritis and MALT lymphoma. **A:** Gastric mucosa with chronic active gastritis with prominent reactive lymphoid follicles in response to *H. pylori* infection (hematoxylin and eosin stain original magnification 100×). **B:** *H. pylori* bacteria are seen within the glandular lumen (*arrow*) (thiazine stain, original magnification 400×).

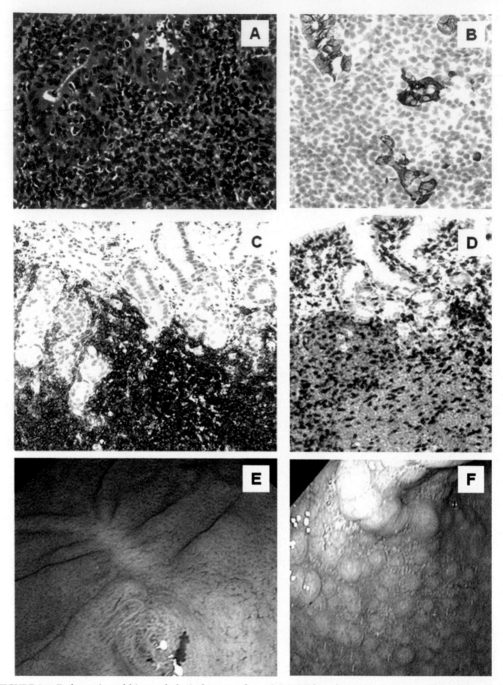

FIGURE 3-4 Endoscopic and histopathologic features of gastric MALT lymphoma. A: Expansion of B-cell lymphoid population with formation of lymphoepithelial lesion (hematoxylin and eosin stain original magnification 100×). **B:** Cytokeratin immunostaining highlights the presence of lymphoepithelial lesions with destruction of gastric glandular epithelium. **C:** Immunohistochemical stain for CD20 demonstrates expansion of a B-cell population that is characteristic of MALT lymphoma. **D:** Immunohistochemical stain demonstrates an admixed population of reactive T lymphocytes associated with the chronic gastritis process in which the MALT lymphoma developed. **E,F:** Endoscopic photographs from a case of MALT lymphoma reveal a linear ulcer with raised borders (**E**) and nodular appearance of the background gastric mucosa (**F**) (immunohistochemical stains original magnification 100×) (Endoscopic images contributed by Dr. Faten Aberra, University of Pennsylvania.)

MALT lymphomas.[53] Since CagA-positive *H. pylori* strains induce a strong inflammatory response through IL-8, a potent chemokine for neutrophil activation, it has been hypothesized that the activated neutrophils generate ROS that lead to DNA damage, including double-strand breaks, and may lead to the occurrence of t(11;18)(q21;q21) in MALT lymphomas.[53]

Only a small proportion of *H. pylori*–infected patients go on to develop MALT lymphoma. As is the case in *H. pylori*–associated gastric carcinogenesis, the specific mechanisms remain poorly understood and may include host susceptibility factors that are yet to be defined.

Molecular Features of *H. pylori*–associated MALT Lymphomas

MALT lymphomas exhibit immunoglobulin heavy and light chain gene rearrangements and somatic hypermutation of variable regions, indicating that they are derived from postgerminal center B cells.[54] Until recently, it was thought that clonality assessment by immunoglobulin heavy chain (IGH) rearrangement analysis by PCR may not be specific enough for lymphoma, as clonal populations may also be detected in gastritis.[55] More recently, Hummel et al.[56] have demonstrated a high sensitivity and specificity of advanced PCR technology to distinguish gastritis from MALT lymphoma in biopsies with ambiguous morphology.

The t(11;18)(q21;q21) translocation is the most common chromosomal abnormality in MALT lymphomas (Fig. 3-5). It is specific for MALT lymphomas and is absent in other types of lymphomas, including nodal or splenic marginal zone lymphomas and nodal or extranodal diffuse large B-cell lymphomas.[46,52] This translocation has been observed in 5% to 40% of gastric MALT lymphomas with the lowest frequency reported in North America.[57] The t(11;18)(q21;q21) results in the fusion of the DNA region encoding the amino terminal of the AP12(apoptosis inhibitor 2) gene at 11q21 and the region encoding the carboxyl terminal of the MALT1

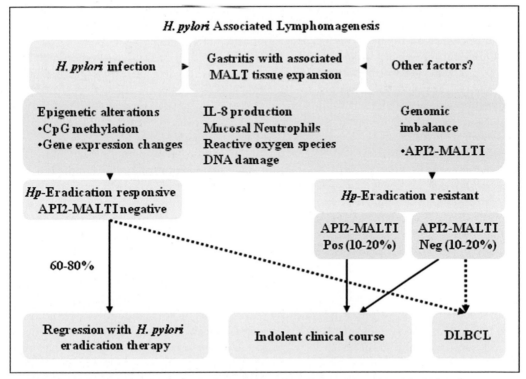

FIGURE 3-5 Diagram representation of *H. pylori*–associated lymphomagenesis. (Adapted from Inagaki H. Mucosa-associated lymphoid tissue lymphoma: molecular pathogenesis and clinicopathological significance. *Pathol Int.* 2007; 57:474–484.)

(MALT lymphoma-associated translocation 1) gene at 18q21 forming a chimeric fusion protein that activates the nuclear factor (NF)-κB signaling pathway. NF-κB is a transcription factor that controls genes promoting cell survival, such as those encoding cytokines, growth factors, cell adhesion molecules, and apoptosis inhibitors and, therefore, promotes tumor development. The NF-κB signaling pathway is activated through B-cell or T-cell antigen receptor stimulation, which assists in the recruitment and oligomerization of three molecules: caspase recruitment domain-containing MAGUK1 (CARMA1), B-cell chronic lymphocytic leukemia/lymphoma 10 (BCL10), and MALT1. This protein complex ubiquitinates and enhances the degradation of NEMO, which is an inhibitor of NF-κB, resulting in activation of the NF-κB pathway. It has been proposed that the API2-MALT1 fusion product bypasses this pathway and directly ubiquitinates NEMO and activates NF-κB.[46] In addition, the API2-MALT1 fusion protein exerts an antiapoptotic effect through its inhibition of the Smac and HtrA2, mitochondrial proteins that are involved in caspase-mediated apoptosis.[46]

The presence of the t(11;18)(q21;q21) translocation is associated with a more advanced tumor stage, predicts resistance to *H. pylori* eradication therapy, and has been found to be significantly associated with infection by CagA-positive strains of *H. pylori*.[58] These lymphomas exhibit resistance to oral alkylating agents but respond to chemotherapy with the nucleoside analog cladribine (2-chlorodeoxyadenosine).[46] Interestingly, lymphomas that harbor API2-MALT1 do not undergo large cell transformation, and in spite of being refractory to *H. pylori* eradication and present at advanced stages, API2-MALT1–positive tumors do not exhibit aggressive behavior (Fig. 3-5).[59]

Gastric MALT lymphomas can be categorized into three groups based on the presence or absence of the t(11;18)(q21;q21) translocation and the response to *H. pylori* eradication therapy: (a) eradication responsive and API2-MALT1–fusion negative, (b) eradication resistant and API2-MALT1 fusion–negative, and (c) eradication resistant and API2-MALT1–fusion positive (Fig. 3-5).[46,59] Factors that are associated with resistance to *H. pylori* eradication include advanced disease stage (stage II and above), API2-MALT1 positivity, and nuclear expression of BCL10.[59] Resistance to *H. pylori* eradication therapy has also been observed in patients with *Fas* gene mutations, which are frequently seen in association with autoimmune disease.[59]

Other chromosomal translocations have been described in MALT lymphomas, including t(1;14)(p22;q32), t(14;18)(q32;q21), and t(3;14)(p14;q32), which deregulate the expression of the *BCL10, MALT1*, and forkhead box protein P1 (*FOXP1*) genes, respectively. The t(1;14)(p22;q32) translocation has been reported in approximately 4% to 5% of gastric MALT lymphomas and also predicts resistance to *H. pylori* eradication therapy.[52] The t(3;14)(p14;q32) and t(14;18)(q32;q21) translocations are rarely observed in gastric MALT lymphomas.[46,57]

Recent studies have revealed epigenetic alterations in MALT lymphoma. CpG-island methylation studies have shown that aberrant hypermethylation of tumor suppressor and other tumor-related genes is associated with *H. pylori* infection in MALT lymphomas. In contrast, the *H. pylori*–independent lymphomas, including those with the t(11;18)(q21;q21) translocation, are associated with a low level of CpG methylation.[60] The frequency of promoter methylation of several genes, such as the death associated protein kinase (*DAPK*) and the E-cadherin (*CDH1*) genes, increases with the progression of MALT lymphoma to diffuse large B-cell lymphoma (DLBCL).[60] The methylation level of the *MGMT* gene was observed to be significantly higher in lymphomas with extragastric involvement than in those without extragastric involvement and may be associated with a better therapeutic response to alkylating agents. Promoter methylation of *p16, MGMT*, and *p21* was higher in low-grade MALT lymphomas than in DLBCL, suggesting that CpG methylation events may occur early in lymphomagenesis. In addition, the methylation levels decrease after *H. pylori* eradication therapy. It has been suggested that *H. pylori* infection brings about these epigenetic alterations through the effects of its various molecules (CagA, VacA, OipA, and DNA methyltransferases) and inflammatory responses that give rise to ROS. The reversibility of DNA methylation with changes in the microenvironment could also contribute to the regression of lymphoma with *H. pylori* eradication therapy.[60]

References

1. Warren JR, Marshall B. Unidentified curved bacilli on gastric epithelium in active chronic gastritis. *Lancet.* 1983;1:1273–1275.
2. International Agency for Research of Cancer. Shistosomes, liver flukes and *Helicobacter pylori. IARC Monogr Eval Carcinog Risks Hum.* 1994;61:177–241.
3. Parsonnet J, Friedman GD, Vandersteen DP, et al. *Helicobacter pylori* and the risk of gastric carcinoma. *N Eng J Med.* 1991;325:1127–1131.
4. Wotherspoon AC, Ortiz-Hidalgo C, Falzon MR, et al. *Helicobacter pylori*-associated gastritis and primary B-cell gastric lymphoma. *Lancet.* 1991;338:1175–1176.
5. Gologan A, Graham DY, Sepulveda AR. Molecular markers in *Helicobacter pylori*-associated gastric carcinogenesis. *Clin Lab Med.* 2005;25:197–222.
6. Dixon MF, Genta RM, Yardley JH, et al. Classification and grading of gastritis. The updated Sydney system. International workshop on the histopathology of gastritis, Houston 1994. *Am J Surg Pathol.* 1996;20:1161–1181.
7. Herrera V, Parsonnet J. *Helicobacter pylori* and gastric adenocarcinoma. *Clin Microbiol Infect.* 2009;15:971–976.
8. Group HaCC. Gastric cancer and *Helicobacter pylori*: a combined analysis of 12 case control studies nested within prospective cohorts. *Gut.* 2001;49:347–353.
9. Uemura N, Okamoto S, Yamamoto S, et al. *Helicobacter pylori* infection and the development of gastric cancer. *N Engl J Med.* 2001;345:784–789.
10. Whiting JL, Sigurdsson A, Rowlands DC, et al. The long term results of endoscopic surveillance of premalignant gastric lesions. *Gut.* 2002;50:378–381.
11. Watanabe T, Tada M, Nagai H, et al. *Helicobacter pylori* infection induces gastric cancer in mongolian gerbils. *Gastroenterology.* 1998;115:642–648.
12. Franco AT, Johnston E, Krishna U, et al. Regulation of gastric carcinogenesis by *Helicobacter pylori* virulence factors. *Cancer Res.* 2008;68:379–387.
13. Wong BC, Lam SK, Wong WM, et al. *Helicobacter pylori* eradication to prevent gastric cancer in a high-risk region of China: a randomized controlled trial. *JAMA.* 2004;291:187–194.
14. Fukase K, Kato M, Kikuchi S, et al. Effect of eradication of *Helicobacter pylori* on incidence of metachronous gastric carcinoma after endoscopic resection of early gastric cancer: an open-label, randomised controlled trial. *Lancet.* 2008;372:392–397.
15. Malfertheiner P, Megraud F, O'Morain C, et al. Current concepts in the management of *Helicobacter pylori* infection: the Maastricht III Consensus Report. *Gut.* 2007;56:772–781.
16. Robinson K, Argent RH, Atherton JC. The inflammatory and immune response to *Helicobacter pylori* infection. *Best Pract Res Clin Gastroenterol.* 2007;21:237–259.
17. Correa P. Human gastric carcinogenesis: a multistep and multifactorial process—First American Cancer Society Award Lecture on Cancer Epidemiology and Prevention. *Cancer Res.* 1992;52:6735–6740.
18. Sepulveda A, Peterson LE, Shelton J, et al. Histological patterns of gastritis in *H. pylori*-infected individuals with a family history of gastric cancer. *Am J Gastroenterol.* 2002;97:1365–1370.
19. Fenoglio-Preiser C, Carneiro F, Correa P, et al. Gastric carcinoma. In: Hamilton S, Aaltonen L, eds. *Pathology and genetics of tumours of the digestive system.* Lyon, IARC Press; 2000:39–52.
20. Sepulveda AR, Wu L, Ota H, et al. Molecular identification of main cellular lineages as a tool for the classification of gastric cancer. *Hum Pathol.* 2000;31:566–574.
21. Kao JY, Zhang M, Miller MJ, et al. *Helicobacter pylori* immune escape is mediated by dendritic cell-induced treg skewing and Th17 suppression in mice. *Gastroenterology.* 2010;138:1046–1054.
22. Correa P, Houghton J. Carcinogenesis of *Helicobacter pylori. Gastroenterology.* 2007;133:659–672.
23. Wen S, Moss SF. *Helicobacter pylori* virulence factors in gastric carcinogenesis. *Cancer Lett.* 2009;282:1–8.
24. Handa O, Naito Y, Yoshikawa T. CagA protein of *Helicobacter pylori*: a hijacker of gastric epithelial cell signaling. *Biochem Pharmacol.* 2007;73:1697–1702.
25. Parsonnet J, Friedman GD, Orentreich N, et al. Risk for gastric cancer in people with CagA positive or CagA negative *Helicobacter pylori* infection [see comments]. *Gut.* 1997;40:297–301.
26. Crabtree JE, Covacci A, Farmery SM, et al. *Helicobacter pylori* induced interleukin-8 expression in gastric epithelial cells is associated with CagA positive phenotype. *J Clin Pathol.* 1995;48:41–45.

27. Sepulveda AR, Yao Y, Yan W, et al. CpG Methylation and reduced expression of O(6)-methylguanine DNA methyltransferase is associated with *Helicobacter pylori* infection. *Gastroenterology*. 2010;138:1836–1844.

28. Ohnishi N, Yuasa H, Tanaka S, et al. Transgenic expression of *Helicobacter pylori* CagA induces gastrointestinal and hematopoietic neoplasms in mouse. *Proc Natl Acad Sci U S A*. 2008;105:1003–1008.

29. Brenner H, Arndt V, Sturmer T, et al. Individual and joint contribution of family history and *Helicobacter pylori* infection to the risk of gastric carcinoma. *Cancer*. 2000;88:274–279.

30. El-Omar EM. Role of host genes in sporadic gastric cancer. *Best Pract Res Clin Gastroenterol*. 2006;20:675–686.

31. Yao Y, Tao H, Park DI, et al. Demonstration and Characterization of mutations induced by *helicobacter pylori* organisms in gastric epithelial cells. *Helicobacter*. 2006;11:272–286.

32. Chiba T, Marusawa H. A novel mechanism for inflammation-associated carcinogenesis; an important role of activation-induced cytidine deaminase (AID) in mutation induction. *J Mol Med*. 2009;87:1023–1027.

33. Umar A, Boland CR, Terdiman JP, et al. Revised Bethesda Guidelines for hereditary nonpolyposis colorectal cancer (Lynch syndrome) and microsatellite instability. *J Natl Cancer Inst*. 2004;96:261–268.

34. Kim JJ, Tao H, Carloni E, et al. *Helicobacter pylori* impairs DNA mismatch repair in gastric epithelial cells. *Gastroenterology*. 2002;123:542–553.

35. Leung WK, Kim JJ, Kim JG, et al. Microsatellite instability in gastric intestinal metaplasia in patients with and without gastric cancer. *Am J Pathol*. 2000;156:537–543.

36. Farinati F, Cardin R, Bortolami M, et al. Oxidative DNA damage in gastric cancer: CagA status and OGG1 gene polymorphism. *Int J Cancer*. 2008;123:51–55.

37. Chan AO, Chu KM, Huang C, et al. Association between *Helicobacter pylori* infection and interleukin 1beta polymorphism predispose to CpG island methylation in gastric cancer. *Gut*. 2007;56:595–597.

38. Kim SY, Kim JH, Lee HS, et al. Meta- and gene set analysis of stomach cancer gene expression data. *Mol Cells*. 2007;24:200–209.

39. Myllykangas S, Junnila S, Kokkola A, et al. Integrated gene copy number and expression microarray analysis of gastric cancer highlights potential target genes. *Int J Cancer*. 2008;123:817–825.

40. Belair C, Darfeuille F, Staedel C. *Helicobacter pylori* and gastric cancer: possible role of microRNAs in this intimate relationship. *Clin Microbiol Infect*. 2009;15:806–812.

41. Zhang Z, Li Z, Gao C, et al. miR-21 plays a pivotal role in gastric cancer pathogenesis and progression. *Lab Invest*. 2008;88:1358–1366.

42. Isaacson PG, Du MQ. MALT lymphoma: from morphology to molecules. *Nat Rev Cancer*. 2004;4:644–653.

43. Wotherspoon AC, Doglioni C, Diss TC, et al. Regression of primary low-grade B-cell gastric lymphoma of mucosa- associated lymphoid tissue type after eradication of *Helicobacter pylori*. *Lancet*. 1993;342:575–577.

44. Zullo A, Hassan C, Andriani A, et al. Eradication therapy for *Helicobacter pylori* in patients with gastric MALT lymphoma: a pooled data analysis. *Am J Gastroenterol*. 2009;104:1932–1937; quiz 1938.

45. Sumida T, Kitadai Y, Hiyama T, et al. Antibodies to *Helicobacter pylori* and CagA protein are associated with the response to antibacterial therapy in patients with *H. pylori*-positive API2-MALT1-negative gastric MALT lymphoma. *Cancer Sci*. 2009;100:1075–1081.

46. Inagaki H. Mucosa-associated lymphoid tissue lymphoma: molecular pathogenesis and clinicopathological significance. *Pathol Int*. 2007;57:474–484.

47. Lehours P, Ruskone-Fourmestraux A, Lavergne A, et al. Which test to use to detect *Helicobacter pylori* infection in patients with low-grade gastric mucosa-associated lymphoid tissue lymphoma? *Am J Gastroenterol*. 2003;98:291–295.

48. Enno A, O'Rourke JL, Howlett CR, et al. MALToma-like lesions in the murine gastric mucosa after long-term infection with Helicobacter felis. A mouse model of *Helicobacter pylori*-induced gastric lymphoma. *Am J Pathol*. 1995;147:217–222.

49. Nakamura T, Seto M, Tajika M, et al. Clinical features and prognosis of gastric MALT lymphoma with special reference to responsiveness to *H. pylori* eradication and API2-MALT1 status. *Am J Gastroenterol*. 2008;103:62–70.

50. Hussell T, Isaacson PG, Crabtree JE, et al. *Helicobacter pylori*-specific tumour-infiltrating T cells provide contact dependent help for the growth of malignant B cells in low-grade gastric lymphoma of mucosa-associated lymphoid tissue. *J Pathol*. 1996;178:122–127.

51. Isaacson PG, Du MQ. Gastrointestinal lymphoma: where morphology meets molecular biology. *J Pathol.* 2005;205:255–274.

52. Todorovic M, Balint B, Jevtic M, et al. Primary gastric mucosa associated lymphoid tissue lymphoma: clinical data predicted treatment outcome. *World J Gastroenterol.* 2008;14:2388–2393.

53. Ye H, Liu H, Attygalle A, et al. Variable frequencies of t(11;18)(q21;q21) in MALT lymphomas of different sites: significant association with CagA strains of *H.pylori* in gastric MALT lymphoma. *Blood.* 2003;102:1012–1018.

54. Isaacson P, Chott A, Nakamura S, et al. *Extranodal marginal zone lymphoma of mucosa-associated lymphoid tissue (MALT lymphoma).* Lyon, IARC Press; 2008.

55. Weston AP, Banerjee SK, Horvat RT, et al. Specificity of polymerase chain reaction monoclonality for diagnosis of gastric mucosa-associated lymphoid tissue (MALT) lymphoma: direct comparison to Southern blot gene rearrangement. *Dig Dis Sci.* 1998;43:290–299.

56. Hummel M, Oeschger S, Barth TF, et al. Wotherspoon criteria combined with B cell clonality analysis by advanced polymerase chain reaction technology discriminates covert gastric marginal zone lymphoma from chronic gastritis. *Gut.* 2006;55:782–787.

57. Remstein ED, Dogan A, Einerson RR, et al. The incidence and anatomic site specificity of chromosomal translocations in primary extranodal marginal zone B-cell lymphoma of mucosa-associated lymphoid tissue (MALT lymphoma) in North America. *Am J Surg Pathol.* 2006;30:1546–1553.

58. Du MQ. MALT lymphoma: recent advances in aetiology and molecular genetics. *J Clin Exp Hematop.* 2007;47:31–42.

59. Inagaki H, Nakamura T, Li C, et al. Gastric MALT lymphomas are divided into three groups based on responsiveness to *Helicobacter pylori* eradication and detection of API2-MALT1 fusion. *Am J Surg Pathol.* 2004;28:1560–1567.

60. Kondo T, Oka T, Sato H, et al. Accumulation of aberrant CpG hypermethylation by *Helicobacter pylori* infection promotes development and progression of gastric MALT lymphoma. *Int J Oncol.* 2009;35: 547–557.

4

Epstein-Barr Virus and Gastric Carcinoma

▶ Masashi Fukayama

▶ Aya Shinozaki

▶ Rumi Hino

INTRODUCTION

Several human neoplasms, including gastric carcinoma (GC), develop in close association with infectious organisms. *Helicobacter pylori* and Epstein-Barr virus (EBV) are now regarded as causative microorganisms of GC.[1,2] Like other human oncogenic microorganisms, these infectious agents cause malignant neoplasms to develop in a limited number of patients out of a large population of healthy or healthy-appearing carriers through unknown mechanisms.[2] However, the roles of *H. pylori* and EBV in the development and progression of GC are quite different (Table 4-1).

EBV was the first human oncogenic virus to be identified when it was discovered in human neoplastic cells (Burkitt lymphoma cell lines) in 1964. Subsequent investigations have identified the virus in nasopharyngeal carcinoma (NPC), Hodgkin lymphoma, B-cell lymphomas with or without immunosuppression, and nasal natural killer/T-cell lymphoma. EBV was identified in GC tissues in 1990 (Fig. 4-1), when the in situ hybridization (ISH) method for detecting EBV-encoded small RNA (*EBER*) had just been introduced to the field of pathology (Fig. 4-1C and D).[3] *EBER* is abundant in latently infected cells (up to 10^7 copies per infected cell) and is identified in nearly all neoplastic cells of tumor tissues when it is present in GC. Thus, detection of *EBER* by ISH is a gold standard for the identification of EBV-associated GC. Furthermore, ISH can be used to identify *EBER* in archived materials, such as formalin-fixed and paraffin-embedded tissues, which can be used to investigate the epidemiology of this type of GC. EBV-associated GC occurs worldwide and its frequency is estimated to be 8.7% (95% confidence interval: 7.5%–10.0%) of all GC cases,[4] which corresponds to an annual incidence of 70,000 to 80,000 patients worldwide.[1]

EBV-ASSOCIATED GC IS A DISTINCT CLINICOPATHOLOGICAL SUBGROUP OF GC

EBV-associated GC is defined as the presence of latent EBV infection in neoplastic cells. This type of GC (Table 4-2)[4-6] affects predominantly males and is usually located in the proximal stomach. Some reports suggest that this carcinoma occurs in patients of a relatively younger age compared to those with non-EBV GC, but meta-analyses did not confirm that observation.[4,5] EBV is involved in 25% of remnant GCs, that is, GC, which occurs in the remnant stomach, at least >5 to 10 years after the initial gastrectomy for either benign or malignant stomach diseases, and several reports have suggested that multiple carcinomas are likely to occur in association with EBV.[6] EBV-associated GC has a lower rate of lymph node involvement, especially during its early stage

Table 4-1	Comparison of *H. pylori* and the EBV as causative agents of GC	
	H. pylori	**Epstein-Barr Virus**
Carriers	More than 75% of people over age 40	More than 95% of people over age 20
Involvement in GC	Most GC (intestinal/diffuse types of histology)	10% of GC, including LE-like GC
	Higher risk of GC in carriers compared to noncarriers	Monoclonal EBV present in all neoplastic cells
Carcinogenic mechanisms	Hummingbird phenomenon by transfection of the *CagA* gene into epithelial cells	Transformation of epithelial cells after transfection of the *LMP2A* gene.
	Activation of ERK mediated by CagA/ SHP2 or Grb2	Abnormal signal transduction mediated by LMP2A
Model animal/ cell line	Mongolian gerbil, CagA transgenic mouse	GC strain (KT), transplantable to SCID mice/GC cell line (SNU-719)
Other related malignancies	MALT lymphoma	Lymphomas (Burkitt lymphoma, Hodgkin lymphoma, T/NK cell lymphoma)
		Nasopharyngeal carcinoma
		Neoplasms in immunocompromised hosts

GC, gastric carcinoma; LE, lymphoepithelioma-like.

within the submucosa, and has a relatively favorable prognosis compared with EBV-negative GC, although both findings remain to be confirmed.[5]

EBV-associated GC often occurs as an ulcerated or saucer-like tumor accompanied by marked thickening of the gastric wall (Fig. 4-1A). These features are easily discernible on endoscopic ultrasonograms and CT scans of the stomach. There are two histological types of EBV-associated GCs, lymphoepithelioma (LE)-like (Fig. 4-1B and C) and ordinary (Fig. 4-1D), although there is a continuum between the types.[6] The typical morphology of LE-like GC is described as poorly

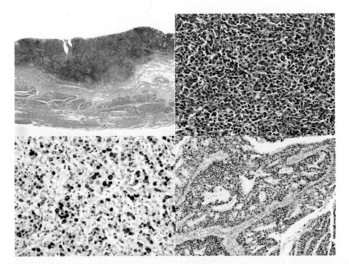

FIGURE 4-1 Histopathology of EBV associated GC. **A** (**left upper**): Low-power view of EBV–associated GC. Lymphoepithelioma (LE)-like carcinoma shows expansive growth with prominent infiltration of lymphocytes. **B** (**right upper**): High-power view of LE-type of EBV-associated GC shown in (**A**). **C** (**left lower**): EBER in situ hybridization of LE-type of EBV-associated GC (**A**). **D** (**right lower**): EBER in situ hybridization of ordinary type of EBV-associated GC.

Table 4-2	Clinicopathological features of EBV-associated GC
Clinical	Nearly 10% of Total GC Male Predominance Remnant Stomach
Macroscopic	Location at gastric cardia/body
	Ulcerated or saucer-like tumor
	Marked thickening of the gastric wall
	Multiple carcinomas[a]
Microscopic	Lymphoepithelioma-like histology
	Moderate to poorly differentiated adenocarcinoma
	Lymphocytic infiltration in various degrees
	Lace pattern within the mucosa
	Lymphoid follicle in the invasive sites
Behavioral	Lower rate of lymph node involvement[a]
	Relatively favorable prognosis[a]

[a]Findings have been suggested, but more evidence is necessary for confirmation.

differentiated carcinoma with dense infiltration of lymphocytes, resembling NPC.[3] LE-like GC is nearly identical to the subgroup that Watanabe et al.[7] reported as "GC with lymphoid stroma (GCLS)," but GCLS is relatively a broad category that includes LE-like GC. The relative ratio of the LE-like/GCLS type to the ordinary type reported in the literature varies considerably from 1:10 to 4:1.[6] This variability is due to interpretation variability in diagnostic criteria of the LE-like/GCLS type, especially when there is heterogeneity within the tumor. More than 80% of the LE-like/GCLS-type tumors were positive for EBV in most reports.[3,6,8] The histopathological features of EBV-positive LE-like/GCLS tumors, which are not seen in EBV-negative LE-like/GCLS tumors, are mild cellular pleomorphism, rare mitotic figures, a marked degree of lymphoid stroma, and lymphoid infiltration within the cancer cell nests.[8]

For EBV-associated GC, the incidence of intramucosal and submucosal carcinomas (early GC) at diagnosis is not statistically different from that of deeply invasive carcinomas (advanced GC). At the intramucosal stage, EBV-associated GC shows a "lace pattern," which is formed by the connection and fusion of neoplastic glands within the mucosa proper. Further invasion of the carcinoma into the submucosa is frequently accompanied by the infiltration of massive lymphocytes (Fig. 4-1A) consisting of CD8-positive T lymphocytes, CD4-positive T lymphocytes, and CD68-positive macrophages, in a ratio of 2:1:1, respectively. EBV infection is observed in only a very limited number of these infiltrating lymphocytes. Infiltrating cells are sometimes variable, and their extreme effect is prominent lymphoplasmacytic infiltration with numerous Mott cells[9] or a granulomatous reaction with many osteoclast-like giant cells (Ushiku et al., *Pathol Int.* 2010;60:551–558).

EBV INFECTION AND DEVELOPMENT OF CARCINOMA

The evidence regarding the lineage of EBV-infected cells, the clonality of EBV in infected cells, and the infection of epithelial cells by EBV, as described below, strongly suggests that stomach epithelial cells initiate clonal growth after they are infected with EBV from the reactivation of EBV-carrying lymphocytes at the mucosa (Fig. 4-2).

Lineage of EBV-infected Cells

Neoplastic cells from EBV-associated GC show characteristic profiles of differentiation markers, which might be associated with the lineage of EBV-infected cells. Claudin (CLDN) proteins

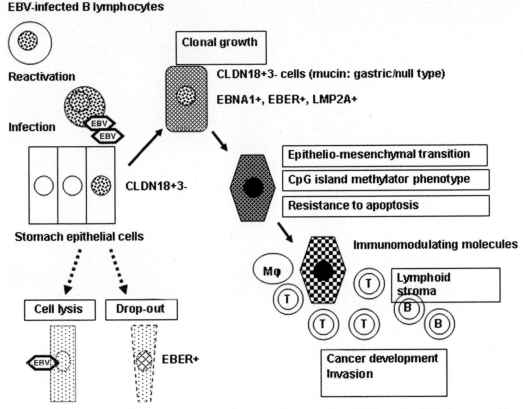

FIGURE 4-2 Schematic representation of the development and progression of EBV–associated GC. Stomach epithelial cells are infected with EBV from the reactivation of EBV-carrying lymphocytes at the mucosa. Some EBV-infected cells begin to grow clonally in the milieu of atrophic gastritis. The neoplastic cells retain the claudin 18–positive/claudin 3–negative (CLDN18+, 3−) gastric phenotype, which may correspond to the phenotype of the original EBV-infected cells. The CpG-island methylation phenotype is the primary abnormality in neoplastic cells of EBV-associated GC. Expression and secretion of immunomodulator molecules induce the characteristic stromal reaction.

constitute the tight junction, and neoplastic cells of EBV-associated GC showed a high frequency of CLDN18 expression (84%) and a low frequency of CLDN3 expression (5%).[10] This expression profile (CLDN18+, 3−) corresponds to that of the normal gastric epithelium in adults and fetuses, but not to that of intestinal metaplasia (CLDN18−, 3+). In accordance with the CLDN expression patterns, almost half of the EBV-associated GC cases in a study by Barua et al.[11] had gastric-type mucin expression (MUC5AC, MUC6), and the other half lacked gastric- or intestinal-type mucin or CD10 expression. These results indicate that EBV-associated GC is very homogenous with regard to cellular differentiation and that it preserves the nature of the cells of origin. Thus, the cells that are targets of EBV infection and their subsequent transformation may be precursor cells with intrinsic differentiation potential toward the gastric cell type.

Clonality of EBV in Infected Cells

EBV is a double-stranded DNA virus (184 kb in size), which is maintained in a linear form in the virus particles. After EBV enters infected cells, the viral DNA circularizes by fusing the terminal repeats (TRs, repetitive 500-bp structures) at both ends of the linear genome and maintains its circular form in the nuclei of latently infected cells.[2] Southern blot analysis of EBV-TRs provides information about the clonality of EBV and the state of viral activation, that is, replicating (linear configuration) versus latent (episomal circular forms). In EBV-associated GC, TR analysis has demonstrated that monoclonal EBV is present in an episomal form without integration into the

FIGURE 4-3 Clonal analysis of EBV derived from virus-associated GC. Southern blot hybridization analysis of TRs of EBV DNA, extracted from EBV-associated GC. DNA is cut with the *Bam*HI restriction enzyme, electrophoresed, and hybridized with an EBV-TR-specific probe (R, R': Raji cell used as a control, 1–5: samples of intramucosal carcinomas, 6–9: samples of submucosal carcinomas). Analysis of the blot shows either one or two bands larger than 6 kb in each sample. When the detected bands are short, it indicates that EBV takes the linear form in viral particles. Smeared signals indicate infection of the tumor with various EBV clones. (From Uozaki H, Fukayama M. *Int J Clin Exp Pathol.* 2008;1:198–216[2], with permission from the Journal.)

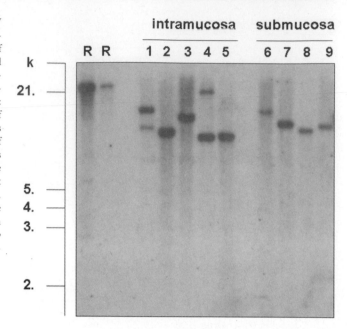

host genome and infection is latent, with no viral replication. Monoclonal or biclonal EBV was observed in carcinoma tissues in the intramucosal stage; however, it was always monoclonal in the submucosal invasion stage (Fig. 4-3) and in more advanced carcinomas.[12,13] Since all carcinoma cells show a positive signal in *EBER*-ISH in all cases of EBV-associated GC, EBV infection must occur at the initial or a very early stage of carcinoma development.

EBV Infection in Epithelial Cells

It is not clear how EBV infection is established in the stomach mucosa, as the viral receptor molecule, CD21, expressed in B lymphocytes is not expressed on epithelial cells.[14] Because the cocultivation of uninfected cells with virus-producing cells shows better infection efficiency (up to 800-fold) than cell-free infection, direct cell-to-cell contact is the most likely mode of viral spread to the epithelial cells in vivo.[15]

In a previous study, we identified EBV infection in a small fraction of the nonneoplastic epithelium of the stomach.[13] More recently, we confirmed that the finding on a larger scale and positive EBER signals were infrequently present in a single cell on the surface of the gastric pits (Otake, et al., manuscript in preparation). We also found that EBER-positive epithelial cells showing regenerated changes with and without cellular atypia formed one or several glands; therefore, EBV-infected epithelial cells, most likely in the neck zone of the fundic glands, are likely to initiate clonal growth leading to EBV-associated GC. In addition, atrophic gastritis[16] might induce the infiltration of EBV-carrying lymphocytes to increase the chance of contact with epithelial cells, or inflammation may produce a cytokine-rich milieu to support the clonal growth of EBV-infected epithelial cells.

CELLULAR AND MOLECULAR ABNORMALITIES IN EBV-ASSOCIATED GC

The cellular and molecular (genetic and epigenetic) abnormalities observed in EBV-associated GC are listed in Table 4-3 and discussed below.[1,2]

Proliferation and Apoptosis

An important cellular abnormality in EBV-associated GC is resistance to apoptosis. The number of apoptotic and proliferating cells is significantly lower in EBV-associated GC than in EBV-negative GC.[17–19]

Table 4-3	Cellular and molecular abnormalities in EBV-associated GC		
Abnormalities	**Comments**	**Methods**	**References**
Apoptosis	Low (1.8%–2.0%) vs. EBV-negative GC (3.3%–4.3%)	TUNEL	17,18
	Low (4.36%) vs. EBV-negative GC (6.50%) in early GC	Morphology	19
Proliferation	Low (23.7%–40%) vs. EBV-negative GC (48.0%–48.5%)	IHC (Ki67, MIB1)	17–19
p53 overexpression/ mutation	Overexpression (>10%, >30%, or 50%): none or rare	IHC, PCR-SSCP	20,21–23
	Sporadic expression: controversial (frequent in GCLS or low in early GC)	IHC	19,23–26
Bcl-2 expression	Controversial	IHC	17,18
Chromosomal aberration	Gain in chromosome 11, loss in 15q15	FISH	29
	Loss of chromosome 4p, 11p, 18q		30
LOH	Rare (5q, 17p, 18q LOH)	PCR-LOH	21,31
	FAL score: low (0.097) vs. EBV-negative GC (0.341)	(21 markers)	21
MSI	None or rare in some reports	PCR, IHC (hMLH1)	22,31–34
	10%–15%, similar frequency to that in EBV-negative GC in other reports	PCR	21,25,35
CIMP	CIMP-high	MSP	22,40
	Loss of expression (P16, E-cadherin, p73)	MSP, IHC	22,32,36–38

CIMP, CpG-island methylation phenotype; FAL, fractional allelic loss, defined as the ratio of number of markers with LOH to total number of informative markers; GC, gastric carcinoma; GCLS, gastric carcinoma with lymphoid stroma; IHC, immunohistochemistry; LOH; loss of heterozygosity; MSI, microsatellite instability; MSP, methylation-specific PCR; PCR-SSCP, PCR-single-strand conformation polymorphism.

p53 and Related Molecules

The definition of p53 overexpression, reflecting the mutation status of *p53*, differs in the literature and includes 10%,[20] 30%,[21,22] and 50%[17,23] of p53-positive cells out of the total number of cells. Although there is a range in the values defining p53 overexpression, all studies agree that diffuse overexpression is rare in EBV-associated GC (<10% of cases), in marked contrast to EBV-negative GC (>30%). On the other hand, sporadic expression of p53 (<10%, probably "wild type") is reportedly increased in EBV-negative GC,[23,24] especially in the GCLS subtype.[25] Ishii et al. reported the opposite result; they found that sporadic p53 expression was lower in the early-carcinoma stage of EBV-associated GC than in EBV-negative GC, and the authors speculated that EBV infection may block p53 expression, suppressing apoptosis of the infected cells.[19]

Immunomodulatory Molecules

The significance of CD8-positive T lymphocytes in EBV-associated GC is not clear. Although infiltrating T cells contain a subpopulation recognizing EBV-infected epithelial cells, T-cell infiltration is also induced by immunomodulatory molecules, which are secreted from carcinoma cells. Using a high-density oligonucleotide array, we observed increased expression of IL1-β in an EBV-associated GC strain in **severe combined immunodeficiency mice** (KT-tumor).[26] IL1-β messages were also identified in the carcinoma cells of surgically resected EBV-associated GC.

Global Analysis of Expression Profiles

The global analysis of gene expression profiles has been applied to various carcinomas, including GC. In one such study,[27] the expression levels of 326 genes were significantly associated with EBV infection, some of which appeared to be related to lymphoid infiltrate. Analysis of the data also confirmed that EBV-associated GC showed a gastric-like gene expression phenotype. Another approach to the global analysis of protein expression using tissue microarrays has been shown to be potentially useful for stratifying patients with EBV-associated GC into different prognostic subgroups.[28]

Cytogenetics and Loss of Heterozygosity

There are few studies of EBV-associated GC using comparative genomic hybridization. According to Chan et al.,[29] gains in chromosome 11 and losses in 15q15 are more common in EBV-associated GC. zur Hausen et al.[30] reported that loss of chromosome 4p and 11p was exclusively restricted to EBV-associated GC and loss of 18q was also significantly more frequent in this type of GC. In addition, studies by our group[31] and van Rees et al.[21] have reported loss of heterozygosity (LOH). LOH on chromosomal regions 5q, 17p, and 18q is rare, and allelic loss is generally rare in EBV-associated GC. The latter finding was represented as the low score of fractional allelic loss using 21 markers (Table 4-3).[21]

Microsatellite Instability

Microsatellite instability (MSI) has been reported to be absent or rare in EBV-associated GC, in contrast to its high frequency in EBV-negative GC,[22,32–35] although similar frequencies in both groups have also been reported.[21,25,36] On the basis of the findings that either MSI is absent or that hMLH1 expression is preserved in EBV-associated GC, some authors have suggested that the contributions of EBV and MSI to gastric carcinogenesis may be mutually exclusive.[34,35]

Aberrant DNA Methylation

Global and nonrandom CpG-island methylation in the promoter region of many cancer-related genes is the primary abnormality in EBV-associated GC.[1] CpG islands are often located in the promoter or 5′-exon sequences of the coding genes, and their methylation leads to the repression of transcription, resulting in the inactivation of downstream genes. Importantly, the subsequent reduction of gene expression has been confirmed in EBV-associated GC for the $p16^{INK4A,22,32,36}$ *E-cadherin*,[37] and *p73*[38] genes, but a link between promoter methylation and gene silencing has not been consistently shown in EBV-negative GC.

Kaneda et al.[39] used methylation-sensitive representational difference analysis and identified five genes whose promoter regions were densely methylated in GC (*LOX, HRASLS, FLNC, HAND1*, and *THBD*). By using these genes as indicators and using the methylation-specific PCR (MSP), Chang et al.[40] classified GC into three subgroups based on its CpG-island methylation phenotype (CIMP), which was defined as CIMP none, intermediate, and high (CIMP-N, -I, and -H) according to the numbers of methylated loci (0, 1–3, and 4 or more, respectively).[40] Nearly all cases (14 of 15) of EBV-associated GC exhibited the CIMP-H phenotype and also showed frequent CpG-island methylation in other cancer-related genes (Fig. 4-4). Of particular interest is the finding that EBV-associated GC had significantly higher frequencies of cancer-related gene methylation (*p14ARF, p15, p16INK4A, p73, TIMP3, E-cadherin, DAPK*, and *GSTP1*) than the EBV-negative/CIMP-H GCs, except for the *hMLH1* and *MGMT* genes. These findings indicate that CpG-island methylation is not random and is compatible with infrequent MSI abnormalities, as described above.

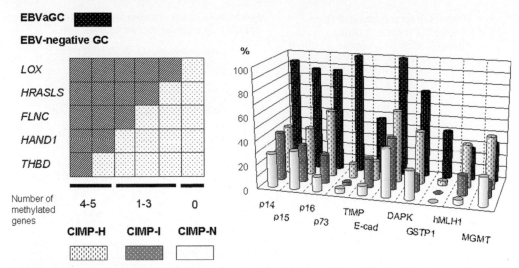

FIGURE 4-4 Frequencies of CpG methylation of cancer-related genes in GCs, with and without association of EBV infection. GC cases were classified into three subgroups according to the methylation status of the indicator genes *LOX*, *HRASLS*, *FLNC*, *HAND1*, and *THBD*. The GCs were classified as CpG-island methylation phenotype (CIMP) none (CIMP-N), intermediate (CIMP-I), and high (CIMP-H) by the numbers of methylated loci: 0, 1–3, and 4 or more, respectively. EBV-associated GCs showed significantly higher frequencies of cancer related–gene methylation than the EBV-negative/CIMP-H GCs. Note that *p73* methylation is highly specific to EBV-associated GCs and that the methylation of *hMLH1* and *MGMT* in EBV-associated GCs is not different from that in EBV-negative/CIMP-H GCs.

VIRAL GENES AND CARCINOGENESIS

EBV infection in EBV-associated malignant neoplasms is latent without the production of viral particles, that is, only a limited number of latent EBV genes are expressed in neoplastic cells. Furthermore, the expression of latent EBV genes is determined by the host cell types and the host immune status. EBV-associated GC is a latency I neoplasm, in which the only latent gene products expressed are EBV nuclear antigen I (*EBNA1*), *EBER*, latent membrane protein 2A (*LMP2A*), and BamHI-A rightward transcripts (*BARTs*).[12,13] The representative viral proteins EBNA2 and LMP1, which have immortalization activity in lymphocytes and transformation in rodent cells, respectively, are not expressed in latency I neoplasms. Therefore, it is challenging to discover how viral latent gene products cause cellular and molecular abnormalities in EBV-associated GC (Figs. 4-5 and 4-6).

Resistance to Apoptosis and LMP2A

To reveal the role of EBV infection in EBV-associated GC in vitro, we systematically compared the biological characteristics (cell growth, apoptosis, and migration) of GC cell lines with and without infection with recombinant EBV,[41] in which the neomycin resistance gene *Neo*[r] was inserted into EBV-DNA (Fig. 4-5). In this screening, we observed that resistance to serum deprivation–induced apoptosis is characteristic of EBV-infected GC cell lines. Subsequent analyses demonstrated that viral latent protein LMP2A upregulates the cellular *survivin* gene through activation of NF-κB and that increased survivin protein is responsible for the survival advantage of EBV-infected cells. Survivin is the smallest member of a protein family known as inhibitors of apoptosis proteins (IAPs), which play a key role in the regulation of apoptosis and cell division. Immunohistochemical studies confirmed survivin expression in carcinoma tissues of GC, which was significantly more frequent in EBV-associated GC than in EBV-negative GC, especially in the advanced stage.[41]

LMP2A consists of a long N-terminal tail, 12 membrane-spanning domains, and a short C-terminal tail and aggregates in patches on the surface of all forms of latently infected cells

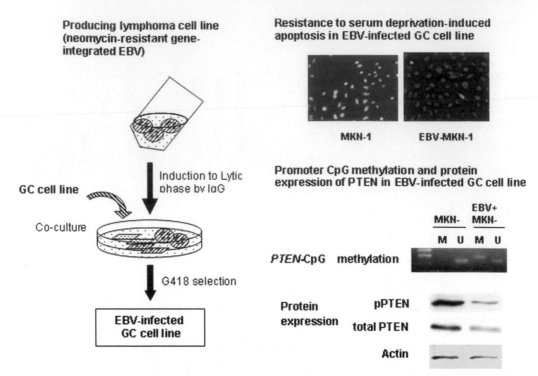

FIGURE 4-5 Experimental system of EBV infection demonstrating resistance to apoptosis and CpG methylation of the **PTEN** gene promoter in an infected GC cell line. Shown is the coculture method used with producer cells containing recombinant EBV in which the neomycin resistance gene *Neo*[r] is inserted into the EBV-DNA. EBV-infected GC cell line (EBV + MKN1) shows resistance to serum deprivation–induced apoptosis. Note the marked decrease of TUNEL-positive cells in the EBV + MKN1 cell line. EBV infection also reproduces the CpG methylation of the *PTEN* gene promoter and repression of PTEN expression.

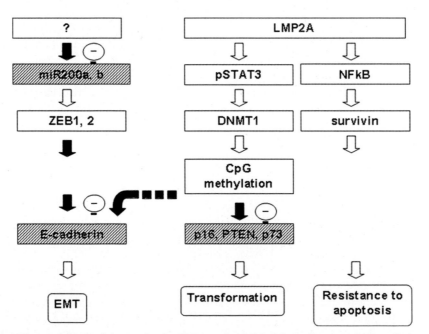

FIGURE 4-6 Virus and host cell interaction in EBV–associated GC. Schematic representation of virus and host cell interaction, causing abnormalities of EBV-associated GC. Viral latent membrane protein 2A (LMP2A) increases phosphorylated STAT3, which upregulates DNMT1 expression. LMP2A also activated τηε NF-κβ/survivin pathway.

(further references for LMP2A were listed in Ref. [1]). LMP2A is related to the survival of B lymphocytes, but its functional role in epithelial cells is not clear. Eight tyrosine residues and ubiquitin ligase–binding regions in the N-terminal tail have been suggested as potential binding sites for LMP2A in cellular signaling pathways.[1]

Aberrant Methylation and LMP2A

Aberrant promoter methylation and loss of PTEN expression were also reproduced in the GC cell lines MKN-1 and MKN-7 infected with recombinant EBV (Fig. 4-5).[42] In this experimental system, viral LMP2A also plays a central role in this abnormality: It induces the phosphorylation of STAT3, which increases the transcription of *DNMT1*. The up-regulation of DNMT1, therefore, causes the loss of PTEN expression through CpG-island methylation of the *PTEN* promoter. Although STAT3 can be phosphorylated through gp130 in an IL6- or IL11-dependent manner,[43] the LMP2A/pSTAT3/DNMT1 pathway appears to be independent of IL6/gp130 in this experimental setting. Immunohistochemical analysis confirmed the concurrent expression of pSTAT3 and DNMT1 in the neoplastic cells of EBV-associated GC in vivo. Thus, transient or constitutive expression of LMP2A is a fundamental mechanism of the development of EBV-associated GC through CpG-island methylation of the host DNA.

Epithelial-Mesenchymal Transition

We recently focused on a characteristic morphological feature, a lace pattern in EBV-associated GC, because of its similarity to the epithelial-mesenchymal transition (EMT) (Shinozaki, et al., *Cancer Res.* 2010;70:4719–4727). The EMT-related miRNAs, *miR-200a* and *miR-200b*, were reduced in EBV-associated GC, as compared with EBV-negative GC. In addition, we found that the *miR-200* family was downregulated in GC cell lines infected with recombinant EBV, which was accompanied by the loss of cell adhesion, a reduction in E-cadherin expression, and up regulation of *ZEB1* and *ZEB2*. The suppression of expression of the miR-200 family was at the transcription level in EBV-infected GC cell lines, and the precise mechanism in relation to EBV latent gene products is under investigation in our laboratory.

Other Abnormalities and Latent Gene Products

EBER-1 and -2 are nonpolyadenylated, noncoding RNAs that form a stem-loop structure by intermolecular base pairing, giving rise to double-stranded RNA (dsRNA)-like molecules. These noncoding RNAs are abundant in EBV-infected cells, as described above. *EBER* upregulates the expression of insulin-like growth factor (IGF) at the transcriptional level, and the secreted IGF-I acts as an autocrine growth factor in the gastric cancer cell line NU-GC-3.[44]

BARF1 has recently been determined to be a transforming and immortalizing EBV gene and encodes a functional homologue of the human colony-stimulating factor (CSF) receptor. *BARF1* was originally thought to be a lytic gene in B lymphocytes, but its expression has been demonstrated in latently infected cells of epithelial malignancies in the absence of lytic genes.[45] BARF1 is secreted from EBV-infected epithelial cells, but its role in resistance to apoptosis remains to be determined.[46]

EPIGENETIC ABNORMALITIES IN EBV-ASSOCIATED GCs

On the basis of the findings of CpG-island methylation and subsequent repression of tumor suppressor genes, we believe that abnormalities in methylation mechanisms play a central role in the carcinogenesis of EBV-associated GC.[1,47] It is of interest to note that latent genes are also repressed by the CpG methylation of EBV DNA through cellular methylation mechanisms.[48] Thus, DNA methylation may act as a host defense mechanism against foreign DNA to suppress the expression of viral genes; however, in contrast, viruses can utilize host cell methylation for their own survival and propagation.[1,47] Blocking the expression of EBV latent proteins by CpG methylation allows EBV-infected cells to escape from cytotoxic T cells.[48] Furthermore, the up-regulation of such DNA-methylation mechanisms may lead to the repression of many cancer-associated genes, which results in the transformation of host cells; thus, this series of events (viral latent infection, up-regualtion of host methylation mechanisms, repression of viral latent proteins and host tumor suppressors, and neoplastic transformation of the host) may be a survival strategy of viruses.

According to the epigenetic progenitor model,[49] "tumor-progenitor genes" promote the epigenetic disruption of stem/progenitor cells as a first step in the development of cancer. Chronic inflammation expands the pools of epigenetically altered progenitor cells, which are prone to carcinoma. Such a hypothetical view can be applied to the early process of GC development in association with infectious agents, such as EBV. However, further studies will be necessary to delineate the epigenetic abnormalities in stem cells that lead to the development of infection-associated carcinoma in the stomach.

Fu et al.[50] recently proposed a therapeutic approach that utilizes the virus–host interactions in EBV-associated neoplasms, that is, the use of a pharmacologic agent to modulate viral replication genes (thymidine kinase) to target radiotherapy to tumor tissue. Because viral replication is inhibited by promoter methylation of EBV DNA, demethylating agents, such as 5-aza cytidine, can induce lytic infection of EBV, leading to lysis of the infected cells. This approach may be particularly useful in EBV-associated GC, where methylation of tumor suppressor genes is also a key abnormality. Therefore, the efficiency of drug delivery and the side effects of demethylating agents should be studied further.

CONCLUDING REMARKS

EBV-associated GC is a distinct subgroup of GC, consisting of the monoclonal growth of neoplastic cells with latent infection by EBV. The possible sequence of events within the stomach mucosa is EBV infection of certain gastric stem cells, the expansion of epigenetically abnormal stem cells through LMP2A, and the growth of the predominant clone as it interacts with other etiologic factors.[1,6] EBV-associated GC represents a particular GC subtype with CIMP-H abnormalities,[47] in which epigenetic therapy might be effective both for correcting cellular abnormalities and for inducing EBV to enter the replication phase.

References

1. Fukayama M, Hino R, Uozaki H. Epstein-Barr virus and gastric carcinoma: virus-host interactions leading to carcinoma. *Cancer Sci.* 2008;99:1726–1733.
2. Uozaki H, Fukayama M. Epstein-Barr virus associated gastric carcinoma-viral carcinogenesis through epigenetic mechanisms. *Int J Clin Exp Pathol.* 2008;1:198–216.
3. Shibata D, Tokunaga M, Uemura Y, et al. Association of Epstein-Barr virus with undifferentiated gastric carcinomas with intense lymphoid infiltration. Lymphoepithelioma-like carcinoma. *Am J Pathol.* 1991; 139:469–474.
4. Murphy G, Pfeiffer R, Camargo MC, et al. Meta-analysis shows that prevalence of Epstein-Barr virus-positive gastric cancer differs based on sex and anatomic location. *Gastroenterology.* 2009;137:824–833.
5. Lee JH, Kim SH, Han SH, et al. Clinicopathological and molecular characteristics of Epstein-Barr virus-associated gastric carcinoma: a meta-analysis. *J Gastroenterol Hepatol.* 2009;24:354–365.
6. Fukayama M, Ushiku T. Epstein-Barr virus-associated gastric carcinoma. *Pathol Res Prac.* In press.
7. Watanabe H, Enjoji M, Imai T. Gastric carcinoma with lymphoid stroma: its morphologic characteristics and prognostic correlations. *Cancer.* 1976;38:232–243.

8. Nakamura S, Ueki T, Yao T, et al. Epstein-Barr virus in gastric carcinoma with lymphoid stroma. Special reference to its detection by the polymerase chain reaction and in situ hybridization in 99 tumors, including a morphologic analysis. *Cancer.* 1994;73:2239–2249.

9. Shinozaki A, Ushiku T, Fukayama M. Prominent Mott cell proliferation in Epstein-Barr virus associated gastric carcinoma. *Hum Pathol.* 2010;41:134–138.

10. Shinozaki A, Ushiku T, Morikawa T, et al. Epstein-Barr virus-associated gastric carcinoma: a distinct carcinoma of gastric phenotype by claudin expression profiling. *J Histochem Cytochem.* 2009;57: 775–785.

11. Barua RR, Uozaki H, Chong JM, et al. Phenotype analysis by MUC2, MUC5AC, MUC6, and CD10 expression in Epstein-Barr virus-associated gastric carcinoma. *J Gastroenterol.* 2006;41:733–739.

12. Imai S, Koizumi S, Sugiura M, et al. Gastric carcinoma: monoclonal epithelial malignant cells expressing Epstein-Barr virus latent infection protein. *Proc Natl Acad Sci U S A.* 1994;91:9131–9135.

13. Fukayama M, Hayashi Y, Iwasaki Y, et al. Epstein-Barr virus-associated gastric carcinoma and Epstein-Barr virus infection of the stomach. *Lab Invest.* 1994;71:73–81.

14. Yoshiyama H, Imai S, Shimizu N, et al. Epstein-Barr virus infection of human gastric carcinoma cells: implication of the existence of a new virus receptor different from CD21. *J Virol.* 1997;71:5688–5691.

15. Imai S, Nishikawa J, Takada K. Cell-to-cell contct as an efficient mode of Epstein-Barr virus infection of diverse human epithelial cells. *J Virol.* 1998;72:4371–4378.

16. Kaizaki Y, Sakurai S, Chong JM, et al. Atrophic gastritis, Epstein-Barr virus infection, and Epstein-Barr virus-associated gastric carcinoma. *Gastric Cancer.* 1999;2:101–108.

17. Ohfuji S, Osaki M, Tsujitani S, et al. Low frequency of apoptosis in Epstein-Barr virus-associated gastric carcinoma with lymphoid stroma. *Int J Cancer.* 1996;68:710–715.

18. Kume T, Oshima K, Shinohara T, et al. Low rate of apoptosis and overexpression of bcl-2 in Epstein-Barr virus-associated gastric carcinoma. *Histopathology.* 1999;34:502–509.

19. Ishii HH, Gobe GC, Yoneyama J, et al. Role of p53, apoptosis, and cell proliferation in early stage Epstein-Barr virus positive and negative gastric carcinomas. *J Clin Pathol.* 2004;57:1306–1311.

20. Kim BM, Byun SJ, Kim YA, et al. Cell cycle regulators, APC/b-catenin, NF-kB and Epstein-Barr virus in gastric carcinomas. *Pathology.* 2010;42:58–65.

21. van Rees BP, Caspers E, zur Hausen A, et al. Different pattern of allelic loss in Epstein-Barr virus-positive gastric cancer with emphasis on the p53 tumor suppressor pathway. *Am J Pathol.* 2002;161:1207–1213.

22. Kang GH, Lee S, Kim WH, et al. Epstein-barr virus-positive gastric carcinoma demonstrates frequent aberrant methylation of multiple genes and constitutes CpG island methylator phenotype-positive gastric carcinoma. *Am J Pathol.* 2002;160:787–794.

23. Ojima H, Fukuda T, Nakajima T, et al. Infrequent overexpression of p53 protein in Epstein-Barr virus-associated gastric carcinomas. *Jnp J Cancer Res.* 1997;88:262–266.

24. Leung SY, Chan KY, Yuen ST, et al. p53 overexpression is different in Epstein-Barr virus-associated and Epstein-Barr virus-negative carcinoma. *Histopathology.* 1998;33:311–317.

25. Wu MS, Shun CT, Wu CC, et al. Epstein-Barr virus-associated gastric carcinomas: relation to *H. pylori* infection and genetic alterations. *Gastroenterology.* 2000;118:1031–1038.

26. Chong JM, Sakuma K, Sudo M, et al. Interleukin-1beta expression in human gastric carcinoma with Epstein-Barr virus infection. *J Virol.* 2002;76:6825–6831.

27. Chen X, Leung SY, Yuen ST, et al. Variation in gene expression patterns in human gastric cancers. *Mol Biol Cell.* 2003;14:3208–3215.

28. Lee HS, Chang MS, Yang HK, et al. Epstein-Barr virus-positive gastric carcinoma has a distinct protein expression profile in comparison with epstein-barr virus-negative carcinoma. *Clin Cancer Res.* 2004;10:1698–1705.

29. Chan WY, Liu Y, Li CY, et al. Recurrent genomic aberrations in gastric carcinomas associated with *Helicobacter pylori* and Epstein-Barr virus. *Diag Mol Pathol.* 2002;11:127–134.

30. zur Hausen A, van Grieken NC, Meijer GA, et al. Distinct chromosomal aberrations in Epstein-Barr virus-carrying gastric carcinomas tested by comparative genomic hybridization. *Gastroenterology.* 2001;121:612–618.

31. Chong JM, Fukayama M, Hayashi Y, et al. Microsatellite instability in the progression of gastric carcinoma. *Cancer Res.* 1994;54:4595–4597.

32. Vo QN, Geradts J, Gulley ML, et al. Epstein-Barr virus in gastric adenocarcinomas: association with ethnicity and CDKN2A promoter methylation. *J Clin Pathol.* 2002;55:669–675.

33. Chang MS, Lee HS, Kim HS, et al. Epstein-Barr virus and microsatellite instability in gastric carcinogenesis. *J Pathol.* 2003;199:447–452.

34. Grogg KL, Lohse CM, Pankratz VS, et al. Lymphocyte-rich gastric cancer; associations with Epstein-Brr virus, microsatellite instability, histology, and survival. *Mod Pathol.* 2003;16:641–651.

35. Leung SY, Yuen ST, Chung LP, et al. Microsatellite instability, Epstein-Barr virus, mutation of type II transforming growth factor b receptor and BAX in gastric carcinomas in Hong Kong Chinese. *Br J Cancer.* 1999;79:582–588.

36. Osawa T, Chong JM, Sudo M, et al. Reduced expression and promoter methylation of *p16* gene in Epstein-Barr virus-associated gastric carcinoma. *Jpn J Cancer Res.* 2002;93:1195–1200.

37. Sudo M, Chong JM, Sakuma K, et al. Promoter hypermethylation of *E-cadherin* and its abnormal expression in Epstein-Barr virus-associated gastric carcinoma. *Int J Cancer.* 2004;109:194–199.

38. Ushiku T, Chong JM, Uozaki H, et al. p73 gene promoter methylation in Epstein-Barr virus-associated gastric carcinoma. *Int J Cancer.* 2007;120:60–66.

39. Kaneda A, Kaminishi M, Yanagihara K, et al. Identification of silencing of nine genes in human gastric cancers. *Cancer Res.* 2002;62:6645–6650.

40. Chang MS, Uozaki H, Chong JM, et al. CpG island methylation status in gastric carcinoma with and without infection of Epstein-Barr virus. *Clin Cancer Res.* 2006;12:2995–3002.

41. Hino R, Uozaki H, Inoue Y, et al. Survival advantage of EBV-associated gastric carcinoma: survivin up-regulation by viral latent membrane protein 2A. *Cancer Res.* 2008;68:1427–1435.

42. Hino R, Uozaki H, Murakami N, et al. Activation of DNA methyltransferase 1 by EBV latent membrane protein 2A leads to promoter hypermethylation of PTEN gene in gastric carcinoma. *Cancer Res.* 2009; 69:2766–2774.

43. Ernst M, Najdovska M, Grail D, et al. STAT3 and STAT1 mediate IL-11-dependent and inflammation-associated gastric tumorigenesis in gp130 receptor mutant mice. *J Clin Invest.* 2008;118:1727–1738.

44. Iwakiri D, Eizuru Y, Tokunaga M, et al. Autocrine growth of Epstein-Barr virus-positive gastric carcinoma cells mediated by an Epstein-Barr virus-encoded small RNA. *Cancer Res.* 2003;63:7062–7067.

45. Seto E, Yang L, Middeldorp J, et al. Epstein-Barr virus (EBV)-encoded BARF1 gene is expressed in nasopharyngeal carcinoma and EBV-associated gastric carcinoma tissues in the absence of lytic gene expression. *J Med Virol.* 2005;76:82–88.

46. Seto E, Ooka T, Middeldrop J, et al. Reconstitution of nasopharyngeal carcinoma-type infection induces tumorigenesis. *Cancer Res.* 2008;68:1030–1036.

47. Fukayama M. Epstein-Barr virus and gastric carcinoma. *Pathol Int.* 2010;60:337–350.

48. Niller HH, Wolf H, Minarovits J. Epigenetic dysregulation of the host cell genome in Epstein-Barr virus-associated neoplasia. *Semin Cancer Biol.* 2009;19:158–164.

49. Feinberg AP, Ohlsson R, Henikoff S. The epigenetic progenitor origin of human cancer. *Nat Rev Genet.* 2006;7:21–33.

50. Fu DX, Tanhehco YC, Chen J, et al. Bortezomib-induced enzyme-targeted radiotherapy in herpesvirus-associated tumors. *Nat Med.* 2008;14:1118–1122.

Histopathology

Gastric Carcinoma: Classifications and Morphologic Variants

5

▶ Do Youn Park
▶ Hye Seung Han
▶ Gregory Y. Lauwers

INTRODUCTION

Several chapters of this book cover the epidemiologic and biologic characteristics of gastric cancer. Others discuss the staging of gastric adenocarcinoma in detail, including its classification into early and advanced gastric cancers. This chapter focuses on the classification of gastric adenocarcinoma, specifically as it relates to anatomic location and especially with regard to cancers of the proximal stomach (i.e., cardia); genetic predisposition; and, most particularly, the various morphologies of gastric cancer.

CARCINOMA OF THE PROXIMAL STOMACH

Worldwide, most gastric adenocarcinomas are diagnosed in the antropyloric region and preferentially on the lesser curvature. Nevertheless, the incidence of proximal stomach cancers has increased, particularly in geographic areas of low risk for gastric cancer.[1] However, this phenomenon has not been noted uniformly worldwide.[2]

Anatomic Controversies

These previous considerations notwithstanding, there is confusion with regard to proximal gastric adenocarcinoma.

First, there is no consensus on the origin of the cardiac-type mucosa that lines the most proximal stomach. This debate is beyond the scope of this chapter, but suffice it to say that this mucosa is variably considered as an original, native lining of the stomach as it connects to the esophagus or as developing (i) secondary to columnar metaplasia of the distal esophageal squamous mucosa due to gastroesophageal reflux and (ii) due to atrophy of the oxyntic mucosa immediately distal to the normal cardia mucosa from *Helicobacter pylori* infection.[3-5]

Just as there is debate about the origin of the cardia, there is no clear anatomic landmark, either. Pragmatically, the term "cancer of the proximal stomach" (cardia cancer) is applied to adenocarcinomas involving primarily the very first centimeters of the stomach near the gastroesophageal junction (GEJ). A complicating issue is that esophageal tumors may grow downward and involve the cardia. Thus, these tumors frequently overlap, and it is challenging to clarify whether a given tumor is an esophageal adenocarcinoma, or a GEJ or cardial tumor. In an attempt to clarify the issue, Siewert and Stein[6] classified tumors of the GEJ region into three types based on the estimated location of the tumor center. Type 1 tumors were classified as true Barrett adenocarcinomas of the distal esophagus, and type 3 tumors represented subcardial gastric tumors. Type 2 tumors were those centered

FIGURE 5-1 Adenocarcinoma of proximal stomach. The ulcerated tumor is located just below the GEJ. (Courtesy of center for Gastric Cancer, National Cancer Center, Korea.)

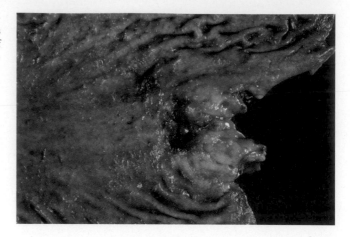

at the GEJ. However, there does not seem to be appropriate justification for separating GEJ tumors from adenocarcinomas of the distal esophagus, especially from a pathophysiologic standpoint. More recently, the International Gastric Cancer Association has endorsed another scheme for classifying these tumors.[7] Type I tumors are defined as those in the distal esophagus, type II are tumors of the true gastric cardia, and type III are those in the gastric mucosa of the subcardia (Fig. 5-1). Finally, the recently published 7th edition of the TNM classification by the American Joint Committee on Cancer proposes a novel classification scheme. Cancers whose epicenter is in the lower thoracic esophagus or EGJ, or within the proximal 5 cm of the stomach (i.e., cardia) and extending into the EGJ or esophagus are to be stage grouped similar to adenocarcinoma of the esophagus, while cancers with an epicenter in the stomach >5 cm distal to the EGJ, as well as those within 5 cm of the EGJ but not extending into the EGJ or esophagus, are to be classified and staged as gastric cancer.[8]

Epidemiologic Characteristics and Risk Factors of Adenocarcinoma of the Proximal Stomach

In geographic areas of low incidence of gastric cancers, proximal stomach tumors are characterized by a higher M/F ratio than distal tumors, and in the United States, they are more common in the white population than in African Americans.[9] Furthermore, a proportion of adenocarcinomas arising in the proximal stomach may have an etiology and pathogenesis similar to esophageal adenocarcinoma, that is, an association with a history of reflux symptoms. However, this association is much weaker than that between reflux symptoms and esophageal adenocarcinoma. High body mass index, smoking, and alcohol intake have not been universally accepted as risk factors of the proximal stomach cancer.[2,10,11] Furthermore, the association between chronic *H. pylori* infection and cancer of the proximal stomach is complex. The prevalence of *H. pylori* infection in patients with cancer of the proximal stomach was the same as in the control population, suggesting that it is not involved in the pathogenesis. However, a trend toward a positive association between *H. pylori* infection and cancers of the proximal stomach is reported in China.[12]

Overall, it appears that cancer of the proximal stomach may be connected to at least two disparate etiologies. This provides an explanation for the differing association between *H. pylori* and cardia cancer in different regions of the world. In regions of the Western world, where *H. pylori* atrophic gastritis is uncommon and gastroesophageal reflux disease common, the majority of these cancers are of esophageal type. In contrast, in China, where *H. pylori* atrophic gastritis is common and reflux disease less prevalent, the majority of cancers of the proximal stomach are of the *H. pylori* atrophic gastritis type and thus resemble distal gastric cancers.

Morphology and Phenotype of Proximal Gastric Adenocarcinoma

Cancers of the proximal stomach share the same morphologic patterns as distal tumors. However, the prevalence of adenocarcinoma has been noted to be higher than for distal tumors at early and late stages.[13] With regard to phenotypic differentiation, differentiated proximal gastric cancers are also more likely to have a gastric immunophenotype. It has been shown that the incidence of human gastric mucin (HGM) expression is significantly higher in proximal tumors at an early stage, whereas in advanced cancers, MUC2 expression is lower than in distal tumors.

HEREDITARY GASTRIC CANCER SYNDROMES

About 10% to 15% of gastric cancers can be qualified as familial.[14] Several syndromes and genes are involved, and usually, several organs are at risk of developing various malignancies (Table 5-1).

Hereditary Diffuse Gastric Cancer

Hereditary diffuse gastric cancer (HDGC) patients typically present with diffuse type gastric cancer with signet ring cells and, at late stage, linitis plastica. In addition to a high susceptibility of developing diffuse gastric carcinoma, an increased risk for lobular breast carcinoma is reported.[15] Germline mutations in the E-cadherin gene (*CDH1*) account for 30% to 40% of HDGC cases.[16–18] The penetrance of the gene varies between 70% and 80%, and the average age for the diagnosis of cancer is 37 years.[18] The lifetime risk of developing a gastric cancer is about 67% in men and 83% in women.[19]

Analysis of prophylactic gastrectomy, the sole preventive treatment, has led to the detection of in situ signet-ring cell carcinomas (SRCCs) and the pagetoid spread of signet ring cells between the foveolar epithelium and basement membrane (Fig. 5-2),[20] as well as the presence of multiple foci of stage T1a SRCC confined to the superficial lamina propria and without nodal

Table 5-1	Hereditary Gastric Cancer Syndromes	
Hereditary Syndromes	**Genes**	**Tumor Types**
HDGC syndrome	CDH1	Lobular Breast Cancer Colorectal Cancer
Hereditary nonpolyposis colorectal cancer syndrome	MLII1, MSH2, MSH6, PMS2	Colorectal Cancer Endometrial Cancer Urinary Tract Cancer Ovarian Cancer
Peutz-Jeghers syndrome	STK11	Colon Cancer Ovarian Cancer Cervical Cancer Breast Cancer Pancreatic Cancer
Juvenile polyposis syndrome	SMAD4, BMPR1A	Colon Cancer
FAP	APC	Colon Cancer Brain Tumors
LFS	Tp53	Osteosarcoma Soft Tissue Sarcoma Breast Cancer Brain tumors Leukemia Adrenal Cortical Carcinoma Lung Cancer Colorectal cancer Lymphoma

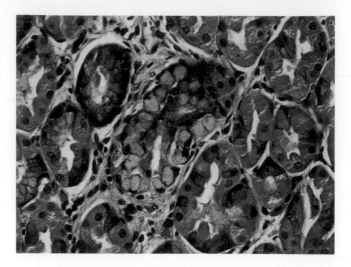

FIGURE 5-2 In situ signet-ring cell carcinoma in a patient with hereditary gastric cancer syndrome. The neoplastic signet ring cells are located within the confines of the pit's basement membrane.

metastases.[20,21] These lesions are not readily identified by endoscopic examination. In most cases, the neoplastic foci spare the antral mucosa, and there is a marked increase in density and size within the transition zone between the antrum and the body.[21] There is wide variation in the number of foci both within and between HDGC kindred, from an average over 100 to <20.[20,22–24] No correlation between patient age and number of foci has been observed. Phenotypic differentiation and proliferation studies support that the neoplasms are developing from the upper isthmus of the neck region of the gastric gland.[25]

Hereditary Nonpolyposis Colorectal Cancer Syndrome

Gastric carcinoma, usually of the intestinal type, accounts for 5% to 11% of all carcinomas in these patients. The lifetime risk is 10% for patients of Western ancestry and up to 30% for patients of Asian ancestry.[26–29] An RER phenotype is present in 65% of these cases.

Familial Adenomatous Polyposis Coli

Familial adenomatous polyposis (FAP) patients frequently develop multiple gastric polyps, with fundic gland polyps more common than adenomas. The former have been proven to be neoplastic in nature, with frequent somatic mutations of the APC gene.[30] However, the development of carcinoma in fundic gland polyps remains extremely rare.[31] Adenomas, which also arise in these patients, are much less common, but at risk for transformation.

Li-Fraumeni Syndrome

Li-Fraumeni syndrome (LFS) is an autosomal dominant hereditary cancer syndrome associated with germline mutations in the *tp53* tumor suppressor gene. Gastrointestinal tract tumors are relatively infrequent in this syndrome, accounting for <10% of all neoplasms that develop; however, among these patients, gastric carcinomas occur more frequently than colon cancers, representing over 50% of the cases.[32]

Peutz-Jeghers Syndrome

Most patients who meet the clinical criteria present with germline mutations of the serine/threonine protein kinase STK11, found on chromosome 19p. Those who are afflicted with this syndrome develop characteristic polyp and have an increased risk of gastric cancer.[33]

HISTOMORPHOLOGIC CLASSIFICATION

Just as gastric cancers represent a biologically and genetically heterogeneous group of tumors, their histology is characterized by marked heterogeneity at the architectural and cellular level, reflected, for example, by a combination of foveolar, intestinal, and endocrine-type cells.[34]

Table 5-2	Gastric Adenocarcinoma Classification Systems				
WHO (2010)	**CARNEIRO (1997)**	**GOSEKI (1992)**	**MING (1977)**	**LAUREN (1965)**	
• Papillary adenocarcinoma • Tubular adenocarcinoma • Mucinous adenocarcinoma	• Glandular carcinoma	• Well-differentiated tubules Intracellular mucin poor • Well-differentiated tubules Intracellular mucin rich	• Pushing	• Intestinal type	
• Signet-ring cell carcinoma and other poorly cohesive carcinomas	• Isolated-cell type carcinoma • Solid carcinoma	• Poorly differentiated tubules Intracellular mucin poor • Poorly differentiated tubules Intracellular mucin rich	• Infiltrating	• Diffuse type	
• Mixed carcinoma	• Mixed carcinoma			• Indeterminate type	
• Adenosquamous carcinoma • Squamous cell carcinoma • Hepatoid adenocarcinoma • Carcinoma with lymphoid stroma • Choriocarcinoma • Carcinosarcoma • Parietal cell carcinoma • Malignant rhabdoid tumour • Mucoepidermoid carcinoma • Paneth cell carcinoma • Undifferentiated carcinoma • Mixed adeno-neuroendocrine carcinoma • Endodermal sinus tumour • Embryonal carcinoma • Pure gastric yolk sac tumour • Oncocytic adenocarcinoma	• Adenosquamous carcinoma • Squamous carcinoma • Choriocarcinoma • Embryonal carcinoma • Hepatoid carcinoma • Parietal cell carcinoma • Others				

Population-based differences may be seen as well. For example, following the Lauren classification, in high-risk regions of the world, intestinal-type adenocarcinoma is more common than the diffuse type that is relatively more common in low-risk areas. A shift in the proportion of subtypes has also been noted, with the incidence of gland-forming adenocarcinoma decreasing mainly in young patients, and an increasing rate of diffuse-type carcinoma localized to the proximal stomach. Finally, in young individuals, a higher proportion of tumors are of the diffuse type that affects females more often than males.[35,36]

WHO Classification

This descriptive classification recognizes four main patterns: tubular, papillary, mucinous, and poorly cohesive (including signet ring cell type), with other variants. Most gastric cancers show significant variability, and the predominant pattern is used to represent the final descriptive diagnosis (Table 5-2).

Tubular Adenocarcinoma

This type of cancer, which tends to form polypoid or fungating masses, is composed of distended and/or anatomizing branching tubules of various sizes (Fig. 5-3A–D). Mucus and cellular

FIGURE 5-3 **A:** Tubular adenocarcinoma, enteric type. This tumor is formed by irregular-shaped glands lined by hyperchromatic pencillate nuclei. **B:** Tubular adenocarcinoma, not otherwise specified. This tumor is composed of irregular-sized and -shaped tubules.

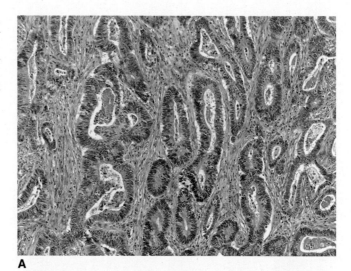

A

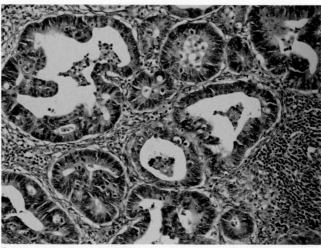

B

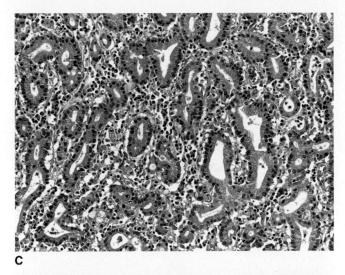

FIGURE 5-3 *(continued)* **C:** Tubular adenocarcinoma, pyloric type. The neoplasm is composed of irregular-shaped tubules lined by columnar tumor cells resembling pyloric gland epithelium. The phenotype is confirmed by MUC6 positivity. **D:** Tubular adenocarcinoma, foveolar type. This lesion is composed by tall tumor cells resembling foveolar-type epithelium. The phenotype is confirmed by MUC5AC positivity.

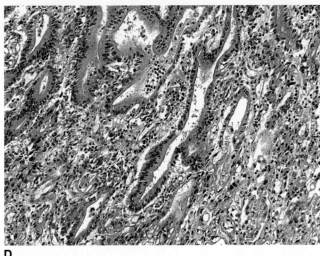

and inflammatory debris can be noted intraluminally. Individual neoplastic cells can be either columnar or cuboidal, or with various degrees of atypia and mitoses. In some well-differentiated cases, the neoplasm can mimic intestinal metaplasia perfectly.[37] A poorly differentiated variant is sometimes called solid carcinoma (Fig. 5-4). Tubular adenocarcinoma is the most common histologic type of early gastric cancers, representing 52% of the cases.

Papillary Adenocarcinoma

These are well-differentiated exophytic carcinomas characterized by epithelial projections scaffolded by a central fibrovascular core (Fig. 5-5). Cellular atypia and mitotic index are variable. The invasive front of this type of carcinoma usually is sharply demarcated from surrounding structures. A dense inflammatory component can be seen. This variant accounts for between 6% and 11% of gastric carcinomas and tends to affect older patients. It has been commonly reported in the proximal stomach and is frequently associated with liver metastases[38] and a higher rate of lymph node metastases. The papillary variant of gastric cancer represents 37% of the cases of early gastric cancers and, like the tubular variant, can be difficult to differentiate from dysplasia.[39] Combined papillotubular variants are also seen.

FIGURE 5-4 Solid variant of gastric adenocarcinoma. This tumor is formed of compact sheets of neoplastic cells with little to no gland formation.

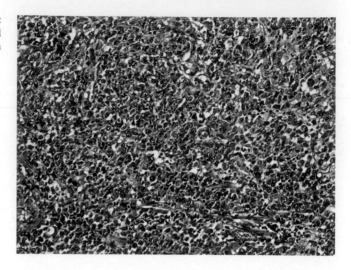

Mucinous Adenocarcinoma

This subtype represents 10% of gastric carcinomas. The extracellular mucinous pools constitute at least 50% of the tumor (Fig. 5-6). The cellular component can be formed of glandular structures and irregular cell clusters, and may even contain scattered signet ring cells floating in the abundant mucin.

Signet-Ring Cell and Other Poorly Cohesive Carcinomas

SRCCs are tumors composed solely of signet ring cells. However, many tumors are composed of a mixture of poorly cohesive non–signet ring cells as well as signet ring cells (Fig. 5-7). In many cases, signet ring cells are restricted to the upper half of the mucosal component of the tumors in combination with poorly cohesive cells within deeper levels of the gastric wall. Poorly cohesive non–signet ring cells include those that resemble plasma cells, histiocytes, or lymphocytes (Fig. 5-8). The tumor cells of poorly cohesive carcinomas can be arranged in lace-like gland or delicate microtrabecular patterns. Usually, they are accompanied by marked desmoplasia in the gastric wall. SRCC and poorly differentiated carcinoma represent 26% and 14% of early gastric cancers, respectively, and are usually depressed or ulcerated.[40–42]

FIGURE 5-5 Papillary-type gastric adenocarcinoma. The projecting anastomosing fibrovascular cores lined by neoplastic cells are the hallmark of this type.

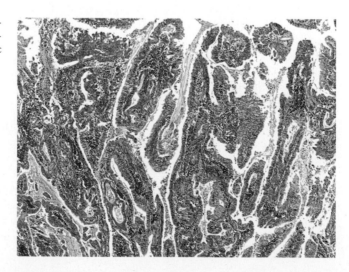

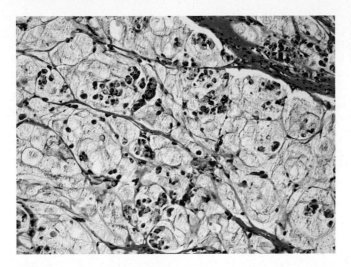

FIGURE 5-6 Gastric mucinous adeno-carcinoma. In this case, scattered signet ring cells are observed in the prominent mucinous lakes.

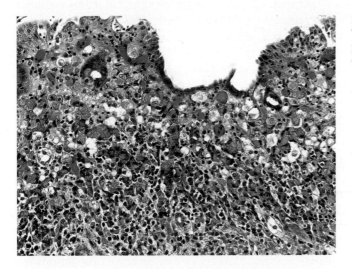

FIGURE 5-7 Signet-ring cell carcinoma. The neoplastic cells are characterized by prominent intracytoplasmic mucin with eccentric flattened nuclei.

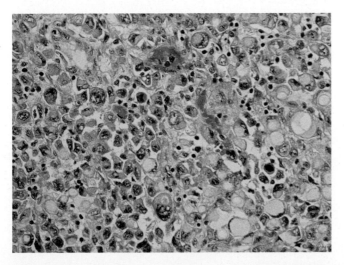

FIGURE 5-8 Poorly cohesive cell variant of gastric carcinoma. This tumor is composed of a mixture of discohesive signet ring cells with other cells that resemble histiocytes and plasma cells.

Tumor Grading

A three-tier grading system based on the resemblance of the neoplasm to gastric or metaplastic intestinal epithelium applies only to tubular and papillary carcinomas. Well-differentiated neoplasms are composed of well-formed glands lined by mature cells of either absorptive or goblet cell types. Moderately differentiated adenocarcinomas display features intermediate between well differentiated and poorly differentiated. Poorly differentiated adenocarcinomas are composed of highly irregular glands, single cells, or irregular cellular clusters. Other subtypes and variants of gastric cancers are not graded.[43]

Uncommon Subtypes of Gastric Adenocarcinoma

Various uncommon histologic varieties of gastric adenocarcinoma have been reported. They represent about 5% of gastric cancers. With the exception of carcinoma with a lymphoid stroma, their prognosis generally is worse than that of common varieties.

Gastric Carcinoma with Lymphoid Stroma (Medullary Carcinoma)

This variant is characterized by a prominent lymphoid infiltration of the stroma (Fig. 5-9). Over 80% of these tumors have been associated with Epstein-Barr virus (EBV) infection. Excluding EBV-infected gastric cancer of usual histology, gastric carcinoma with lymphoid stroma (GCLS) represents about 8% of gastric carcinomas.[44,45] This type of tumor is more common in the proximal stomach and in the remnant stomach. GCLS characteristically has a pushing microscopic interface and is composed of irregular sheets of small to medium size polygonal cells associated with a prominent lymphocytic infiltrate (predominantly CD8 positive) with occasional lymphoid follicles.[46] Whether EBV plays a direct role in the carcinogenesis or merely tags the neoplastic cells is debated.[46] However, it is likely an early process, since EBV can be found in the surrounding dysplastic epithelium.[47] EBV-positive GCLS also has been shown to represent a CpG island methylator phenotype with frequent aberrant methylation of multiple genes.[48] The prognosis of this variety of gastric cancer is reportedly better than that of the ordinary type's, with over 75% survival rate at 5 years, although this remains controversial and is possibly related to differences on the pattern of the inflammatory response.[49–51]

Hepatoid- and Alpha-Fetoprotein–Producing Carcinomas

Two histologic types of alpha-fetoprotein (AFP)-producing tumors are recognized, both of which can be detected by high AFP serum levels. Hepatoid carcinomas are formed of large polygonal cells with distinct eosinophilic cytoplasm (Fig. 5-10A and B).[52] Bile and PAS-positive and diastase-resistant intracytoplasmic eosinophilic globules can be observed. The lesions are rarely pure and frequently are intermixed within typical adenocarcinomas. A second type of

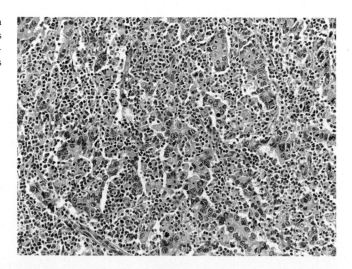

FIGURE 5-9 Gastric adenocarcinoma with lymphoid stroma. This variant is composed of irregular sheets of polygonal tumor cells infiltrated by numerous lymphocytes.

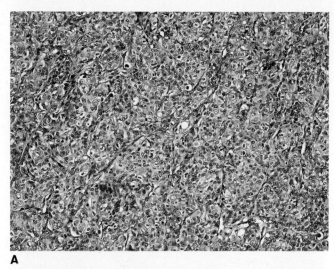

A

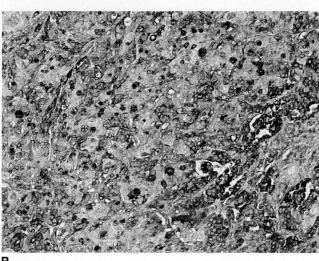

B

FIGURE 5-10 A,B: Gastric hepatoid carcinoma. This tumor shows trabecular growth patterns and is composed of polygonal cells with abundant eosinophilic cytoplasm. Rare gland-like spaces are also noted. Positive AFP immunoreaction. (Courtesy of Center for Gastric Cancer, National Cancer Center, Korea.)

AFP-producing tissue is a well-differentiated tubular or papillary adenocarcinoma with clear cytoplasm.[52] Special techniques have been shown to highlight albumin, AFP, alpha 1-antichymotrypsin, and bile production. Of note, a combination of both hepatoid and clear types can be seen. AFP-producing yolk sac tumor–like carcinoma has been reported as well. This variety of neoplasm is particularly aggressive, particularly the hepatoid variant.[53]

Adenosquamous and Squamous Cell Carcinomas

Adenosquamous carcinomas are tumors in which the squamous neoplastic component comprises at least 25% of the carcinoma (Fig. 5-11).[54] These tumors are usually deeply invasive and associated with lymphovascular invasion and carry a poor prognosis.[55] The exceedingly rare pure squamous cell carcinoma may vary from moderately differentiated with keratin pearl formation to poorly differentiated. The exact pathogenesis is unknown; it has not been established whether the squamous component arises from squamous metaplasia of adenocarcinomatous cells, from a focus of heterotopic squamous epithelium, or from multipotential stem cells.[56] Interestingly, it affects men four times as often as women. In the proximal stomach, the caudal extension of an esophageal squamous cell carcinoma should be ruled out. Gastric squamous cell carcinomas are usually diagnosed at a late stage.[56]

FIGURE 5-11 Gastric squamous cell carcinoma with moderate differentiation.

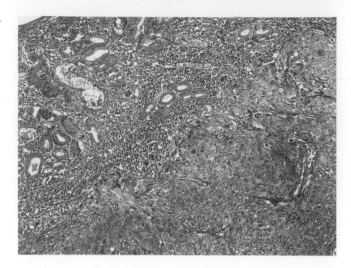

Gastric Choriocarcinoma

Adenocarcinomas with choriocarcinomatous elements are usually exophytic and characterized by prominent necrosis and hemorrhage at the macroscopic and microscopic level. Pure gastric choriocarcinomas demonstrate a combination of syncytiotrophoblast and cytotrophoblast elements with an otherwise variably differentiated adenocarcinoma from which they likely develop (Fig. 5-12).[57,58] Yolk sac and hepatoid carcinoma components can also be seen. Human chorionic gonadotropin (HCG) is usually detected by immunohistochemistry and in the patient's serum as well. Disseminated hematogenous and lymphatic metastases are common.[59]

Gastric Carcinosarcoma

Gastric carcinosarcomas are neoplasms composed of various proportions of adenocarcinomatous elements and either uncommitted sarcomatous elements or cells demonstrating features of chondrosarcomatous, osteosarcomatous, rhabdomyosarcomatous, or leiomyosarcomatous differentiation.[60–62] Combination with adenosquamous and neuroendocrine components also has been reported.[63]

Gastric Neuroendocrine Carcinoma

Neoplasms of this variant are frequently diagnosed at an advanced stage.[64,65] Histologically, they commonly present a sheet-like infiltrative growth pattern with frequent rosette-like arrangement

FIGURE 5-12 Gastric choriocarcinoma showing predominant cytotrophoblast elements with hemorrhage. The immunohistochemical staining for β-HCG revealed diffuse reactivity (not shown). (Courtesy of center for Gastric Cancer, National Cancer Center, Korea.)

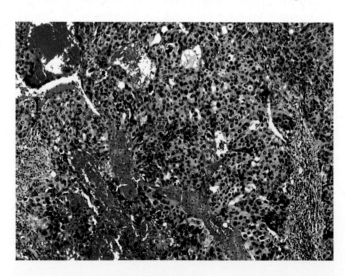

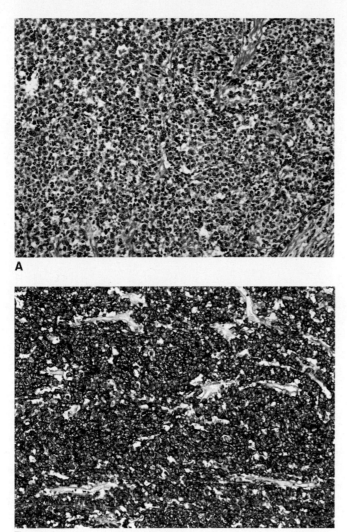

FIGURE 5-13 A,B: Gastric small cell carcinoma. This variant is characterized by sheets of small polygonal cells in rosette-like arrangements. Positive chromogranin immunoreactivity. (Courtesy of Center for Gastric Cancer, National Cancer Center, Korea.)

A

B

(Figs. 5-13A, B and 5-14). Neuron-specific enolase (NSE) and chromogranin A immunohistochemical stains are usually positive, and CEA is commonly negative.[66,67]

Gastric Parietal Cell Carcinomas and Oncocytic Carcinomas

Parietal cell carcinomas are composed of solid sheets of polygonal cells with abundant, finely granular eosinophilic cytoplasm that stains with phosphotungstic acid-hematoxylin. Immunohistochemically, the tumor cells are positive for parietal cell–specific antibodies to H/K-ATPase and human milk fat globule-2 (HMFG-2). Few cases of oncocytic adenocarcinomas, which are morphologically similar to parietal cell carcinomas but negative for antiparietal cell antibodies, have been recently reported.[68]

Gastric Micropapillary Carcinoma

This is a newly recognized variant, morphologically characterized by small papillary clusters composed of tumor cells but devoid of fibrovascular core and surrounded by empty spaces (Fig. 5-15). The proportion of micropapillary component necessary to establish the diagnosis is unclear, as it usually coexists with a conventional adenocarcinoma and is found at the advancing edge. Interestingly, a gastric phenotype (MUC5AC+, MUC6+) is predominant. The prognostic significance is not determined.[69]

FIGURE 5-14 Example of collision tumor with coexisting tubular adenocarcinoma and well-differentiated endocrine carcinoma. (Courtesy of center for Gastric Cancer, National Cancer Center, Korea.)

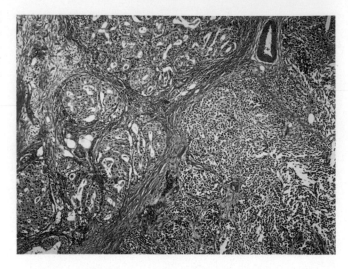

Gastric Mucoepidermoid and Paneth Cell Carcinomas

Mucoepidermoid carcinomas show the typical admixture of mucus-producing and squamous epithelia.[70] The few examples of Paneth cell carcinomas reported have been characterized by a predominance of intracytoplasmic eosinophilic granules positive for lysozyme by immunohistochemistry.[71]

Gastric Malignant Rhabdoid Tumor

These neoplasms are composed of poorly cohesive round to polygonal cells with an eosinophilic or clear cytoplasm and large nuclei with predominant nucleoli. These cells are strongly immunoreactive for vimentin, cytokeratin, and epithelial membrane antigen, and also may have focal NSE positivity and, frequently, negativity for CEA.[72,73]

Finally, *undifferentiated gastric carcinomas* that lack any differentiated features have been reported. Such cases need to be differentiated from lymphomas, squamous cell carcinomas, or sarcomas.

FIGURE 5-15 Micropapillary adenocarcinoma. This rare variant type is characterized by small papillary clusters of tumor cells that are devoid of fibrovascular core and surrounded by empty spaces.

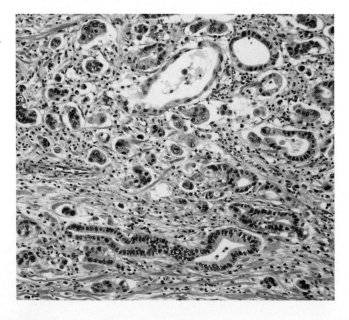

Other Classifications

Over the years, various histopathological classifications have reflected the difficulty of satisfactorily classifying a neoplasm by architectural diversity, pattern of growth, cell differentiation, and histogenesis.

The historic Lauren classification that recognizes *intestinal type, diffuse type*, and *indeterminate/unclassified type* has been cardinal in helping to understand the role of environmental factors and epidemiological trends.[74] Diffuse carcinomas consist of poorly cohesive cells with little or no gland formation. Intestinal carcinomas form glands of various degrees of differentiation. Tumors that contain approximately equal quantities of intestinal and diffuse components are termed mixed. Undifferentiated tumors are classified as indeterminate. However, more recent studies using lines of differentiation have demonstrated, for example, that many intestinal tumors have a mixed or gastric phenotype.

The Ming classification is a two-tier scheme based on the tumors' pattern of growth and invasiveness.[75] The expanding type is characterized by growth by expansion of cohesive tumor masses with a well-defined interface with the stroma. Conversely, the infiltrative type is characterized by single infiltrative cells growing independently or aggregated in small nests.

Goseki presented a four-type classification based on tubular differentiation and mucus production, including well-differentiated tubules in intracellular mucin-poor and mucin-rich subgroups and poorly differentiated type divided into mucin-rich and mucin-poor groups.[76]

Finally, the Carneiro system recognizes four categories (glandular, isolated cell, solid, and mixed) based first on morphology but also on the line of differentiation.[77] This author also has emphasized that tumors that were designated as "intestinal" in the Lauren classification include tumors with intestinal, gastric, and mixed differentiation.

It is important to point out that beyond morphologic classification, the use of mucin phenotypic markers, is useful in highlighting the different cellular components. Various lines of differentiation can be established using gastric markers (MUC5AC [gastric foveolar marker], MUC6 [antral/pyloric gland marker], and HGM [human gastric mucin], and trefoil peptide TFF1); intestinal markers (MUC2 [goblet cell marker], CDX2, and CD10 [brush border marker]); and others (pepsinogen-1). This has led to phenotype classification of gastric cancer into tumors of G type (gastric phenotype), I type (intestinal phenotype), and GI type (mixed phenotype), while those with neither pattern are classified as N (null) type.[77,78] G-type tumors have been noted to account for over 25% of all papillary/tubular carcinomas, while about 10% of all undifferentiated-type tumors have an I phenotype (Fig. 5-16).[13] For each histologic type, a shift from gastric to intestinal phenotype is observed with progression (see Chapter 6, by S. Ban).

Clinical Relevance of Histologic Typing with Reference to Spread and Prognosis

Based on their phenotype, gastric adenocarcinoma can spread by direct extension, lymphovascular metastasis, or peritoneal dissemination. Interestingly, the patterns of extension are different for gland-forming cancers and discohesive neoplasms. For example, tumors of so-called intestinal type preferentially disseminate hematogenously and develop hepatic metastases, while diffuse carcinomas commonly develop peritoneal seeding.[79,80] Bilateral ovarian involvement (Krukenberg tumor), commonly associated with discohesive neoplasms, can result from transperitoneal or hematogenous spread. Of note, mixed tumors exhibit the metastatic patterns of both types.

The combination of tumor location and histologic type should prompt specific concerns. For example, diffuse-type cancers of the antropyloric region have a high frequency of serosal and lymphovascular invasion, and lymph node metastases. These tumors also have the propensity to invade the duodenum via submucosal or subserosal routes, or via the submucosal lymphatics. In practice, frozen section of the surgical margins of distal gastrectomy for such a tumor should be performed in order to exclude submucosal extension that is macroscopically inapparent.

FIGURE 5-16 Tubular adenocarcinoma. Immunohistochemical staining reveals MUC5AC zonal
reactivity in the upper half of the neoplasm and
MUC6 in the lower half.

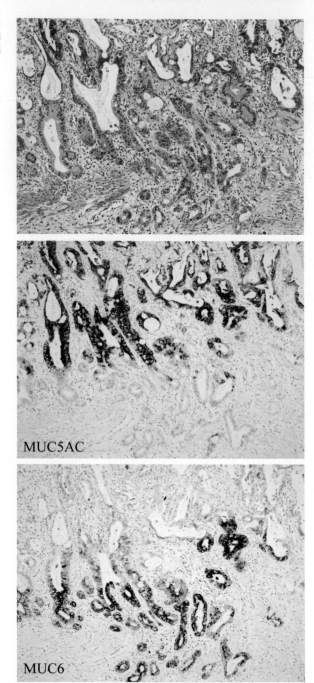

The value of the histological type in predicting tumor prognosis is variable and controversial. Whether diffuse carcinomas carry a worse prognosis than gland-forming carcinomas is debated. It has been suggested that diffuse-type carcinomas encompass lesions with a different prognosis, that is, a low-grade desmoplastic subtype (with no or scarce angio-lympho-neuroinvasion) and a high-grade subtype (with anaplastic cells).[81] The density of tumor-infiltrating lymphocytes, particularly peritumoral regulatory T cells, has been shown to be predictive of regional lymph node metastasis with improved outcome.[82–84] Scirrhous stromal reaction also has been reported as a predictor of peritoneal seeding and poor outcome.[84]

The prognosis of poorly cohesive carcinoma is particularly bad for children and young adults, in whom the diagnosis is often delayed.[85] Stage-matched survival analyses have shown that neuroendocrine carcinoma has a significantly worse prognosis than gastric adenocarcinoma.[67]

Expanding adenocarcinoma of the Ming classification (usually well-differentiated tubular cancers) has a better prognosis than the infiltrative carcinomas (usually composed of poorly cohesive types).[41] Also, retrospective studies have shown that advanced (pT3) mucus-rich tumors of Goseki types II and IV usually have a worse prognosis than mucus-poor (Goseki types I and III) T3 tumors (18% vs. 53%; p <0.003). This likely results from a more advanced tumor status at the time of diagnosis, rather than from the mucinous histology.[86] Finally, phenotypic classification has been shown to have prognostic value; however, conflicting results are reported. [87–89]

References

1. Blot WJ, Devesa SS, Kneller RW, et al. Rising incidence of adenocarcinoma of the esophagus and gastric cardia. *JAMA*. 1991;265:1287–1289.
2. Okabayashi T, Gotoda T, Kondo H, et al. Early carcinoma of the gastric cardia in Japan: is it different from that in the West? *Cancer*. 2000;89:2555–2559.
3. Chandrasoma PT, Der R, Ma Y, et al. Histology of the gastroesophageal junction: an autopsy study. *Am J Surg Pathol*. 2000;24:402–409.
4. De Hertogh G, Van Eyken P, Ectors N, et al. On the existence and location of cardiac mucosa: an autopsy study in embryos, fetuses, and infants. *Gut*. 2003;52:791–796.
5. Genta RM, Huberman RM, Graham DY. The gastric cardia in *Helicobacter pylori* infection. *Hum Pathol*. 1994: 25:915–919.
6. Siewert JR, Stein HJ. Carcinoma of the cardia: carcinoma of the gastroesophageal junction; classification, pathology, and extent of resection. *Dis Esophagus*. 1996;9:173–182.
7. Siewert JR, Stein HJ. Classification of adenocarcinoma of the oesophagogastric junction. *Br J Surg*. 1998;85:1457–1459.
8. Edge SB, Byrd DR, Compton CC, et al., eds. *AJCC cancer staging manual*. 7th ed. New York: Springer; 2010.
9. Morales TG. Adenocarcinoma of the gastric cardia. *Dig Dis*. 1997;15:346–356.
10. Lagergren J, Bergstrom R, Nyren O. Association between body mass and adenocarcinoma of the esophagus and gastric cardia. *Ann Intern Med*. 1999;130:883–890.
11. Chow WH, Blot WJ, Vaughan TL, et al. Body mass index and risk of adenocarcinomas of the esophagus and gastric cardia. *J Natl Cancer Inst*. 1998;90:150–155.
12. Helicobacter and Cancer Collaborative Group. Gastric cancer and *Helicobacter pylori*: a combined analysis of 12 case control studies nested within prospective cohorts. *Gut*. 2001;49:347–353.
13. Tajima Y, Yamazaki K, Makino R, et al. Differences in the histological findings, phenotypic marker expressions and genetic alterations between adenocarcinoma of the gastric cardia and distal stomach. *Br J Cancer*. 2007;96:631–638.
14. Zanghieri G, Di Gregorio C, Sacchetti C, et al. Familial occurrence of gastric cancer in the 2-year experience of a population-based registry. *Cancer*. 1990;66:2047–2051.
15. Keller G, Vogelsang H, Becker I, et al. Diffuse type gastric and lobular breast carcinoma in a familial gastric cancer patient with an E-cadherin germline mutation. *Am J Pathol*. 1999;155:337–342.
16. Kaurah P, MacMillan A, Boyd N, et al. Founder and recurrent CDH1 mutations in families with hereditary diffuse gastric cancer. *JAMA*. 2007;297:2360–2372.
17. Guilford P, Hopkins J, Harraway J, et al. E-cadherin germline mutations in familial gastric cancer. *Nature*. 1998;392:402–405.
18. Caldas C, Carneiro F, Lynch HT, et al. Familial gastric cancer: overview and guidelines for management. *J Med Genet*. 1999;36:873–880.
19. Pharoah PD, Guilford P, Caldas C, et al. Incidence of gastric cancer and breast cancer in CDH1 (E-cadherin) mutation carriers from hereditary diffuse gastric cancer families. *Gastroenterology*. 2001;121:1348–1353.
20. Huntsman DG, Carneiro F, Lewis FR, et al. Early gastric cancer in young, asymptomatic carriers of germ-line E-cadherin mutations. *N Engl J Med*. 2001;344:1904–1909.

21. Charlton A, Blair V, Shaw D, et al. Hereditary diffuse gastric cancer: predominance of multiple foci of signet ring cell carcinoma in distal stomach and transitional zone. *Gut.* 2004;53:814–820.

22. Barber ME, Save V, Carneiro F, et al. Histopathological and molecular analysis of gastrectomy specimens from hereditary diffuse gastric cancer patients has implications for endoscopic surveillance of individuals at risk. *J Pathol.* 2008;216:286–294.

23. Carneiro F, Huntsman DG, Smyrk TC, et al. Model of the early development of diffuse gastric cancer in E-cadherin mutation carriers and its implications for patient screening. *J Pathol.* 2004;203:681–687.

24. Rogers WM, Dobo E, Norton JA, et al. Risk-reducing total gastrectomy for germline mutations in E-cadherin (CDH1): pathologic findings with clinical implications. *Am J Surg Pathol.* 2008;32:799–809.

25. Humar B, Blair V, Charlton A, et al. E-cadherin deficiency initiates gastric signet-ring cell carcinoma in mice and man. *Cancer Res.* 2009;69:2050–2056.

26. Aarnio M, Salovaara R, Aaltonen LA, et al. Features of gastric cancer in hereditary non-polyposis colorectal cancer syndrome. *Int J Cancer.* 1997;74:551–555.

27. Mecklin JP, Jarvinen HJ, Peltokallio P. Cancer family syndrome. Genetic analysis of 22 Finnish kindreds. *Gastroenterology.* 1986;90:328–333.

28. Chung DC, Rustgi AK. The hereditary nonpolyposis colorectal cancer syndrome: genetics and clinical implications. *Ann Intern Med.* 2003;138:560–570.

29. Park YJ, Shin KH, Park JG. Risk of gastric cancer in hereditary nonpolyposis colorectal cancer in Korea. *Clin Cancer Res.* 2000;6:2994–2998.

30. Abraham SC, Nobukawa B, Giardiello FM, et al. Fundic gland polyps in familial adenomatous polyposis: neoplasms with frequent somatic adenomatous polyposis coli gene alterations. *Am J Pathol.* 2000;157:747–754.

31. Hofgartner WT, Thorp M, Ramus MW, et al. Gastric adenocarcinoma associated with fundic gland polyps in a patient with attenuated familial adenomatous polyposis. *Am J Gastroenterol.* 1999;94:2275–2281.

32. Kleihues P, Schauble B, zur Hausen A, et al. Tumors associated with p53 germline mutations: a synopsis of 91 families. *Am J Pathol.* 1997;150:1–13.

33. Beggs AD, Latchford AR, Vasen HF, et al. Peutz-Jeghers syndrome: a systematic review and recommendations for management. *Gut.* 2010;59:975–986.

34. Fiocca R, Villani L, Tenti P, et al. Characterization of four main cell types in gastric cancer: foveolar, mucopeptic, intestinal columnar and goblet cells. An histopathologic, histochemical and ultrastructural study of "early" and "advanced" tumours. *Pathol Res Pract.* 1987;182:308–325.

35. Kaneko S, Yoshimura T. Time trend analysis of gastric cancer incidence in Japan by histological types, 1975–1989. *Br J Cancer.* 2001;84:400–405.

36. Miyahara R, Niwa Y, Matsuura T, et al. Prevalence and prognosis of gastric cancer detected by screening in a large Japanese population: data from a single institute over 30 years. *J Gastroenterol Hepatol.* 2007;22:1435–1442.

37. Endoh Y, Tamura G, Motoyama T, et al. Well-differentiated adenocarcinoma mimicking complete-type intestinal metaplasia in the stomach. *Hum Pathol.* 1999;30:826–832.

38. Yasuda K, Adachi Y, Shiraishi N, et al. Papillary adenocarcinoma of the stomach. *Gastric Cancer.* 2000;3:33–38.

39. Hirota T, Itabashi M, Suzuki K, et al. Clinicopathologic study of minute and small early gastric cancer. Histogenesis of gastric cancer. *Pathol Annu.* 1980;15:1–19.

40. Everett SM, Axon AT. Early gastric cancer in Europe. *Gut.* 1997;41:142–150.

41. Lewin KJ, Appelman HD. Carcinoma of the stomach. Tumors of the esophagus & stomach. *Atlas of tumor pathology.* 3rd Series, vol. 18. Washington, DC: American Registry of Pathology, 1996.

42. Xuan ZX, Ueyama T, Yao T, et al. Time trends of early gastric carcinoma. A clinicopathologic analysis of 2846 cases. *Cancer.* 1993;72:2889–2894.

43. Lauwers GY, Carneiro F, Graham DY. Gastric carcinoma. In: Bowman FT, Carneiro F, Hruban RH, et al., eds. *Classification of tumours of the digestive system.* World Health Organization, 2010. In press.

44. zur Hausen A, van Grieken NC, Meijer GA, et al. Distinct chromosomal aberrations in Epstein-Barr virus-carrying gastric carcinomas tested by comparative genomic hybridization. *Gastroenterology.* 2001;121:612–618.

45. Herrera-Goepfert R, Reyes E, Hernandez-Avila M, et al. Epstein-Barr virus-associated gastric carcinoma in Mexico: analysis of 135 consecutive gastrectomies in two hospitals. *Mod Pathol.* 1999;12:873–878.

46. Fukayama M, Chong JM, Kaizaki Y. Epstein-Barr virus and gastric carcinoma. *Gastric Cancer.* 1998;1:104–114.

47. Gulley ML, Pulitzer DR, Eagan PA, et al. Epstein-Barr virus infection is an early event in gastric carcinogenesis and is independent of bcl-2 expression and p53 accumulation. *Hum Pathol.* 1996;27:20–27.

48. Kang GH, Lee S, Kim WH, et al. Epstein-barr virus-positive gastric carcinoma demonstrates frequent aberrant methylation of multiple genes and constitutes CpG island methylator phenotype-positive gastric carcinoma. *Am J Pathol.* 2002;160:787–794.

49. Nakamura S, Ueki T, Yao T, et al. Epstein-Barr virus in gastric carcinoma with lymphoid stroma. Special reference to its detection by the polymerase chain reaction and in situ hybridization in 99 tumors, including a morphologic analysis. *Cancer.* 1994;73:2239–2249.

50. dos Santos NR, Seruca R, Constancia M, et al. Microsatellite instability at multiple loci in gastric carcinoma: clinicopathologic implications and prognosis. *Gastroenterology.* 1996;110:38–44.

51. Song HJ, Srivastava A, Lee J, et al. Host inflammatory response predicts survival of patients with Epstein-Barr virus-associated gastric carcinoma. *Gastroenterology.* 2010;139:84–92.e2.

52. Motoyama T, Aizawa K, Watanabe H, et al. Alpha-Fetoprotein producing gastric carcinomas: a comparative study of three different subtypes. *Acta Pathol Jpn.* 1993;43:654–661.

53. Nagai E, Ueyama T, Yao T, et al. Hepatoid adenocarcinoma of the stomach. A clinicopathologic and immunohistochemical analysis. *Cancer.* 1993;72:1827–1835.

54. Namatame K, Ookubo M, Suzuki K, et al. A clinicopathological study of five cases of adenosquamous carcinoma of the stomach. *Jpn J Cancer Clin.* 1986;32:170–175.

55. Mori M, Iwashita A, Enjoji M. Adenosquamous carcinoma of the stomach. A clinicopathologic analysis of 28 cases. *Cancer.* 1986;57:333–339.

56. Marubashi S, Yano H, Monden T, et al. Primary squamous cell carcinoma of the stomach. *Gastric Cancer.* 1999;2:136–141.

57. Wurzel J, Brooks JJ. Primary gastric choriocarcinoma: immunohistochemistry, postmortem documentation, and hormonal effects in a postmenopausal female. *Cancer.* 1981;48:2756–2761.

58. Liu Z, Mira JL, Cruz-Caudillo JC. Primary gastric choriocarcinoma: a case report and review of the literature. *Arch Pathol Lab Med.* 2001;125:1601–1604.

59. Imai Y, Kawabe T, Takahashi M, et al. A case of primary gastric choriocarcinoma and a review of the Japanese literature. *J Gastroenterol.* 1994;29:642–646.

60. Nakayama Y, Murayama H, Iwasaki H, et al. Gastric carcinosarcoma (sarcomatoid carcinoma) with rhabdomyoblastic and osteoblastic differentiation. *Pathol Int.* 1997;47:557–563.

61. Sato Y, Shimozono T, Kawano S, et al. Gastric carcinosarcoma, coexistence of adenosquamous carcinoma and rhabdomyosarcoma: a case report. *Histopathology.* 2001;39:543–544.

62. Tsuneyama K, Sasaki M, Sabit A, et al. A case report of gastric carcinosarcoma with rhabdomyosarcomatous and neuroendocrinal differentiation. *Pathol Res Pract.* 1999;195:93–7; discussion 98.

63. Yamazaki K. A gastric carcinosarcoma with neuroendocrine cell differentiation and undifferentiated spindle-shaped sarcoma component possibly progressing from the conventional tubular adenocarcinoma; an immunohistochemical and ultrastructural study. *Virchows Arch.* 2003;442:77–81.

64. Namikawa T, Kobayashi M, Okabayashi T, et al. Primary gastric small cell carcinoma: report of a case and review of the literature. *Med Mol Morphol.* 2005;38:256–261.

65. Takaku H, Oka K, Naoi Y, et al. Primary advanced gastric small cell carcinoma: a case report and review of the literature. *Am J Gastroenterol.* 1999;94:1402–1404.

66. Kusayanagi S, Konishi K, Miyasaka N, et al. Primary small cell carcinoma of the stomach. *J Gastroenterol Hepatol.* 2003;18:743–747.

67. Jiang SX, Mikami T, Umezawa A, et al. Gastric large cell neuroendocrine carcinomas: a distinct clinicopathologic entity. *Am J Surg Pathol.* 2006;30:945–953.

68. Takubo K, Honma N, Sawabe M, et al. Oncocytic adenocarcinoma of the stomach: parietal cell carcinoma. *Am J Surg Pathol.* 2002;26:458–465.

69. Roh JH, Srivastava A, Lauwers GY, et al. Micropapillary carcinoma of stomach: a clinicopathologic and immunohistochemical study of 11 cases. *Am J Surg Pathol.* 2010;34:1139–1146.

70. Hayashi I, Muto Y, Fujii Y, et al. Mucoepidermoid carcinoma of the stomach. *J Surg Oncol.* 1987;34:94–99.

71. Ooi A, Nakanishi I, Itoh T, et al. Predominant Paneth cell differentiation in an intestinal type gastric cancer. *Pathol Res Pract.* 1991;187:220–225.

72. Pinto JA, Gonzalez Alfonso JE, Gonzalez L, et al. Well differentiated gastric adenocarcinoma with rhabdoid areas: a case report with immunohistochemical analysis. *Pathol Res Pract.* 1997;193:801–5; discussion 806–808.

73. Ueyama T, Nagai E, Yao T, et al. Vimentin-positive gastric carcinomas with rhabdoid features. A clinicopathologic and immunohistochemical study. *Am J Surg Pathol.* 1993;17:813–819.

74. Lauren P. The two histological main types of gastric carcinoma: diffuse and so-called intestinal-type carcinoma: an attempt at a histo-clinical classification. *Acta Pathol Microbiol Scand.* 1965;64:31–49.

75. Ming SC. Gastric carcinoma. A pathobiological classification. *Cancer.* 1977;39:2475–2485.

76. Goseki N, Takizawa T, Koike M. Differences in the mode of the extension of gastric cancer classified by histological type: new histological classification of gastric carcinoma. *Gut.* 1992;33:606–612.

77. Carneiro F. Classification of gastric carcinomas. *Curr Diagn Pathol.* 1997;4:51–59.

78. Machado JC, Nogueira AM, Carneiro F, et al. Gastric carcinoma exhibits distinct types of cell differentiation: an immunohistochemical study of trefoil peptides (TFF1 and TFF2) and mucins (MUC1, MUC2, MUC5AC, and MUC6). *J Pathol.* 2000;190:437–443.

79. Mori M, Sakaguchi H, Akazawa K, et al. Correlation between metastatic site, histological type, and serum tumor markers of gastric carcinoma. *Hum Pathol.* 1995;26:504–508.

80. Esaki Y, Hirayama R, Hirokawa K. A comparison of patterns of metastasis in gastric cancer by histologic type and age. *Cancer.* 1990;65:2086–2090.

81. Chiaravalli AM, Klersy C, Tava F, et al. Lower- and higher-grade subtypes of diffuse gastric cancer. *Hum Pathol.* 2009;40:1591–1599.

82. Haas M, Dimmler A, Hohenberger W, et al. Stromal regulatory T-cells are associated with a favourable prognosis in gastric cancer of the cardia. *BMC gastroenterology.* 2009;9:65.

83. Lee HE, Chae SW, Lee YJ, et al. Prognostic implications of type and density of tumour-infiltrating lymphocytes in gastric cancer. *Br J Cancer.* 2008;99:1704–1711.

84. Huang KH, Chen JH, Wu CW, et al. Factors affecting recurrence in node-negative advanced gastric cancer. *J Gastroenterol Hepatol.* 2009;24:1522–1526.

85. Umeyama K, Sowa M, Kamino K, et al. Gastric carcinoma in young adults in Japan. *Anticancer Res.* 1982;2:283–286.

86. Martin IG, Dixon MF, Sue-Ling H, et al. Goseki histological grading of gastric cancer is an important predictor of outcome. *Gut.* 1994;35:758–763.

87. Lee OJ, Kim HJ, Kim JR, et al. The prognostic significance of the mucin phenotype of gastric adenocarcinoma and its relationship with histologic classifications. *Oncol Rep.* 2009;21:387–393.

88. Han HS, Lee SY, Lee KY, et al. Unclassified mucin phenotype of gastric adenocarcinoma exhibits the highest invasiveness. *J Gastroenterol Hepatol.* 2009;24:658–666.

89. Wakatsuki K, Yamada Y, Narikiyo M, et al. Clinicopathological and prognostic significance of mucin phenotype in gastric cancer. *J Surg Oncol.* 2008;98:124–129.

Early and Advanced Gastric Carcinomas

6

▶ Shinichi Ban

INTRODUCTION

If untreated, gastric adenocarcinomas, which develop first in the epithelial component of the mucosa, will infiltrate the deeper layers of the gastric wall. The level of infiltration is important, since it influences prognosis, and the layers of the gastric wall are used as landmarks to define the T factor of the International Union Against Cancer (UICC) TNM-staging system of gastric carcinoma.[1] However, it is only in the last several decades, with advances in radiologic and endoscopic diagnostic modalities, that an increasing number of early stage gastric carcinomas (pT1) have been detected, a shift that has prompted a division of gastric carcinomas into two groups, early and advanced, on the basis of the depth of invasion of the gastric wall. This division is convenient because the two categories differ in not only prognosis but also morphology and various clinicopathological aspects. Consequently, the recognition of these differences, in which pathologists have played a significant role, has contributed to the increasing improvement in the early detection and treatment of gastric carcinomas. Given this background, this chapter reviews various aspects of early and advanced gastric carcinomas, including their macroscopic appearances, the progression patterns from early to advanced stage, histologic characteristics, and prognostic relevance.

DEFINITIONS AND RELATIVE INCIDENCE OF EARLY AND ADVANCED GASTRIC CARCINOMA

Early gastric carcinoma has been defined as any invasive adenocarcinoma confined to either the mucosa or submucosa, irrespective of the presence of lymph node metastases.[2] Importantly, the term "early" does not necessarily refer to the size or age of the lesion.[3] Conversely, gastric adenocarcinomas infiltrating into the muscularis propria or beyond are termed advanced gastric carcinoma.[2] The concept of early gastric carcinoma was first established in Japan in 1962 by the (now defunct) Japanese Endoscopic Society (currently the Japan Gastroenterological Endoscopy Society), which included endoscopists, surgeons, radiologists, and pathologists. The defining concept was that this group of gastric carcinomas could be successfully treated by surgery.[4] It since has been confirmed that gastric carcinomas limited to the mucosa and submucosa generally have an excellent prognosis, with a 5-year survival rate exceeding 90%.[5,6] In contrast, the 5-year survival rate of advanced gastric carcinomas is around 60% or lower.[7]

Early and advanced gastric carcinomas differ in not only their prognosis but various biologic characteristics as well, which guarantee the validity of separately defining early and advanced gastric carcinomas. One difference is in the growth rate of these neoplasms. Although the infiltration of the gastric wall by neoplastic cells morphologically appears to be a continuous process, it has been shown that the progression is not constant. Gastric carcinomas often remain in the early stage for a long time, in contrast to advanced stages, which often progress rapidly. A retrospective radiologic follow-up study estimated that the doubling time of early gastric carcinomas is several years, but less than a year for advanced ones.[8] Another long-term prospective follow-up study of early gastric carcinomas similarly revealed that many cases remained stable for a median duration of 3.7 years.[9] A second, important distinction between the stages of gastric cancer is in macroscopic appearance. This was illustrated in a retrospective study by Nishizawa et al.[10] who suggested that the radiological changes noted in gastric carcinomas reflected deep submucosal invasion.

Although the detection of early gastric carcinomas has become increasingly common, the ratio of early to advanced tumors still differs significantly between Japan and the West. In some Japanese institutions, early gastric carcinomas account for approximately half or more of all treated cases, whereas in the West, the incidence is only up to 25%.[2,5,11,12] The difference can be attributed to the availability of endoscopic surveillance in Japan combined with mass screening of asymptomatic patients. Furthermore, the differences between Japanese and Western diagnostic criteria for gastric intramucosal neoplasms also are likely to influence the incidence rate of early gastric carcinomas. Classically, Japanese pathologists render a diagnosis of intramucosal carcinoma based solely on the cytologic atypia of neoplastic cells with various degrees of architectural atypia, whereas Western pathologists make a point of identifying a breach of basement membrane and stromal invasion.[13] This difference commonly results in a diagnosis of carcinoma by Japanese pathologists for lesions that Western pathologists frequently would classify as high-grade dysplasia (high-grade intraepithelial neoplasm).[14] Consequently, there have been several international efforts aimed at resolving the differences, such as the Vienna and Padova classifications.[15–17]

MACROSCOPIC CLASSIFICATION OF GASTRIC CARCINOMA

In an effort to provide some consistency in the description of gastric cancers, the Japanese Gastric Cancer Association has established a macroscopic scheme.[18] This system derives from two sources: one is the Borrmann classification, well known for advanced gastric carcinomas,[19] and the other is a classification for early gastric carcinomas, originally proposed by the Japanese Endoscopic Society.[4] The latter was proposed because the Borrmann classification is based mainly on the invasive patterns of carcinomas beyond the mucosal layer, and is not applicable to superficial lesions, whose macroscopic appearance usually changes markedly during progression. Combining these two classifications, gastric carcinomas are macroscopically classified following the scheme shown in Figure 6-1,[18] and a reported percentage of each macroscopic type is shown in Table 6-1.[20]

In this system, in addition to the four types of the Borrmann classification, Type 5 has been added to describe tumors whose appearance cannot be properly classified using Types 1 to 4.

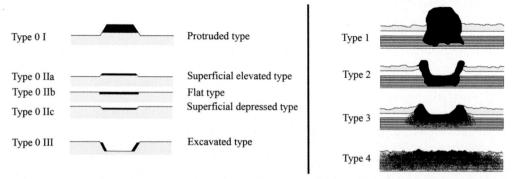

FIGURE 6-1 Macroscopic types of gastric carcinoma according to the rule of the Japanese Gastric Cancer Association.[18] The classification of early gastric cancer (**left**) is a 5-tier system with Type 0 corresponding to superficial, flat tumors with or without minimal elevation or depression. For advanced neoplasms (**right**) the Borrmann classification is followed. The subtypes are defined as follows: Type 1: Polypoid tumors, sharply demarcated from the surrounding mucosa, usually with a broad base; Type 2: Ulcerated carcinomas with sharply demarcated and raised margins; Type 3: Ulcerated carcinomas without well-defined borders, infiltrating into the surrounding wall; Type 4: Diffusely infiltrating carcinomas in which ulceration is usually not a marked feature; Type 5: Nonclassifiable carcinomas that cannot be classified into any of the other types.

Table 6-1	Percentages of gastric carcinomas by macroscopic type		
Early Gastric Carcinoma	**Percentage (%)**	**Advanced Gastric Carcinoma**	**Percentage (%)**
Type 0 I	3.6	Type 1	2.7
Type 0 IIa	16.1	Type 2	21.6
Type 0 IIb	5.6	Type 3	35.8
Type 0 IIc	45.4	Type 4	16.3
Type 0 III	0.1	Type 5	23.6
Combined type	29.1		

Source: From Takizawa T, Iwasaki Y, Iino H, et al. Macro- and microscopic features of gastric cancers. *Stomach Intestine*. 1991;26:1135–1148 [in Japanese with English summary].

Furthermore, Type 0 primarily describes the appearance of early gastric carcinomas, although it also can include advanced carcinomas macroscopically simulating early lesions.[18] Type 0 is divided into five subtypes (I, IIa, IIb, IIc, and III) (Fig. 6-1). In addition, tumors with a combined macroscopic appearance are recognized, and terms such as IIa + IIc, or IIc + III are used. The subtypes of Type 0 are based on elevation, evenness, or depression of tumors in relation to the surrounding mucosa (Fig. 6-1). The classification is applicable to radiological and endoscopic images, as well as the macroscopic appearance of resected specimens.[4] Adoption of this scheme, especially the delineation of Type 0, has greatly improved communication among surgeons, endoscopists, radiologists, and pathologists in Japan. Recently, the usefulness of the subclassification, especially for endoscopic diagnosis and treatment, has been reconfirmed at the Paris Workshop.[21]

One important change that modifies the macroscopic appearance of early gastric carcinomas is secondary ulceration, which leads to scarring (submucosal fibrosis) when it heals (Fig. 6-2). Hirota et al.[6] reported the frequency of secondary ulcer as 64.5% of all early gastric carcinomas, whereas Takizawa et al.[20] observed this process less frequently (15.8%). It should be emphasized that Type 0 III originally meant an ulcer lesion with carcinoma just on its edge, previously referred to as an "ulcer cancer."[4,6]

The histologic types of gastric carcinoma influence the macroscopic appearance. For more than half a century, except for rare variants, ordinary gastric adenocarcinomas have been divided into intestinal and diffuse types by the Laurén classification.[22] Independently, Nakamura proposed classifying gastric carcinomas into differentiated and undifferentiated types, the former being gland-forming carcinomas (e.g., papillary and tubular adenocarcinomas), and the latter being adenocarcinomas with no or little glandular formation (i.e., signet ring cell carcinoma and poorly differentiated adenocarcinoma).[23,24] However, although Laurén and Nakamura classifications were established based on the respective analysis of advanced carcinomas and minute carcinomas, differentiated lesions mostly correspond to intestinal type and undifferentiated lesions to diffuse type.

Although the most common macroscopic pattern of early gastric carcinoma is Type 0 IIc, there are some differences between differentiated and undifferentiated tumors, especially when intramucosal.[25] Differentiated Type 0 IIc tumors tend to be reddish lesions with ill defined margins or mild elevation at the edge corresponding to the replacement of nonneoplastic glands by neoplastic epithelium. In contrast, undifferentiated Type 0 IIc lesions are characterized by an abruptly depressed margin due to atrophy and/or erosions of the neoplastic mucosa, often with residual islands of nonneoplastic regenerative crypts (Fig. 6-3). Undifferentiated Type 0 IIc lesions also are associated with secondary ulcers more often than are differentiated tumors, which tend to form elevated lesions (Type 0 I, Type 0 IIa).[20] Of note, differences are also seen at the stage of advanced gastric carcinoma, with Type 4 tumors predominantly composed of undifferentiated carcinoma.[20]

FIGURE 6-2 Ulcer or ulcer scar occurred in depressed type early gastric carcinomas: **A:** Type 0 IIc + III, measuring 4.5 × 3.5 cm, limited to the mucosa. **B:** Type 0 IIc with ulcer scar depicted by convergence of the folds into the center, measuring 1.9 × 1.5 cm, intramucosal carcinoma with submucosal invasion in the very limited area. **C:** Low power histology of the center of (**B**), showing submucosal scarring involving the muscularis propria.

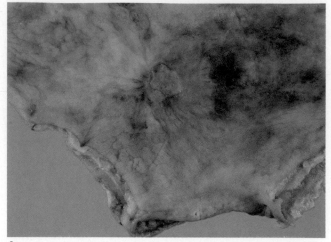

A

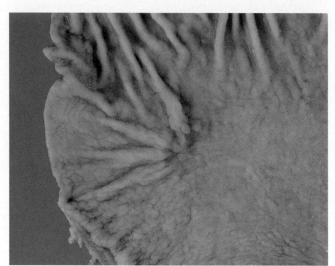

B

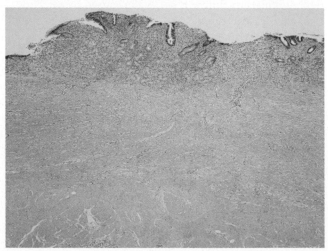

C

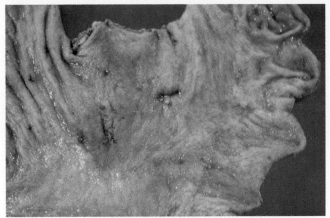

A

FIGURE 6-3 Difference of macroscopic appearance between differentiated and undifferentiated types gastric carcinoma limited to the mucosa: **A:** Type 0 IIc differentiated carcinoma showing an obscure margin and reddish in color. **B:** Type 0 IIc undifferentiated carcinoma characterized by an abruptly depressed margin and islands of nonneoplastic regenerative mucosa.

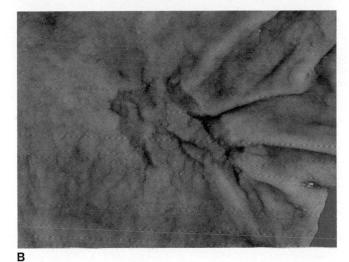
B

The depth of invasion is another factor influencing the macroscopic appearance of early gastric carcinomas. Most Type 0 IIb carcinomas are intramucosal, although a few cases show submucosal invasion (Fig. 6-4). Mixed patterns, that is, IIa + IIb or IIc + IIb, also can be seen. In that group are signet ring cell carcinomas spreading in atrophic mucosa. However, once the tumor extends into the submucosa, the frequency of combined macroscopic types increases, and even simple Type 0 IIc lesions tend to show an uneven dull depressed surface[20] (Table 6-1).

PROGRESSION FROM EARLY TO ADVANCED GASTRIC CARCINOMA

Incipient Phase Gastric Adenocarcinomas

As previously mentioned, the concept of "early" gastric carcinoma does not refer to a chronologically incipient phase. Cases that are small enough in size to be regarded as incipient (<5 mm in diameter) have been termed minute gastric carcinomas (Fig. 6-5). A large series of minute carcinomas (*n* = 145) was first examined by Nakamura et al.,[23,24] and has been collectively examined by several authors.[26–30] The topographic distribution of these cases was similar to that of larger early gastric carcinomas and advanced tumors, and they often display Type 0 IIb pattern, which can barely be recognized macroscopically, and consequently are usually found during the examination

FIGURE 6-4 EBV-related gastric carcinoma, with submucosal invasion: **A:** Type 0
IIb gross pattern, approximately 1 cm in
diameter (*left*). Synchronous multiple
carcinomas (also EBV-related) indicated
are noted. **B:** Loupe view of the lesion,
showing massive submucosal invasion
without apparent elevation or depression
of the mucosal surface. **C:** Middle power
histology showing the so-called medullary carcinoma with lymphoid stroma
with very limited intramucosal spread
and massive submucosal invasion. MM,
muscularis mucosa.

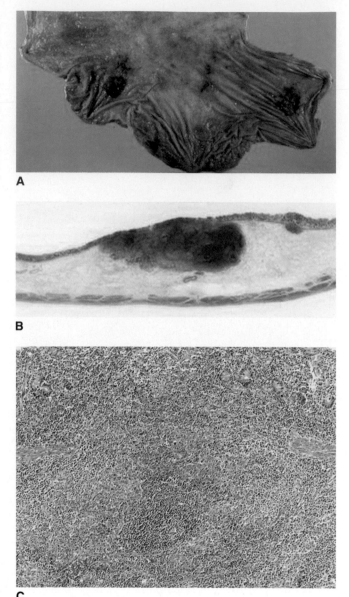

of a gastrectomy performed for other lesions.[24] Minute carcinomas can be either differentiated or
undifferentiated, but the former are six times more common.[24,27] As small as these neoplasms are,
infiltration into the submucosa occurs in 3.3%[23,30] to 9%[27] of cases. Several routes of invasion can
be observed: (a) invasion of the stroma around the vessels that penetrate the muscularis mucosa,
(b) infiltration of the vasculature that penetrates the muscularis mucosa, (c) direct invasion and
destruction of the muscularis mucosa, and (d) infiltration developing from rare cases of submucosal heterotopic mucosa.[31]

The Natural Course of Gastric Carcinomas

Few retrospective and prospective follow-up studies have evaluated the course of untreated gastric
carcinomas. In a prospective follow-up study of 56 cases, the cumulative 5-year risk for progression to advanced stage was 63.0%.[9] This suggests that most untreated early gastric carcinomas, if
not all, progress, although they remain at an early stage for several years (median 3.7 years).[9] Yet
the growth rate can vary considerably. An endoscopic retrospective follow-up study of 72 cases

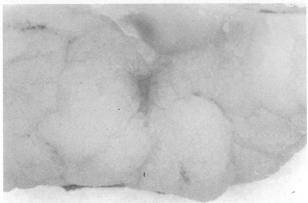

A

FIGURE 6-5 Minute gastric carcinoma: **A:** Stereoscopic view of a Type 0 IIc lesion <5 mm in the largest diameter. **B:** Loupe view of the lesion occupying the entire thickness of the mucosa involving the muscularis mucosa. **C:** Histology of the lesion showing differentiated type carcinoma (tubular adenocarcinoma).

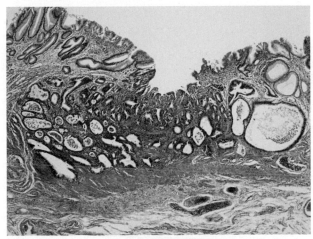
B

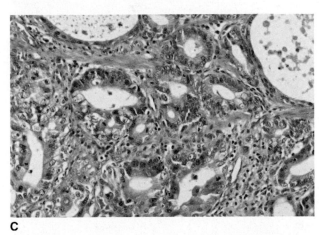
C

suggested that the growth of Type 0 IIc early gastric carcinoma was often gradual for 2 to 6 years, whereas some Type 0 IIa + IIc early gastric carcinomas (as well as Borrmann Type 2 or 3 advanced carcinomas) seemed to develop within a few years from nonulcerative, subtle erythematous discoloration, or slightly elevated granular mucosa, or a shallow depression.[32] Relatively rapid progression (within 2 years) from endoscopically subtle lesions to Type 4 carcinomas also has been seen.[8,32] However, another study reported a longer course (of several years) before Type 4 is seen.[33] Rapid growth (within 2 years) of some elevated type carcinomas without obvious, radiologically demonstrated preceding lesions also has been reported.[34]

FIGURE 6-6 A: Gross appearance of superficially spreading Type 0 IIc gastric carcinoma, limited to the mucosa and measuring 17 × 9 cm. **B:** Type 0 IIc gastric carcinoma measuring 2 × 2 cm and with massive submucosal invasion. **C:** Low power histology of (**B**) showing submucosal invasion of tubular adenocarcinoma.

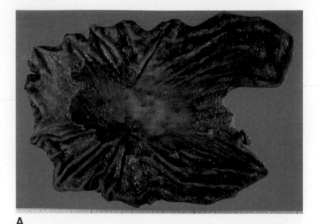

Variable rate of progression from early to advanced carcinoma also is implied by the analysis of resection specimens. Kodama et al. classified the growth patterns of early gastric carcinomas into two types: The superficially spreading type, which is over 4 cm in diameter and confined to the mucosa or with very limited invasion to the submucosa. The second type, on the other hand, the penetrating growth type is <4 cm in diameter with wide submucosal invasion (Fig. 6-6).[35]

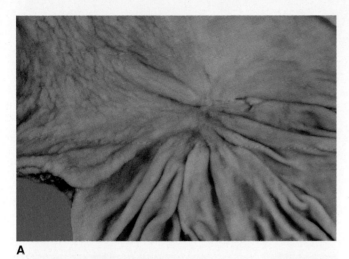

A

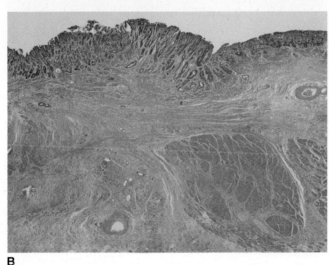

B

FIGURE 6-7 Advanced gastric carcinoma simulating early gastric carcinoma: **A:** Type 0 IIc gross appearance with ulcer scar, measuring 3.5 × 3 cm. Invasion into the muscularis propria is very limited. **B:** Low power histology showing preserved intramucosal growth of tubular adenocarcinoma and a small number of neoplastic glands infiltrating into the muscularis propria with fibrosis.

The clonal origin of superficial widely spreading depressed-type gastric carcinomas was demonstrated with the HUMARA assay, implying that the lesions remained in the mucosa for a long time and do not represent the coalescence of several lesions.[36]

As previously noted, secondary peptic ulceration commonly occurs in depressed type early gastric carcinomas, and a recurrent cycle of ulceration, healing, and reulceration can be observed. Such carcinomas tend to remain at an early stage for an extended period, which is partly explained by tumor cell loss and the deterrent effect of fibrous scarring against invasion.[3,8] Of note, although ulceration is more frequent in undifferentiated neoplasms, differentiated type neoplasms are more likely to show submucosal invasion.[20]

As they progress to advanced stages, some early gastric carcinomas, especially those of depressed type, retain the same endoscopic appearance and do not acquire a macroscopic appearance that could be classified by using the Borrmann classification.[8,37] These tumors account for approximately 10% of resected advanced carcinomas. The dominant macroscopic types of these tumors (accounting for >80% of the cases) are IIc, IIc + III, and III + IIc, with the latter two accounting for 50% of the cases, suggesting a high frequency of association with ulceration. More than half of these cases are of diffuse type (Laurén classification) and about 50% of the cases are limited to the muscularis propria. The overall prognosis of these cases is relatively favorable, with a 73% 5-year survival rate[37] (Fig. 6-7).

FIGURE 6-8 Type 4 diffusely infiltrating gastric carcinomas: **A:** tumor involving the entire antropyloric regions circumferentially, causing severe pyloric stenosis. **B:** carcinoma involving almost all the stomach with enlarged folds of the body and fundus, referred to as linitis plastica. Note, the primary small depressed (IIc) lesion centrally situated within the enlarged folds in the mid body.

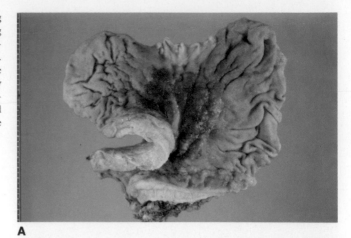

A

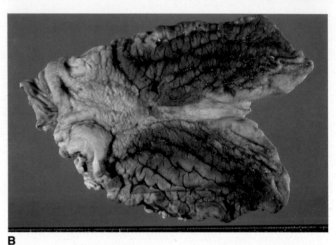

B

Type 4 diffusely infiltrating advanced carcinomas spread widely through the gastric wall and are usually composed of poorly differentiated neoplastic cells, often with signet ring cell element distributed in a dense collagenous stroma with marked thickening of the organ (scirrhous carcinoma). They have been thought to progress from small Type 0 IIc carcinomas (Fig. 6-8) over several years, but some may spread more rapidly (within 2 years).[8,33,38] Analyses of chromosomal copy number alterations demonstrated that submucosal infiltrating poorly differentiated cells shared the same lineage as intramucosal signet ring cells, suggesting that they represent different stages of progression.[39] These cases commonly involve the entire antropyloric region in a circumferential fashion, causing pyloric stenosis (Fig. 6-8). When they involve almost the entire stomach, with enlarged gastric folds of the body/fundus, these neoplasms commonly produce the appearance of linitis plastica (Fig. 6-8). However, some retain a flattened atrophic mucosa.[33] Of note, typical linitis plastica type carcinomas can be missed on endoscopic biopsy because the mucosal lesions can be small, depressed, and hidden between enlarged folds.

Histologic Types and Progression of Gastric Carcinomas

The broad histologic types, Laurén's intestinal and diffuse types, or Nakamura's differentiated and undifferentiated types, are distributed differently depending on the age and gender of the patients. Furthermore, the mode of extragastric progression in advanced stages varies among these types.[22,40,41] Differentiated (intestinal) type carcinomas tend to arise in older males and show

Table 6-2	Mucin phenotype of gastric carcinomas						
		Markers		Frequency of Each Mucin Phenotype (%)			
Reporter	Carcinoma Type	Histochemistry	Immunohistochemistry	Gastric	Mixed Gastric and Intestinal	Intestinal	Null
Tatematsu et al. (1990)[42]	D and U	GCS, s-GOS, PCS	Pg I, Pg II	41.3	29.1	27.8	1.8
Yamachika et al. (1997)[43]	Sig, Early, and Advanced	GOS, s-GOS, PCS	Pg II, SH-7, TKH2	64.0	34.0	2.0	—
Bamba et al. (2001)[44]	Sig, Early, and Advanced	MUC2, PCS	HGM	27.8	68.5	3.7	—
Saito et al. (2001)[45]	D and U, Early	PCS, HID-AB	HGM	16* 18**	58* 60**	23* 17**	3* 5**
Tajima et al. (2001)[46]	D and U, Advanced	—	HGM, MUC6, MUC2, CD10	36.8	41.2	15.4	6.6
Kawachi et al. (2003)[29]	D, minute carcinoma	—	HGM, M-GGMC-1, MUC2, CD10	20	8	20	52
Shiroshita et al. (2004)[30]	D, minute carcinoma	PCS	HGM, MUC5AC, MUC6, MUC2, M-GGMC-1, CD10	33.3	36.3	30.3	—

* <10 mm.

** ≥10 mm.

D, differentiated type carcinoma; U, undifferentiated type carcinoma; Sig, signet ring cell carcinoma; Early, early gastric carcinoma; Advanced, advanced gastric carcinoma; GOS, galactose oxidase-Schiff; s-GOS, sialidase-galactose oxidase-Schiff; PCS, paradoxical concanavalin A staining; HID-AB, high-iron diamine-Alcian blue (pH2.5); Pg, pepsinogen; HGM, human gastric mucin.

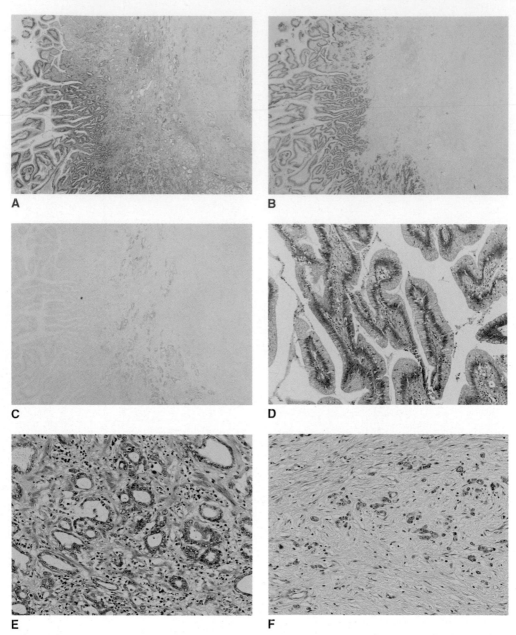

FIGURE 6-9 Differentiated type carcinoma with a complete gastric phenotype showing undifferentiated type appearance (nonsolid type poorly differentiated adenocarcinoma) in the area of submucosal invasion: **A:** Low power view showing the transition from intramucosal papillotubular growth to submucosal poorly differentiated component. **B:** MUC5AC immunoreactivity in the superficial papillotubular pattern. **C:** MUC6 immunoreactivity in the deeper invasive area. The tumor was negative for MUC2 or CD10 (not shown). **D:** High power view of the intramucosal papillotubular pattern showing extremely well-differentiated low-grade appearance similar to gastric foveolar epithelium. **E:** High power view of the deeper intramucosal area showing microtubular growth pattern. **F:** High power view of the submucosal invasion showing nonsolid type poorly differentiated adenocarcinoma with scirrhous stroma.

hematogenous metastases, whereas undifferentiated (diffuse) type carcinomas are prone to occur in younger female patients and to develop lymph node metastases and peritoneal dissemination. Not uncommonly, undifferentiated type carcinomas will develop in the fundic region of a young adult female, first as IIc lesions, and progress to scirrhous carcinomas in the advanced stage (Fig. 6-8).

Using mucin histochemistry and electron microscopy, Nakamura reported that differentiated type carcinomas tend to phenotypically resemble intestinal metaplastic epithelium, whereas undifferentiated type carcinoma cells tend to have a gastric phenotype.[40] Using mucin immunohistochemical markers, carcinomas have been classified into several variants, lineages, or phenotypes in more detail. The three types are gastric (including foveolar, pyloric, and mucinous neck cell subcategories), intestinal (including goblet cell, Paneth cell, and absorptive cell categories), and mixed gastric and intestinal type. Although the frequency of each type varies according to the markers and the criteria used for classification[29,30,42-46] (see Table 6-2), a significant number of differentiated type adenocarcinomas display a gastric phenotype (10% to 30% of cases).[29,30,42,45,46] The same is true for undifferentiated type carcinomas, particularly signet ring cell variant.[42-45]

These recent studies call attention to the alteration of the histologic appearance of gastric carcinomas with their progression in relation to the tumor phenotype. For example, undifferentiated type carcinomas represent only about 20% of intramucosal carcinomas, but >50% of advanced carcinomas.[20] This also may be partly related to the lower detection rate of undifferentiated early gastric carcinomas because of their tendency to arise at a young age, and partly to a higher miss rate in radiologic and endoscopic detection.[47] Another possibility is that early differentiated type carcinomas dedifferentiate as they invade more deeply.[20] In fact, a cell lineage analysis using comparative genomic hybridization has suggested the possibility of an interchangeable transition between tubular and signet ring cell and/or poorly differentiated morphologies.[48] Notably, differentiated type early carcinomas that transform to an undifferentiated morphotype commonly display a gastric immunophenotype (Fig. 6-9).[45,49-51] Furthermore, these cases share clinicopathological features characteristic of undifferentiated type carcinomas.[49] That is, they tend to occur in relatively younger females and in the proximal stomach.

Another situation in which the morphotype can change with progression is in solid type poorly differentiated adenocarcinomas of elder patients, which can derive from differentiated type tumors.[52] Furthermore, these carcinomas often reveal microsatellite instability (MSI) and hMLH1 promoter hypermethylation.[52]

Many carcinomas, either differentiated or undifferentiated, have a mixed phenotype.[42,45,46] In fact, they may be committed to both phenotypes in the incipient phase, since minute carcinomas of differentiated type may display a mixed phenotype.[29,30] However, the phenotype of gastric carcinomas changes with neoplastic growth. Intestinalization occurs independently of the histologic type as the tumor progresses.[53,54] For example, they may acquire acidic mucin as they grow.[43,44] Conversely, reversible environmental induction of the intestinal phenotype has been reported in some undifferentiated type carcinomas as well.[55]

It is particularly noteworthy that some differentiated carcinomas with very low grade cytologic atypia may present with either a gastric or an intestinal phenotype (Fig. 6-10).[51,56-58] Of note, different molecular characteristics have been reported, depending on whether they have a completely gastric or intestinal phenotype.[59]

PROGNOSTIC INDICATORS OF EARLY AND ADVANCED GASTRIC CARCINOMAS

Multiple factors, not always independent of one another, influence the prognosis of gastric cancer patients after resection. One study reported that univariate analysis revealed six clinicopathological factors that influenced 5-year survival.[60] They are lymphatic and/or capillary microinvasion, proximal location, extension beyond the gastric wall, lymph node metastases, diffuse type (Laurén classification),[22] and infiltrative type (Ming classification).[61] However, multivariate analysis revealed lymphatic and/or capillary microinvasion as the only independent prognostic factor. Yet, when vascular microinvasion was omitted, extension beyond the gastric wall and lymph node metastases were statistically significant variables.[60]

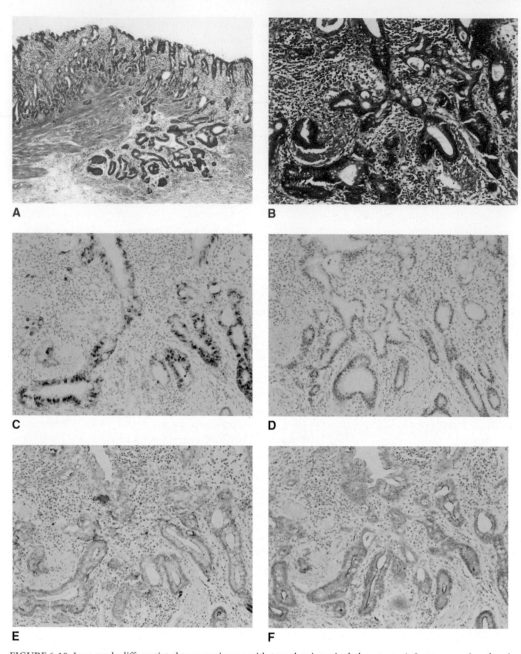

FIGURE 6-10 Low-grade differentiated type carcinoma with complete intestinal phenotype. **A:** Low power view showing intramucosal growth with focal submucosal invasion. **B:** High power view showing proliferation of very low grade neoplastic epithelium with goblet cells and Paneth cells, resembling intestinal metaplasia. The neoplastic epithelium is immunoreactive to MUC2 (**C**), CDX2 (**D**), CD10 (**E**), and villin (**F**), but negative for MUC5AC, MUC6, or M-GGMC-1 (not shown).

Local extent and lymph node metastases represent T and N factors of the TNM-staging system[1] according to which the prognosis of gastric carcinoma patients is usually estimated. Additionally, the pathologic evaluation of resected specimens according to the rule of the Japanese Gastric Cancer Association includes the assessment of lymphatic and venous microinvasions, the carcinoma stroma (medullary or scirrhous), and infiltrating growth patterns.[18] Invasion of the lymphatics in particular has been proven to be an independent predictor of lymph node metastasis in a study using LYVE-1 antibody.[62] Furthermore, ongoing studies have been performed with

Table 6-3	Risk factors of lymph node metastasis for early gastric carcinomas				
Risk Factor	Yamao et al. (1996)[64] (M)	Satou et al. (2001)[66] (M) and (SM)	Gotoda et al. (2000)[65] (M) and (SM)	Ohashi et al. (2007)[67] (SM)	Tajima et al. (2010)[68+] (SM)
Young age	○(<57 y)				
Depressed type	○		○		
Large size	○* (>30 mm)	○++ (average 5.3 cm)	○ (>30 mm)	○*	○* (>20 mm)
Undifferentiated type histology	○	○++	○		○* (and mixed D type and U type carcinoma)
Ulcer association+++	○*	○++	○		
Lymphatic invasion	○*		○ (or invasion of venules)	○*	○*
Submucosal invasion	NA	○	○ (submucosal invasion >500 μm)	○* (relatively deeper submucosal invasion)	○* (submucosal invasion >500 μm)

+Including micrometastasis and isolated carcinoma cells detected by cytokeratin immunohistochemistry.
(M), targeting intramucosal carcinomas; (SM), targeting carcinomas infiltrating into the submucosa.
○ reported risk factors; ○*, independent risk factors by a multivariate analysis; ○++, risk factors of intramucosal carcinoma.
+++Including microscopic ulcers and ulcer scars.
D type, differentiated type; U type, undifferentiated type; NA, not applicable.

regard to the prognostic significance of sentinel lymph node metastases and of micrometastasis (measuring <2 mm in diameter or composed of isolated tumor cell foci <0.2 mm in diameter) detected by either immunohistochemistry or molecular biology.[63]

Early gastric cancers metastasize to lymph nodes with an incidence of 2% to 3% for intramucosal neoplasms[64–66] and 20% to 30% for carcinomas with submucosal invasion.[65,67,68] The prediction of lymph node metastases is particularly important because of the potential for endoscopic therapy.[69] Reportedly, risk factors for lymph node metastasis from early gastric carcinomas include age (<60 years), depressed macroscopic type and ulceration (including histological ulcer or ulcer scars), large size (>2–3 cm), undifferentiated histologic type, lymphatic invasion, and deep submucosal invasion (invasion >500 μm)[64–68] (Table 6-3). Additionally, a gastric mucin phenotype may be associated with an increased risk of nodal metastasis,[66] a finding that can be explained by the predominance of undifferentiated tumors in these cases.

Although the prognosis of early gastric carcinomas is excellent overall, approximately 2% recur after curative resection, with intervals ranging from 4 months to over 10 years.[70] Submucosal invasion, lymph node metastasis, or differentiated type is associated with an increased risk of recurrence.[70] One noteworthy risk factor is differentiated histology, for which the major mode of recurrence is through hematogenous metastases.[70] The recurrence rate of early gastric carcinomas with lymph node metastasis has been reported at 8%.[71] In those cases, the most common site of recurrence was naturally a lymph node, and the number of positive nodes has been noted as independent risk factor.[71] Thus, these patients should be closely monitored, and those who are at high risk should be considered for adjuvant chemotherapy. Also, synchronous and metachronous multiple occurrence of gastric carcinomas should be considered after local excision.[72,73]

The relationship between prognosis and histologic type is not straightforward. In the original description of Laurén,[22] intestinal type carcinomas had a more favorable prognosis than diffuse type. However, in recent reports,[74,75] this morphotype has not always been prognostically informative. Interestingly, using Nakamura's classification, differentiated type carcinomas confined to the submucosa or muscularis propria showed 5-year survival rates lower than those for undifferentiated type carcinomas,[40] possibly because of their tendency to develop hematogenous metastasis. However, for cases that invade beyond the muscularis propria, the prognosis for undifferentiated type tumors is worse.[40]

There have been multiple attempts to identify the histologic patterns of gastric carcinomas that have a prognostic impact.[74,75] For example, papillary adenocarcinoma has a prognosis worse than any other histologic type at almost every level of invasion,[7] with a particularly higher frequency of lymphatic and venous invasion, and nodal metastases.[76,77] Interestingly, the immunophenotype is variable, with a gastric mucin phenotype predominant in one report,[77] but intestinal or mixed in another report.[78] It has been reported that papillary adenocarcinomas tended to show a high frequency of MSI and methylation of hMLH1 promoter regions,[78] characteristics that others reported to be associated with a better prognosis.[79,80]

Differentiated type carcinomas with very low grade cytological atypia and completely gastric or intestinal phenotype have an improved prognosis.[56] Also, prominent tumor infiltrating lymphocytes, as seen in carcinoma with "lymphoid stroma," which often shows a medullary carcinoma with lymphoid stroma, is associated with a better prognosis (Fig. 6-4).[81,82] Most of these cases overlap with Epstein-Barr virus (EBV)-associated gastric carcinomas, which also have a lower tendency toward lymph node metastasis and so a better prognosis.[83,84] Finally, some recent studies have reported a relatively better prognosis for a group of mucinous and diffuse type adenocarcinomas,[85,86] which is noteworthy, since these subtypes generally have been thought to have a worse prognosis.[7]

EARLY GASTRIC CARCINOMA IN THE ERA OF ESD AND THE IMPORTANCE OF PATHOLOGICAL EXAMINATION

Endoscopic treatment of early gastric carcinomas has become standard practice. There has been a recent shift from endoscopic mucosal resection (EMR) to endoscopic submucosal dissection (ESD), enabling en bloc resection of larger carcinomas.[69] Consequently, the indication criteria for endoscopic treatment of early gastric carcinomas have been challenged, as they were initially established for EMR (endoscopically intramucosal differentiated type carcinoma, 20 mm or less in size, and without findings of ulceration),[69] and the indication criteria for endoscopic treatment have been expanded.[87,88] At present, the proposed expanded criteria in the forthcoming gastric cancer treatment guidelines to be published in Japan are (a) endoscopically intramucosal differentiated type carcinoma over 20 mm in size but without ulcer or ulcer scar, (b) endoscopically intramucosal differentiated type carcinoma with ulcer or ulcer scar but 30 mm or less in size, and (c) endoscopically intramucosal undifferentiated carcinoma, 20 mm or less in size and without ulcer or ulcer scar. With regard to these lesions, the risk of lymph node metastasis is very low if they are without lymphatic or vascular invasion. However, evaluation of long-term prognosis is needed to validate the expanded criteria. In these circumstances, the role of pathologists in assessing resected specimens is particularly important, since the precise evaluation of pathological variables relating to the risk of metastasis and prognosis will determine patient management (Fig. 6-11).

Since the establishment of the concept of early gastric carcinoma, many aspects of clinicopathological features of these neoplasms and their progression to advanced carcinomas have been clarified. Although many molecular biological studies are ongoing, assessment of conventional pathological factors is still mandatory for patient management, and advances in endoscopic treatment of early gastric carcinomas have required more precise pathological diagnoses.

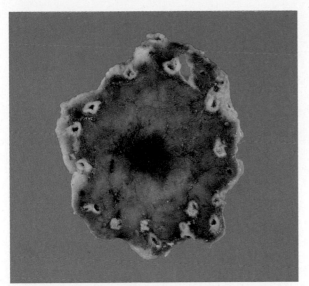

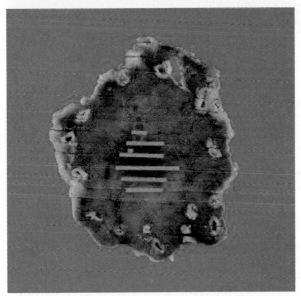

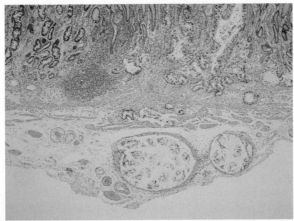

FIGURE 6-11 A: Type 0 IIc carcinoma, 1 cm in the largest diameter, resected by ESD. **B:** The specimen is entirely step sectioned at 2-mm intervals followed by mapping of the microscopic finding on the photograph. Submucosal lymphatic infiltration is noted spreading beyond the extent of the mucosal carcinoma. *Orange line*: mucosal carcinoma, *Double orange line*: submucosal direct invasion, *Pink line*: submucosal lymphatic invasion. **C:** Low power histology of the lesion showing submucosal lymphatic invasion.

References

1. Sobin LH, Gospodarowicz MK, Wittekind CH, eds. *International Union against Cancer (UICC): TNM classification of malignant tumors.* 7th ed. Oxford: Wiley-Blackwell; 2009.
2. Hamilton R, Aaltonen LA, eds. *Tumors of the digestive system.* Lyon: IARC; 2000:39–52.
3. Yoshimori M. The natural history of early gastric cancer. *Jpn J Clin Oncol.* 1989;19:89–93.
4. Murakami T. Patholomorphological diagnosis. Definition and gross classification of early gastric cancer. *Gann Monogr Cancer Res.* 1971;11:53–55.
5. Everett SM, Axon AT. Early gastric cancer in Europe. *Gut.* 1997;41:142–150.
6. Hirota T, Ming SC, Itabashi M. Pathology of early gastric cancer. In: Nishi M, Ichikawa H, Nakajima Y, et al., eds. *Gastric cancer.* Tokyo: Springer-Verlag; 1993:66–85.
7. Hirota T, Ochiai A, Itabashi M, et al. Significance of histological type of gastric carcinoma as a prognostic factor. *Stomach Intestine.* 1991;26:1149–1158 [in Japanese with English summary].
8. Kohli Y, Kawai K, Fujita S. Analytical studies on growth of human gastric cancer. *J Clin Gastroenterol.* 1981;3:129–133.
9. Tsukuma H, Oshima A, Narahara H, et al. Natural history of early gastric cancer: a non-concurrent, long term, follow up study. *Gut.* 2000;47:618–621.
10. Nishizawa M, Nomoto K, Ueno M, et al. Natural history of gastric cancer in a fixed population - with emphasis on depressed sm cancer. *Stomach Intestine.* 1992;27:16–24 [in Japanese with English summary].
11. Everett SM, Axon AT. Early gastric cancer: disease or pseudo-disease? *Lancet.* 1998;351(9112): 1350–1352.
12. Noguchi Y, Yoshikawa T, Tsuburaya A, et al. Is gastric carcinoma different between Japan and the United States? *Cancer.* 2000;89:2237–2246.
13. Schlemper RJ, Itabashi M, Kato Y, et al. Differences in diagnostic criteria for gastric carcinoma between Japanese and western pathologists. *Lancet.* 1997;349(9067):1725–1729.
14. Lauwers GY, Shimizu M, Correa P, et al. Evaluation of gastric biopsies for neoplasia: differences between Japanese and Western pathologists. *Am J Surg Pathol.* 1999;23:511–518.
15. Schlemper RJ, Riddell RH, Kato Y, et al. The Vienna classification of gastrointestinal epithelial neoplasia. *Gut.* 2000;47:251–255.
16. Dixon MF. Gastrointestinal epithelial neoplasia: Vienna revisited. *Gut.* 2002;51:130–131.
17. Rugge M, Correa P, Dixon MF, et al. Gastric dysplasia: the Padova international classification. *Am J Surg Pathol.* 2000;24:167–176.
18. Japanese Gastric Cancer Association. Japanese classification of gastric carcinoma, 2nd English ed. *Gastric Cancer.* 1998;1:10–24.
19. Borrmann R. HandBuch der speziellen pathologischen Anatomie und Histologie. In: von Henke FU, Lubarch O, eds. *IV/erster Teil.* Berlin: Julius Springer Verlag; 1926:864–871.
20. Takizawa T, Iwasaki Y, Iino H, et al. Macro- and microscopic features of gastric cancers. *Stomach Intestine.* 1991;26:1135–1148 [in Japanese with English summary].
21. The Paris endoscopic classification of superficial neoplastic lesions: esophagus, stomach, and colon: November 30 to December 1, 2002. *Gastrointest Endosc.* 2003;58 (6 Suppl):S3–S43.
22. Laurén P: The two histological main types of gastric carcinoma: diffuse and so-called intestinal-type carcinoma. An attempt at a histo-clinical classification. *Acta Pathol Microbiol Scand.* 1965;64:31–49.
23. Nakamura K, Sugano H, Takagi K. Carcinoma of the stomach in incipient phase: its histogenesis and histological appearances. *Gann.* 1968;59:251–258.
24. Nakamura K, Sugano H. Microcarcinoma of the stomach measuring less than 5 mm in the largest diameter and its histogenesis. *Prog Clin Biol Res.* 1983;132D:107–116.
25. Nakamura K. Histogenesis of gastric carcinoma and its clinicopathological significance. In: Nishi M, Ichikawa H, Nakajima Y, et al., eds. *Gastric cancer.* Tokyo: Springer-Verlag; 1993112–132.
26. Hirota T, Itabashi M, Suzuki K, et al. Clinical study of minute and small early gastric cancer. Histogenesis of gastric cancer. *Pathol Ann.* 1980;15:1–19.
27. Mori M, Enjoji M, Sugimachi K. Histopathologic features of minute and small human gastric adenocarcinomas. *Arch Pathol Lab Med.* 1989;113:926–931.
28. Sasaki I, Yao T, Nawata H, et al. Minute gastric carcinoma of differentiated type with special reference to the significance of intestinal metaplasia, proliferative zone, and p53 protein during tumor development. *Cancer.* 1999;85:1719–1729.

29. Kawachi H, Takizawa T, Eishi Y, et al. Absence of either gastric or intestinal phenotype in microscopic differentiated gastric carcinomas. *J Pathol.* 2003;199:436–446.

30. Shiroshita H, Watanabe H, Ajioka Y, et al. Re-evaluation of mucin phenotypes of gastric minute well-differentiated-type adenocarcinomas using a series of HGM, MUC5AC, MUC6, M-GGMC, MUC2 and CD10 stains. *Pathol Int.* 2004;54:311–321.

31. Shinohara N, Mochizuki M. The mode of initial invasion of gastric mucosal carcinoma to the submucosal layer. *Stomach Intestine.* 1990;25:1469–1475 [in Japanese with English summary].

32. Yoshida S, Yoshimori M, Hirashima T, et al. Nonulcerative lesion detected by endoscopy as an early expression of gastric malignancy-retrospective observation of 72 cases of gastric carcinoma. *Jpn J Clin Oncol.* 1981;11:495–506.

33. Mai M, Mibayashi Y, Okumura Y, et al. The natural history of gastric carcinoma viewed from prospective or retrospective follow-up studies-in relation to histological type and growth patterns. *Stomach Intestine.* 1992;27:39–50 [in Japanese with English summary].

34. Miwa H, Iwazaki R, Ohkura R, et al. Radiological retrospective study of gastric cancer in humans: two patterns of development in elevated type gastric cancer. *J Gastroenterol Hepatol.* 1997;12:599–605.

35. Kodama Y, Inokuchi K, Soejima K, et al. Growth patterns and prognosis in early gastric carcinoma. Superficially spreading and penetrating growth types. *Cancer.* 1983;51:320–326.

36. Bamba M, Sugihara H, Okada K, et al. Clonal analysis of superficial depressed-type gastric carcinoma in humans. *Cancer.* 1998;83:867–875.

37. Mori M, Adachi Y, Nakamura K, et al. Advanced gastric carcinoma simulating early gastric carcinoma. *Cancer.* 1990;65:1033–1040.

38. Nakamura K. Linitis plastica. *Stomach Intestine.* 1980;15:225–234 [in Japanese with English abstract].

39. Peng DF, Sugihara H, Mukaisho K, et al. Alterations of chromosomal copy number during progression of diffuse-type gastric carcinomas: metaphase- and array-based comparative genomic hybridization analyses of multiple samples from individual tumours. *J Pathol.* 2003;201:439–450.

40. Sugano H, Nakamura K, Kato Y. Pathological studies of human gastric cancer. *Acta Pathol Jpn.* 1982;32(Suppl 2):329–347.

41. Esaki Y, Hirayama R, Hirokawa K. A comparison of patterns of metastasis in gastric cancer by histologic type and age. *Cancer.* 1990;65:2086–2090.

42. Tatematsu M, Ichinose M, Miki K, et al. Gastric and intestinal phenotypic expression of human stomach cancers as revealed by pepsinogen immunohistochemistry and mucin histochemistry. *Acta Pathol Jpn.* 1990;40:494–504.

43. Yamachika T, Inada K, Fujimitsu Y, et al. Intestinalization of gastric signet ring cell carcinomas with progression. *Virchows Arch.* 1997;431:103–110.

44. Bamba M, Sugihara H, Kushima R, et al. Time-dependent expression of intestinal phenotype in signet ring cell carcinomas of the human stomach. *Virchows Arch.* 2001;438:49–56.

45. Saito A, Shimoda T, Nakanishi Y, et al. Histologic heterogeneity and mucin phenotypic expression in early gastric cancer. *Pathol Int.* 2001;51:165–171.

46. Tajima Y, Shimoda T, Nakanishi Y, et al. Gastric and intestinal phenotypic marker expression in gastric carcinomas and its prognostic significance: immunohistochemical analysis of 136 lesions. *Oncology.* 2001;61:212–220.

47. Ohyama T, Baba Y, Morita H, et al. The actual stage of diagnosis of the small undifferentiated type cancer of the stomach. *Stomach Intestine.* 1996;31:1469–1481 [in Japanese with English abstract].

48. Peng DF, Sugihara H, Mukaisho K, et al. Genetic lineage of poorly differentiated gastric carcinoma with a tubular component analysed by comparative genomic hybridization. *J Pathol.* 2004;203:884–895.

49. Kubo K, Yanagisawa A, Ninomiya Y, et al. Characteristics of differentiated type carcinoma with gastric phenotype of the stomach. *Stomach Intestine.* 1999;34:487–494 [in Japanese with English summary].

50. Nishikura K, Watanabe H, Ajioka Y, et al. Differentiated type adenocarcinoma with gastric phnotype—its new classification and histopathological characteristics. *Stomach Intestine.* 1999;34:495–506 [in Japanese with English summary].

51. Kushima R, Vieth M, Borchard F, et al. Gastric-type well-differentiated adenocarcinoma and pyloric gland adenoma of the stomach. *Gastric Cancer.* 2006;9:177–184.

52. Arai T, Takubo K. Clinicopathological and molecular characteristics of gastric and colorectal carcinomas in the elderly. *Pathol Int.* 2007;57:303–314.

53. Nakamura W, Inada K, Hirano K, et al. Increased expression of sucrase and intestinal-type alkaline phosphatase in human gastric carcinomas with progression. *Jpn J Cancer Res.* 1998;89:186–191.

54. Kushima R, Jancic S, Hattori T. Association between expression of sialosyl-Tn antigen and intestinalization of gastric carcinomas. *Int J Cancer*. 1993;55:904 908.

55. Natsagdorj L, Sugihara H, Bamba M, et al. Intratumoural heterogeneity of intestinal expression reflects environmental induction and progression-related loss of induction in undifferentiated-type gastric carcinomas. Histopathology 2008;53:685–97.

56. Yao T, Utsunomiya T, Oya M, et al. Extremely well-differentiated adenocarcinoma of the stomach: clinicopathological and immunohistochemical features. *World J Gastroenterol*. 2006;12:2510–2516.

57. Endoh Y, Tamura G, Motoyama T, et al. Well-differentiated adenocarcinoma mimicking complete-type intestinal metaplasia in the stomach. *Hum Pathol*. 1999;30:826–832.

58. Ban S, Horigichi H, Ogawa F, et al. Gastric adenocarcinoma with low histologic grade simulating intestinal metaplasia. *Lab Invest*. 2006;86(Suppl 1):102A.

59. Endoh Y, Sakata K, Tamura G, et al. Cellular phenotypes of differentiated-type adenocarcinomas and precancerous lesions of the stomach are dependent on the genetic pathways. *J Pathol*. 2000;191: 257–263.

60. Michelassi F, Takanishi DM Jr, Pantalone D, et al. Analysis of clinicopathologic prognostic features in patients with gastric adenocarcinoma. *Surgery*. 1994;116:804–9.

61. Ming S-C. Gastric carcinoma. A pathobiological classification. *Cancer*. 1977;39:2475–2485.

62. Morita H, Ishikawa Y, Akishima-Fukasawa Y, et al. Histopathological predictor for regional lymph node metastasis in gastric cancer. *Virchows Arch*. 2009;454:143–151.

63. Ishii K, Kinami S, Funaki K, et al. Detection of sentinel and non-sentinel lymph node micrometastases by complete serial sectioning and immunohistochemical analysis for gastric cancer. *J Exp Clin Cancer Res*. 2008;27:7.

64. Yamao T, Shirao K, Ono H, et al. Risk factors for lymph node metastasis from intramucosal gastric carcinoma. *Cancer*. 1996;77:602–606.

65. Gotoda T, Yanagisawa A, Sasako M, et al. Incidence of lymph node metastasis from early gastric cancer: estimation with a large number of cases at two large centers. *Gastric Cancer*. 2000;3:219–225.

66. Satou K, Shimoda T, Ikegami M. Clinicopathological and mucin histochemical examination of gastric intramucosal carcinoma with lymphnode metastasis. *Jikeikai Med J*. 2001;48:63–71.

67. Ohashi S, Okamura S, Urano F, et al. Clinicopathological variables associated with lymph node metastasis in submucosal invasive gastric cancer. *Gastric Cancer*. 2007;10:241–250.

68. Tajima Y, Murakami M, Yamazaki K, et al. Risk factors for lymph node metastasis from gastric cancers with submucosal invasion. *Ann Surg Oncol*. 2010;17:1597–604.

69. Ono H. Early gastric cancer: diagnosis, pathology, treatment techniques and treatment outcomes. *Eur J Gastroenterol Hepatol*. 2006;18:863–866.

70. Sano T, Sasako M, Kinoshita T, et al. Recurrence of early gastric cancer. Follow-up of 1475 patients and review of the Japanese literature. *Cancer*. 1993;72:3174–3178.

71. Saka M, Katai H, Fukagawa T, et al. Recurrence in early gastric cancer with lymph node metastasis. *Gastric Cancer*. 2008;11:214–218.

72. Nasu J, Doi T, Endo H, et al. Characteristics of metachronous multiple early gastric cancers after endoscopic mucosal resection. *Endoscopy*. 2005;37:990–993.

73. Nitta T, Egashira Y, Akutagawa H, et al. Study of clinicopathological factors associated with the occurrence of synchronous multiple gastric carcinomas. *Gastric Cancer*. 2009;12:23–30.

74. Martin IG, Dixon MF, Sue-Ling H, et al. Goseki histological grading of gastric cancer is an important predictor of outcome. *Gut*. 1994;35:758–763.

75. Songun I, van de Velde CJ, Arends JW, et al. Classification of gastric carcinoma using the Goseki system provides prognostic information additional to TNM staging. *Cancer*. 1999;85:2114–2118.

76. Yasuda K, Adachi Y, Shiraishi N, et al. Papillary adenocarcinoma of the stomach. *Gastric Cancer*. 2000;3:33–38.

77. Koseki K, Takizawa T, Koike M, et al. Distinction of differentiated type early gastric carcinoma with gastric type mucin expression. *Cancer*. 2000;89:724–732.

78. Guo RJ, Arai H, Kitayama Y, et al. Microsatellite instability of papillary subtype of human gastric adenocarcinoma and hMLH1 promoter hypermethylation in the surrounding mucosa. *Pathol Int*. 2001;51:240–247.

79. Yamamoto H, Perez-Piteira J, Yoshida T, et al. Gastric cancers of the microsatellite mutator phenotype display characteristic genetic and clinical features. *Gastroenterology*. 1999;116:1348–1357.

80. Falchetti M, Saieva C, Lupi R, et al. Gastric cancer with high-level microsatellite instability: target gene mutations, clinicopathologic features, and long-term survival. *Hum Pathol.* 2008;39:925–932.
81. Watanabe H, Enjoji M, Imai T. Gastric carcinoma with lymphoid stroma. Its morphologic characteristics and prognostic correlations. *Cancer.* 1976;38:232–243.
82. Minamoto T, Mai M, Watanabe K, et al. Medullary carcinoma with lymphocytic infiltration of the stomach. Clinicopathologic study of 27 cases and immunohistochemical analysis of the subpopulations of infiltrating lymphocytes in the tumor. *Cancer.* 1990;66:945–952.
83. Nakamura S, Ueki T, Yao T, et al. Epstein-Barr virus in gastric carcinoma with lymphoid stroma. Special reference to its detection by the polymerase chain reaction and in situ hybridization in 99 tumors, including a morphologic analysis. *Cancer.* 1994;73:2239–2249.
84. van Beek J, zur Hausen A, Klein Kranenbarg E, et al. EBV-positive gastric adenocarcinomas: a distinct clinicopathologic entity with a low frequency of lymph node involvement. *J Clin Oncol.* 2004;22:664–670.
85. Solcia E, Luinetti O, Tava F, et al. Identification of a lower grade muconodular subtype of gastric mucinous cancer. *Virchows Arch.* 2004;445:572–579.
86. Chiaravalli AM, Klersy C, Tava F, et al. Lower- and higher-grade subtypes of diffuse gastric cancer. *Hum Pathol.* 2009;40:1591–1599.
87. Isomoto H, Shikuwa S, Yamaguchi N, et al. Endoscopic submucosal dissection for early gastric cancer: a large-scale feasibility study. *Gut.* 2009;58:331–336.
88. Hirasawa T, Gotoda T, Miyata S, et al. Incidence of lymph node metastasis and the feasibility of endoscopic resection for undifferentiated-type early gastric cancer. *Gastric Cancer.* 2009;12:148–152.

Neuroendocrine Tumors and Nonneoplastic Neuroendocrine Cell Changes

7

▶ Guido Rindi
▶ Enrico Solcia

INTRODUCTION

Over the last few decades gastric neuroendocrine neoplasms have risen in incidence, in both surgical and endoscopic series. This has been paralleled by a better understanding of the origin and biology of these tumors. In this chapter, we review the normal endocrine cells population of the stomach, their nonneoplastic pathology (hyperplasia and dysplasia), and neoplastic growths, which have traditionally been called "carcinoid" when well-differentiated and "small cell carcinoma" when poorly differentiated. Herein we use the term "neuroendocrine tumor" (NET), which corresponds to neoplasms composed of cells expressing neural antigens, and is now widely used by clinicians for its noncommittal significance regarding malignancy. For consistency, "NET" is used as a synonym of "carcinoid" throughout this chapter. Along the same lines, the term "neuroendocrine carcinoma" (NEC) is used as a synonym for small or large cell neuroendocrine carcinoma to indicate malignant and aggressive poorly differentiated neoplasms.

GASTRIC ENDOCRINE CELLULAR CONTINGENT

Five endocrine cell types are detected in the human gastric mucosa. In the oxyntic mucosa, the most common are the histamine-producing, enterochromaffin-like (ECL) cells, and in the antrum, the gastrin-producing G cells.[1,2] Other relatively minor cell populations scattered in both the acidopeptic and the antral mucosa include the serotonin-producing enterochromaffin (EC) cells, the somatostatin D cells, and the ghrelin-producing cells, corresponding to the previously described P/D_1 cells.[3]

PATHOGENESIS AND PREDISPOSING CONDITIONS

Pathogenesis

Long-standing hypergastrinemia is recognized as one of the most important factors leading to endocrine cell hyperplasia and neoplasia in the stomach. Hypergastrinemia is most commonly due to (a) achlorhydria in nonantral (often autoimmune) chronic atrophic gastritis (A-CAG); (b) functioning gastrin cell tumors (gastrinoma) in Zollinger-Ellison syndrome (ZES), with or without the multiple endocrine neoplasia syndrome type 1 (MEN1); and (c) long-term proton pump inhibitor (PPI) treatment.[4-6]

Several lines of evidence support the central role of hypergastrinemia in sustaining ECL cell proliferation. Hypergastrinemia induces increased ECL cell volume density and granule ultrastructure change in CAG patients.[6] Alternatively, the cessation of hypergastrinemia following antrectomy induces a dramatic shrinkage of proliferating ECL cells, sometimes with complete disappearance of hyperplastic changes.[7]

However, hypergastrinemia appears insufficient to promote ECL cell transformation: ECL cell NETs develop in 13% to 43% of MEN1 gastrinoma patients, while developing in <1% of sporadic ZES patients.[8] In addition, the absence of proliferative activity in hyperplastic changes, together with follow-up studies in CAG patients, indicates a lack of progression to neoplasia for hyperplastic changes.[9] Thus, other factors are probably involved, such as active mediators (cytokines) and growth factors participating in A-CAG inflammatory changes of the gastric mucosa.

Predisposing Conditions

A-CAG and ZES are the conditions most frequently associated with gastric endocrine cell growths. Yet, except in a background of MEN1, ZES patients rarely fail to develop ECL cell dysplastic changes and NETs.[10] Pernicious anemia and A-CAG are well-known risk factors for both gastric adenocarcinoma and NETs.[11] The frequency of gastric NETs in pernicious anemia/A-CAG patients may range between 1.6% and 10%, with a comparable rate of ECL dysplasia.[12]

Finally, for sporadic NECs and NETs, that is, developing in nonhypergastrinemic conditions, no specific pathogenetic condition or genetic background has been demonstrated.

NONNEOPLASTIC CHANGES

Observation of gastric endocrine cell changes that do not fit the definition of neoplasia has become more common with increased endoscopic monitoring of dyspepsia, gastritis, and *Helicobacter pylori* infection, together with the widespread use of PPIs with consequent mild hypergastrinemia. Changes can be observed in both the corpus-fundus and the antrum, often complementing the variable inflammation and atrophy observed in the exocrine mucosa. Mostly, though not exclusively, ECL and G cells changes fit into the categories of hyperplasia and dysplasia.

OXYNTIC MUCOSA

ECL cell hyperplasia and dysplasia have been defined in reference to gastrin-dependent ECL neoplasia as part of a continuum of changes or as precursor lesions (Fig. 7-1A and Table 7-1).[13]

ECL cell hyperplastic changes (Fig. 7-1A), which lack significant neoplastic potential, are observed within the basal membrane of the gland or in the lamina propria. They are defined as (a) *simple (diffuse) hyperplasia*, with an increased number of endocrine cells (more than twice Standard Deviation (SD) above normal values) retaining their scattered distribution; (b) *linear or chain-forming hyperplasia*, characterized by at least five cells in a line along the basal membrane, with a minimum of two chains per linear millimeter of mucosa; (c) *micronodular*, clusters of at least five cells (30–150 μm in size), either within the basal membrane of the glands or in the lamina propria, with a minimum of one micronodule per linear millimeter of mucosa; and (d) *adenomatoid*, located within the lamina propria and composed of a minimum of five adjacent micronodules with intervening basal membrane.[13]

ECL cell dysplastic changes are preneoplastic (precarcinoid) lesions, larger in size (150–500 μm), located in the lamina propria, and defined as (a) *enlarging micronodules*, which are cellular clusters >150 mm in size; (b) *fusing micronodules*, apparently resulting from the

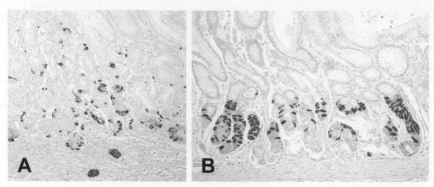

FIGURE 7-1 Gastric hyperplastic changes. **A:** ECL cell changes of the oxyntic mucosa, complex type with diffuse, chain-forming, and micronodular features (**lower part of the micrograph**), in a patient with multiple Type I ECL NETs; anti-chromogranin A immunoperoxidase, hematoxylin counterstain. **B:** Same patient as in (**A**), patchy antral gastrin cell hyperplasia (**right and left part of the micrograph**) with increased number of G cells extending in the deeper part of the gland and above the neck zone (antigastrin immunoperoxidase, hematoxylin counterstain).

disappearance of the basal membranes between adjacent micronodules; (c) *microinvasive lesions*, infiltrating the lamina propria and filling the space between glands; or (d) *nodules with newly formed stroma*, displaying a microlobular or trabecular structure.[13] ECL cell dysplasia is commonly observed in the mucosa adjacent to ECL cell neoplasia.

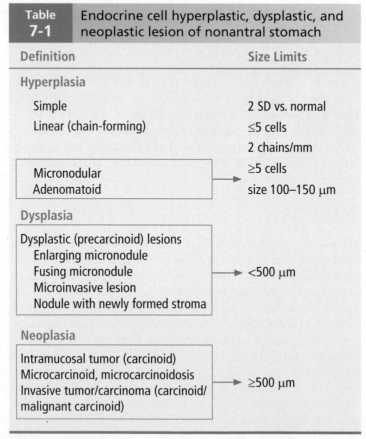

Table 7-1	Endocrine cell hyperplastic, dysplastic, and neoplastic lesion of nonantral stomach
Definition	**Size Limits**
Hyperplasia	
Simple	2 SD vs. normal
Linear (chain-forming)	≤5 cells
	2 chains/mm
Micronodular	≥5 cells
Adenomatoid	size 100–150 μm
Dysplasia	
Dysplastic (precarcinoid) lesions	
Enlarging micronodule	
Fusing micronodule	<500 μm
Microinvasive lesion	
Nodule with newly formed stroma	
Neoplasia	
Intramucosal tumor (carcinoid)	
Microcarcinoid, microcarcinoidosis	
Invasive tumor/carcinoma (carcinoid/	≥500 μm
malignant carcinoid)	

Source: Solcia E, Bordi C, Creutzfeldt W, et al. Histopathological classification of nonantral gastric endocrine growths in man. *Digestion.* 1988;41:185–200.

ANTRAL MUCOSA

No dysplastic changes of antral endocrine cells have been described to date; and only hyperplastic alterations are observed.

Antral gastrin cell hyperplasia (Fig. 7-1B) occurs in achlorhydric conditions and has no neoplastic potential. G cell hyperplasia is observed in patients with chronic atrophic gastritis, hypergastrinemia, and hypochlorhydria.[14] The lesion is characterized by G cells palisading toward the upper and lower parts of the antral gland. Increased G cells (140–250 per linear mm of mucosa vs. 40–90 in controls) often are associated with reduced D cells, resulting in an abnormal antral G/D cell ratio.[15] G cell hyperplasia/hyperfunction and increased G/D cell ratio have been described in children with or without *H. pylori* infection,[16] similar to the changes seen in adults with *H. pylori* gastritis.[17]

D cell hyperplasia has been observed in the stomach and duodenum of a patient with dwarfism, obesity, dryness of the mouth, and goiter.[18]

EC cell hyperplasia with linear or micronodular features has been described in atrophic antral mucosa.[15,19]

NEUROENDOCRINE NEOPLASIA

Incidence

Gastric neuroendocrine neoplasms have risen in incidence in recent series, both surgical and endoscopic. In three large US cancer databases covering from 1950 to 1999, mainly from surgical series, gastric NETs increased from 0.5% to 1.77% of all gastric malignancies (sharply decreasing in absolute figures) and from 2.4% to 8.7% of all gastrointestinal NETs.[20] Similarly, a survey of cancer registries of Florida from 1981 to 2000 showed an increase in incidence.[21] This increased incidence of gastric NETs fits the incremental trend observed for all types of gastrointestinal NETs in recent years.[22,23] Nonetheless, as with nonneoplastic ECL cell changes, the increased figures of gastric NETs may be explained by increased endoscopy and clinical awareness of such lesions. A potentiating role for PPIs still remains to be demonstrated.

Neoplasm Type

NETs represent the largest portion of gastric neuroendocrine neoplasms, while only a minority are NECs. Neoplastic cells with ECL cell characteristics, and, more rarely, G, EC, or ghrelin cells, compose most NETs; other gastric endocrine cell types may also be observed as minor populations.[24,25] In a series of 205 gastric neuroendocrine neoplasms, 193 (94%) were NETs, while 12 only were NECs; and 191 out of 193 NETs (98%) were mainly composed of ECL cells, with only 2 representing G cell tumors.[26] Rare EC cell tumors[27] and, more recently, one "ghrelinoma" have also been described.[28] ECL cell NETs are usually located in the corpus-fundus or in the adjacent mucosa extending into the antrum.[29]

Histology and Grading

Using a series of 102 gastric NETs, a three-tier grading system based on histology and proliferation, has been recently proposed.[30] Most cases in this series (81/102), as well as in general practice, display a monomorphic structure with solid nests and tubules, mild cellular atypia, and very few (0–2/10 high power field [HPF]) typical mitoses (Fig. 7-2). Prevalent solid aggregates, scant punctate necrosis, relatively elevated mitotic count (≥7/10 HPF), and moderate cell atypia were observed in rare (5/102) gastric NETs (Fig. 7-2B). Poorly differentiated NECs (Fig. 7-3), which accounted for 16 of 102 cases in this series, are characterized by solid structure, sometimes organoid, with abundant "geographical chart" necrosis and small to intermediate, overtly atypical cells with numerous, often atypical, mitoses.[30] In addition, gastric high-grade NECs may show medium-sized or even large cell cytologic features (Fig. 7-3A).[31] Limited awareness of gastric NECs, their undifferentiated high-grade features, and the frequent admixture with ordinary

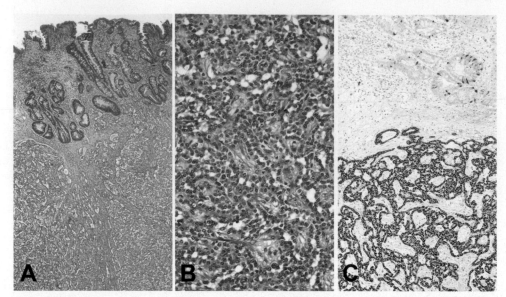

FIGURE 7-2 Gastric NET. Type I ECL cell NET, with severe atrophy and diffuse, complete intestinal metaplasia (**A,** top of the micrograph), the typical solid nest and tubule structure (**B**) and diffuse and intense chromogranin A immunoreactivity (**C,** compare the pattern of endocrine cells of metaplastic mucosa and hyperplastic ECL cell changes in Fig. 7-1**A**). (**A,B:** hematoxylin and eosin; **C:** chromogranin A immunoperoxidase, hematoxylin counterstain.)

adenocarcinoma components may lead to their misdiagnosis as poorly differentiated adenocarcinoma, likely contributing to the relative rarity of reported gastric NECs.[32] Indeed, in our collection of gastric neuroendocrine neoplasms, NECs account for >20% of all cases (unpublished data). NECs should be distinguished from anaplastic nonneuroendocrine cancers,[33] with which they share the highest malignancy behavior of all gastric neoplasms.[34]

This classification scheme of gastric endocrine neoplasms served as a framework for the grading system of gastrointestinal neuroendocrine neoplasms proposed by the European Neuroendocrine Tumor Society (ENETS) (Table 7-2).[35] This system has been since proven to be

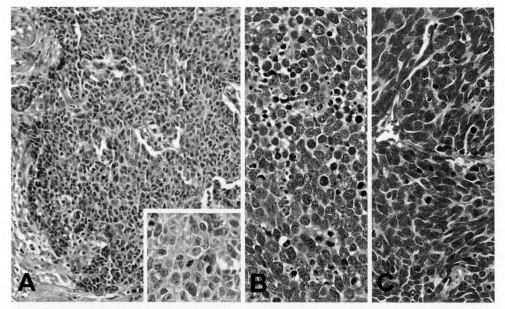

FIGURE 7-3 Gastric NEC. High grade, NEC histology: organoid structure (**A**) with large cell type cytology (**inset**); small cell type, with regular (**B**) or fused cell cytology (**C**) (hematoxylin and eosin.)

Table 7-2	Proposed grading of NETs	
Grade	Mitotic Count (10 HPF)*	Ki-67 Index (%)**
G1	<2	≤2
G2	2–20	3–20
G3	>20	>20

Source: Rindi G, Kloppel G, Alhman H, et al. TNM staging of foregut (neuro)endocrine tumors: a consensus proposal including a grading system. *Virchows Arch.* 2006;449(4): 395–401.
*10 HPF = 2 mm², at least 50 fields (at 40× magnification) evaluated in areas of highest mitotic density.
**MIB1 antibody; % of 500–2,000 tumor cells in areas of highest nuclear labeling.

effective in a series of 202 foregut neoplasms including 48 from the stomach and has been embraced by the American Joint Committee on Cancer (AJCC).[36,37]

NETS

Clinicopathologic Typing

ECL cell NETs are classified into three clinicopathologic types of proven utility in patient management.[24,38] Type I ECL tumors are associated with diffuse, corpus-restricted (A-type), chronic atrophic gastritis (A-CAG) (Fig. 7-2); type II are associated with hypertrophic gastropathy and MEN of type 1, ZES (MEN1-ZES); and type III, or sporadic, are not associated with any distinctive gastric pathology.

A potential novel gastrin-dependent type IV has been proposed for two cases of multiple ECL cell NETs arising in a background of hypergastrinemia, achlorhydria, corpus mucosa hypertrophy, and hyperplasia, in the absence of MEN1-ZES.[39,40] In such cases, ineffective acid production by parietal cells is hypothesized to be at the root of hypergastrinemia, as also suggested by the presence of cystic and engorged oxyntic glands.

Hypergastrinemia is the common basis for both type I and type II NETs, and is associated with hyperplastic and dysplastic changes. Conversely, type III NETs arise independently from gastrin levels and inflammation.[24]

Type I ECL cell NETs are the most common type, have a predilection for older female patients, and are associated with antral gastrin cell hyperplasia. Multiple, multicentric, and small in size (usually <1 cm), type I NETs display well-differentiated G1 histology. In addition to the mucosa, they may invade the muscularis mucosae and the submucosa, while the muscularis propria is rarely involved, and only in larger neoplasms. Metastases are exceptional and associated with deeper wall invasion, and survival is usually excellent, with only occasional lethal cases reported.[24,41]

Type II ECL cell NETs are rare, and in a large study accounted for 12 of 191 cases (6%) with no sex prevalence.[26] Data are scant but general, and type II histology is similar to that of type I NETs. Metastases to local lymph nodes have been reported. Survival is usually excellent and death rare, though reported in an unusually aggressive neoplasm with mixed G1 and G2/G3 histology.[42,43]

Type III ECL cell NETs are the second most common form, accounting for 27 of 191 cases (14%), typically as a single lesion in relatively younger males (sixth decade of life).[26] Hypergastrinemia and gastrin-dependent ECL cell changes are not associated with these large (mean 3.2 cm, vs. 0.7 cm and 1.2 cm for type I and type II NETs), deeply invasive neoplasms.[24,26,30] Their histology may display G1 features, though often with solid aggregates, broader trabeculae, moderate cellular atypia, and mitoses. Some type III NETs (5/17) are G2 with a more obviously solid structure, round to spindle cells, large nuclei, prominent nucleoli, and frequent mitoses (median 9, range 7–18). Metastases are frequent (58% of 17),[30] and tumor-related death did occur (7 out of 26 patients).[26]

NECS

These aggressive carcinomas generally display large size (mean 4.2 cm, range 3–5.5 cm), deep wall invasion, and G3 poorly-differentiated histology with a high proliferation rate (≥20 mitotic count per 10 HPF and ≥20% Ki67 index). Composed of epithelial cells of small to intermediate or even large size,[31] with scarce electron-dense granules (large dense core vesicles), NECs diffusely express the markers of neuroendocrine differentiation of small synaptic-like vesicles (synaptophysin), membrane N-CAM (CD56), and cytosol (e.g., NSE, PGP9.5), more than chromogranin A. An adenocarcinomatous component may be observed.[24,31,32]

Gastric NECs are typically reported in any part of the stomach of patients in the seventh decade, with no sex prevalence, and a high stage at diagnosis.[30] Survival is poor, with most patients dying within few months. Usually, gastric NECs develop without hypergastrinemia, although a few may be associated with A-CAG and ECL cell changes or NETs. The overexpression of p53, the substantially diverse genetic background,[44,45] and the frequent observation of adenocarcinoma foci within NECs suggest a pathogenesis for NECs different from gastrin-dependent NETs, possibly closer to type III NETs and even adenocarcinoma. Conversely, progression to NEC from NET is also possible, and is suggested by some rare cases with coexisting NECs and NETs in a background of either A-CAG or MEN1/ZES.[24,42]

Hormone Hypersecretion

Gastric neuroendocrine neoplasms rarely are associated with hormone hyperfunction and its consequent clinical syndrome. A few, usually sporadic, type III ECL cell NETs have been reported as the cause of the so-called atypical carcinoid syndrome due to 5-hydroxytryptophane and/or histamine hypersecretion.[24] Rare gastrin-producing neoplasms may determine a gastrinoma syndrome.[46] Finally, other and more rare hyperfunctional syndromes have been described in association with NECs as well.[15]

TNM Staging

A novel TNM-staging classification system has been developed for gastric neuroendocrine neoplasms, including NETs and NECs (Table 7-3).[35] Its efficacy has been demonstrated,[36] though validation on larger series is needed. Recently, a substantially similar TNM system has been proposed by AJCC and the Union Internationale Contre le Cancer (UICC), though limited to NETs only.[37,47]

Diagnostic Tools

The *bona fide* ECL cell nature of gastric NETs is implied by strong immunoreactivity for chromogranin A (Fig. 7-2C) and the vesicular monoamine transporter 2 (VMAT2)[48] with no or scant immunoreactivity for other gastric-type hormones (ghrelin, somatostatin, gastrin, and serotonin). Other techniques are of limited usefulness in today's diagnostic practice, including argyrophil (Grimelius and Sevier-Munger silver stains), argentaffin, or diazonium tests for serotonin and transmission electron microscopy, while histochemical testing for histamine, the most specific product of ECL cells, is unsuccessful in ordinary formalin-fixed paraffin sections. It is worth mentioning that ultrastructural studies of ECL cell neoplasms can demonstrate a variety of electron-dense granules with irregular to round cores and adherent to detached, smooth to wavy membranes, whose pattern often mimics that of typical ECL cell granules.[49]

For practical diagnostic purposes, immunohistochemistry for chromogranin A, synaptophysin, and Ki67 is sufficient and recommended.[50,51] In addition, the demonstration of G cell hyperplasia in antral samples also may be of help in defining the clinical type.

Table 7-3	European Neuroendocrine Tumor Society: TNM classification and disease staging for gastric NETs and NECs		
TNM			
T: Primary Tumor			
TX	Primary tumor cannot be assessed.		
T0	No evidence of primary tumor		
Tis	In situ tumor/dysplasia (<0.5 mm)		
T1	Tumor invades lamina propria or submucosa and <1 cm.		
T2	Tumor invades muscularis propria or subserosa or >1 cm.		
T3	Tumor penetrates serosa.		
T4	Tumor invades adjacent structures.		
	Any T add (**m**) for multiple tumors.		
N: Regional Lymph Nodes			
NX	Regional lymph nodes cannot be assessed.		
N0	No regional lymph node metastasis		
N1	Regional lymph node metastasis		
M: Distant Metastasis			
MX	Distant metastasis cannot be assessed.		
M0	No distant metastases		
M1	Distant metastasis		
Stage			
Disease Stages			
Stage 0	Tis	N0	M0
Stage I	T1	N0	M0
Stage IIa	T2	N0	M0
IIb	T3	N0	M0
Stage IIIa	T4	N0	M0
IIIb	any T	N1	M0
Stage IV	any T	any N	M1

For neoplasms, the mitotic count per 2 mm^2 area (10 HPF) and the Ki67 index per 100 cells are mandatory to assess grading. When possible, the TNM stage should also be defined.[35,50–52]

Extensive mapping of the surrounding mucosa is also recommended for NETs to assign a specific subtype and to define the background condition of the gastric mucosa. Biopsy samples from the antrum (two biopsies) and the oxyntic mucosa (four biopsies from corpus and fundus) are recommended to assess endocrine cell changes.[52] Since the number and the severity of the endocrine cell changes directly correlate with the number of biopsies taken, more extensive sampling is justified when there is a suspicion of NET development in patients with ZES.[53]

References

1. Solcia E, Capella C, Vassallo G, et al. Endocrine cells of the gastric mucosa. *Int Rev Cytol*. 1975;42: 223–286.
2. Solcia E, Rindi G, Buffa R, et al. Gastric endocrine cells: types, function and growth. *Regul Pept*. 2000;93 (1–3):31–35.
3. Rindi G, Necchi V, Savio A, et al. Characterisation of gastric ghrelin cells in man and other mammals: studies in adult and fetal tissues. *Histochem Cell Biol*. 2002;117(6):511–519.
4. Solcia E, Capella C, Fiocca R, et al. Gastric argyrophil carcinoidosis in patients with Zollinger-Ellison syndrome due to type 1 multiple endocrine neoplasia. A newly recognized association. *Am J Surg Pathol*. 1990;14(6):503–513.
5. Lamberts R, Creutzfeldt W, Struber HG, et al. Long-term omeprazole therapy in peptic ulcer disease: gastrin, endocrine cell growth, and gastritis. *Gastroenterology*. 1993;104(5):1356–1370.
6. Bordi C, D'Adda T, Azzoni C, et al. Hypergastrinemia and gastric enterochromaffin-like cells. *Am J Surg Pathol*. 1995;19(Suppl 1):S8–S19.
7. Richards AT, Hinder RA, Harrison AC. Gastric carcinoid tumours associated with hypergastrina-emia and pernicious anaemia—regression of tumors by antrectomy. A case report. *S Afr Med J*. 1987;72(1):51–53.
8. Jensen RT. Consequences of long-term proton pump blockade: insights from studies of patients with gastrinomas. *Basic Clin Pharmacol Toxicol*. 2006;98(1):4–19.
9. Roucayrol AM, Cattan D. Evolution of fundic argyrophil cell hyperplasia in nonantral atrophic gastritis. *Gastroenterology*. 1990;99(5):1307–1314.
10. Feurle GE. Argyrophil cell hyperplasia and a carcinoid tumour in the stomach of a patient with sporadic Zollinger-Ellison syndrome. *Gut*. 1994;35(2):275–277.
11. Kokkola A, Sjoblom SM, Haapiainen R, et al. The risk of gastric carcinoma and carcinoid tu-mours in patients with pernicious anaemia. A prospective follow-up study. *Scand J Gastroenterol*. 1998;33(1):88–92.
12. Annibale B, Azzoni C, Corleto VD, et al. Atrophic body gastritis patients with enterochromaffin-like cell dysplasia are at increased risk for the development of type I gastric carcinoid. *Eur J Gastroenterol Hepatol*. 2001;13(12):1449–1456.
13. Solcia E, Bordi C, Creutzfeldt W, et al. Histopathological classification of nonantral gastric endocrine growths in man. *Digestion*. 1988;41:185–200.
14. Arnold R, Hulst MV, Neuhof CH, et al. Antral gastrin-producing G-cells and somatostatin-producing D-cells in different states of gastric acid secretion. *Gut*. 1982;23(4):285–291.
15. Solcia E, Capella C, Fiocca R, et al. Disorders of the endocrine system. In: Ming SC, Goldman H, eds. *Pathology of the gastrointestinal tract*. Philadelphia, PA: Williams & Wilkins; 1998:295–322.
16. Oderda G, Fiocca R, Villani L, et al. Gastrin cell hyperplasia in childood *Helicobacter pylori* gastritis. *Eur J Gastroenterol Hepatol*. 1993;5:13–16.
17. Liu Y, Vosmaer GD, Tytgat GN, et al. Gastrin (G) cells and somatostatin (D) cells in patients with dyspeptic symptoms: *H. pylori* associated and non-associated gastritis. *J Clin Pathol*. 2005;58(9):927–931.
18. Holle GE, Spann W, Eisenmenger W, et al. Diffuse somatostatin-immunoreactive D-cell hyperplasia in the stomach and duodenum. *Gastroenterology*. 1986;91:733–739.
19. Solcia E, Capella C, Vassallo G, et al. Endocrine cells of the stomach and pancreas in states of gastric hypersecretion. *Gastroenterology*. 1970;2:147–158.
20. Modlin IM, Lye KD, Kidd M. A 50-year analysis of 562 gastric carcinoids: small tumor or larger pro-blem? *Am J Gastroenterol*. 2004;99(1):23–32.
21. Hodgson N, Koniaris LG, Livingstone AS, et al. Gastric carcinoids: a temporal increase with proton pump introduction. *Surg Endosc*. 2005;19(12):1610–1612.
22. Hemminki K, Li X. Incidence trends and risk factors of carcinoid tumors: a nationwide epidemiologic study from Sweden. *Cancer*. 2001;92(8):2204–2210.
23. Modlin IM, Kidd M, Latich I, et al. Current status of gastrointestinal carcinoids. *Gastroenterology*. 2005;128(6):1717–1751.

24. Rindi G, Luinetti O, Cornaggia M, et al. Three subtypes of gastric argyrophil carcinoid and the gastric neuroendocrine carcinoma: a clinicopathologic study. *Gastroenterology*. 1993;104(4):994–1006.

25. Papotti M, Cassoni P, Volante M, et al. Ghrelin-producing endocrine tumors of the stomach and intestine. *J Clin Endocrinol Metab*. 2001;86(10):5052–5059.

26. Rindi G, Bordi C, Rappel S, et al. Gastric carcinoids and neuroendocrine carcinomas: pathogenesis, pathology, and behavior. *World J Surg*. 1996;20(2):168–172.

27. Quinonez G, Ragbeer MS, Simon GT. A carcinoid tumor of the stomach with features of a midgut tumor. *Arch Pathol Lab Med*. 1988;112(8):838–841.

28. Tsolakis AV, Portela-Gomes GM, Stridsberg M, et al. Malignant gastric ghrelinoma with hyperghrelinemia. *J Clin Endocrinol Metab*. 2004;89(8):3739–3744.

29. Bordi C, Corleto VD, Azzoni C, et al. The antral mucosa as a new site for endocrine tumors in multiple endocrine neoplasia type 1 and Zollinger-Ellison syndromes. *J Clin Endocrinol Metab*. 2001;86(5): 2236–2242.

30. Rindi G, Azzoni C, La Rosa S, et al. ECL cell tumor and poorly differentiated endocrine carcinoma of the stomach: prognostic evaluation by pathological analysis. *Gastroenterology*. 1999;116(3):532–542.

31. Jiang SX, Mikami T, Umezawa A, et al. Gastric large cell neuroendocrine carcinomas: a distinct clinicopathologic entity. *Am J Surg Pathol*. 2006;30(8):945–953.

32. Brenner B, Tang LH, Klimstra DS, et al. Small-cell carcinomas of the gastrointestinal tract: a review. *J Clin Oncol*. 2004;22(13):2730–2739.

33. Chiaravalli AM, Klersy C, Tava F, et al. Lower- and higher-grade subtypes of diffuse gastric cancer. *Hum Pathol*. 2009;40(11):1591–1599.

34. Solcia E, Klersy C, Mastracci L, et al. A combined histologic and molecular approach identifies three groups of gastric cancer with different prognosis. *Virchows Arch*. 2009;455(3):197–211.

35. Rindi G, Kloppel G, Alhman H, et al. TNM staging of foregut (neuro)endocrine tumors: a consensus proposal including a grading system. *Virchows Arch*. 2006;449(4):395–401.

36. Pape UF, Jann H, Muller-Nordhorn J, et al. Prognostic relevance of a novel TNM classification system for upper gastroenteropancreatic neuroendocrine tumors. *Cancer*. 2008;113(2):256–265.

37. AJCC. *AJCC cancer staging manual*. 7th ed. New York, NY: Springer-Verlag; 2010.

38. Hou W, Schubert ML. Treatment of gastric carcinoids. *Curr Treat Options Gastroenterol*. 2007;10(2): 123–133.

39. Ooi A, Ota M, Katsuda S, et al. An unusual case of multiple gastric carcinoids associated with diffuse endocrine cell hyperplasia and parietal cell hypertrophy. *Endocr Pathol*. 1995;6(3):229–237.

40. Abraham SC, Carney JA, Ooi A, et al. Achlorhydria, parietal cell hyperplasia, and multiple gastric carcinoids: a new disorder. *Am J Surg Pathol*. 2005;29(7):969–975.

41. Wangberg B, Grimelius L, Granerus G, et al. The role of gastric resection in the management of multicentric argyrophil gastric carcinoids. *Surgery*. 1990;108(5):851–857.

42. Bordi C, Falchetti A, Azzoni C, et al. Aggressive forms of gastric neuroendocrine tumors in multiple endocrine neoplasia type I. *Am J Surg Pathol*. 1997;21(9):1075–1082.

43. Norton JA, Melcher ML, Gibril F, et al. Gastric carcinoid tumors in multiple endocrine neoplasia-1 patients with Zollinger-Ellison syndrome can be symptomatic, demonstrate aggressive growth, and require surgical treatment. *Surgery*. 2004;136(6):1267–1274.

44. Pizzi S, Azzoni C, Bassi D, et al. Genetic alterations in poorly differentiated endocrine carcinomas of the gastrointestinal tract. *Cancer*. 2003;98(6):1273–1282.

45. Furlan D, Bernasconi B, Uccella S, et al. Allelotypes and fluorescence in situ hybridization profiles of poorly differentiated endocrine carcinomas of different sites. *Clin Cancer Res*. 2005;11(5):1765–1775.

46. Royston CM, Brew DS, Garnham JR, et al. The Zollinger-Ellison syndrome due to an infiltrating tumour of the stomach. *Gut*. 1972;13(8):638–642.

47. Sobin LH, Gospodarowicz M, Wittekind C. *TNM classification of malignant tumours*. Chichester, UK: Wiley & Sons Ltd.; 2010.

48. Rindi G, Paolotti D, Fiocca R, et al. Vesicular monoamine transporter 2 as a marker of gastric enterochromaffin-like cell tumors. *Virchows Arch*. 2000;436(3):217–223.

49. Capella C, Polak JM, Timson CM, et al. Gastric carcinoids of argyrophil ECL cells. *Ultrastruct Pathol*. 1980;1(3):411–418.

50. Kloppel G, Couvelard A, Perren A, et al. ENETS Consensus Guidelines for the Standards of Care in Neuroendocrine Tumors: towards a standardized approach to the diagnosis of gastroenteropancreatic neuroendocrine tumors and their prognostic stratification. *Neuroendocrinology*. 2009;90(2):162–166.

51. Klimstra D, Modlin IR, Adsay NV, et al. Pathologic reporting of neuroendocrine tumors: application of the Delphic Consensus Process to the development of a minimum pathologic data set. *Am J Surg Pathol.* 2010;34(3):300–313.

52. Ruszniewski P, Delle Fave G, Cadiot G, et al. Well-differentiated gastric tumors/carcinomas. *Neuroendocrinology.* 2006;84(3):158–164.

53. Berna MJ, Annibale B, Marignani M, et al. A prospective study of gastric carcinoids and enterochromaffin-like cell changes in multiple endocrine neoplasia type 1 and Zollinger-Ellison syndrome: identification of risk factors. *J Clin Endocrinol Metab.* 2008;93(5):1582–1591.

Secondary Tumors

8

▶ Mikhail Lisovsky

▶ Amitabh Srivastava

INTRODUCTION

Secondary epithelial tumors may involve the stomach through direct contiguous spread, hematogenous metastasis or as a result of peritoneal seeding. Metastasis to the stomach due to hematogenous spread is uncommon and the reported prevalence varies from 1.7% to 5.4%.[1-4] The higher prevalence reported in more recent studies is possibly a reflection of increased use of upper endoscopy and biopsy for evaluation of solid tumor patients with upper gastrointestinal symptoms. Malignant melanoma appears to have the highest propensity for gastric metastasis among solid tumors. Other common primary tumor sites include the breast, lung, and esophagus. Metastasis to the stomach is reported in 22% to 30% of malignant melanomas, 2.4% to 15.2% of esophageal cancers, 5.9% to 11.6% of breast carcinomas, and 2.4% to 6.8% of lung carcinoma patients.[3,5-10] However, since the prevalence of lung and breast cancer in the general population is much higher than that of malignant melanoma, breast and pulmonary carcinomas are the most common primary sites of gastric metastasis encountered in daily practice.[11,12] Metastases originating from other organs have also reported as rare case reports and small series and include the kidney, ovary, liver, pancreaticobiliary tract, uterus, bladder, colon, prostate, testis, head and neck, and bone and soft tissue tumors.[2,3,13-18]

CLINICAL PRESENTATION

In autopsy studies of gastric metastases from solid tumors, slightly over half of all cases were clinically symptomatic.[2] Diffuse abdominal pain was the commonest presenting symptom, but patients also presented with nausea and vomiting, anorexia, guaiac-positive stools, or upper gastrointestinal bleeding. In most patients, the diagnosis is usually straightforward when a prior diagnosis of another solid tumor is known. Pulmonary and esophageal metastases are usually diagnosed within a year of the diagnosis of the primary malignancy. However, the latency may be longer in cases of breast carcinoma where nearly half of the gastric metastatic lesions are diagnosed after >3 years.[3] In nearly 50% of patients with gastric metastasis, there is also concomitant involvement of another site.[17] In rare instances, the gastric metastasis may be the initial manifestation of a visceral malignancy.[3] The distinction between primary and metastatic gastric tumors is critical because it affects the choice of chemotherapeutic regimen and the patient prognosis. Metastasis to the stomach is typically a marker of advanced malignant disease, and the median survival for these patients is <12 months.[14,17]

Metastatic lesions often produce a characteristic "bull's-eye" or "target" appearance with a bridging mucosal fold on radiographic examination. The filling defect with a central collection of barium is often related to central necrosis in the tumor and the bridging mucosal fold is indicative of the submucosal tumor location. However, this sign is not highly sensitive and in one series it was present in only 44% of the cases.[3] Nevertheless, if multiple "bull's-eye" lesions of varying sizes are present, the diagnosis is most likely to be a metastatic tumor. Other lesions that may produce a similar appearance on radiology include a lymphoma, heterotopic pancreas, carcinoid tumor, submucosal mesenchymal tumors or hemorrhage, and even primary carcinoma of the stomach. On endoscopy, metastatic tumors show surface ulceration and are often described as "volcano-like," "umbilicated," or "heaped-up" lesions. When solitary, this may mimic the appearance of a primary gastric carcinoma.[3,17] Metastatic lesions may sometimes be completely submucosal with a smooth overlying mucosal surface similar to the appearance seen in gastric gastrointestinal stromal tumors or show diffuse gastric infiltration without a visible mass lesion mimicking linitis plastica. Diagnosis may be difficult in these latter instances and multiple, deep biopsies may be necessary for definite diagnosis. It is, therefore, not surprising that up to 30% of endoscopic biopsies are reported to be false negative in some studies, especially in the setting of metastatic breast cancer with diffusely infiltrative pattern of invasion.[14] However, others have shown that endoscopy with biopsy can confirm the diagnosis of a metastatic tumor in 90% of cases.[3]

PATHOLOGY

Macroscopic Features

Macroscopic features of metastatic tumors to the stomach are often nonspecific and may mimic a primary gastric malignancy. Some subtle findings may, at times, point to a specific diagnosis. Multiple, small black spots may be visible in cases of metastatic malignant melanoma but can easily be mistaken for old intratumoral hemorrhage unless the observer is aware of the clinical history. The usual gross appearance of metastatic tumors is that of an ulcerating or fungating mass lesion that mimics Borrmann Type II or III patterns of primary gastric cancer. The diffusely infiltrative Borrmann Type IV pattern is also sometimes seen in cases of metastatic breast or lung cancer. Almost two thirds of metastases present as solitary lesions, which enhances the likelihood of misdiagnosis as a primary gastric tumor. The greater curvature is a common site of involvement, regardless of whether one or multiple metastatic lesions are present in the stomach.[17] Most lesions are present in the middle or upper third of the stomach, which contrasts with the predominant antral location of primary gastric cancer in the setting of *Helicobactor pylori* gastritis seen in endemic regions. Submucosal involvement is always present and large tumors may show transmural spread involving the mucosa and serosa. Gynecological malignancies may spread to the stomach by way of peritoneal seeding. Multiple serosal deposits of tumor are present in these cases that may extend into the wall of the stomach all the way up to the mucosa.

Microscopic Features

The common intestinal type of gastric cancer arises through an inflammation-atrophy-metaplasia-dysplasia-cancer pathway. *H. pylori* gastritis and, to a lesser extent, autoimmune gastritis are the most common inflammatory conditions associated with increased risk of gastric adenocarcinoma. Thus, the lack of inflammation or atrophy in the background nonneoplastic mucosa and the absence of a dysplastic precursor lesion adjacent to the tumor should raise suspicion for a metastatic carcinoma. Multiple serosal deposits or predominant submucosal or intramural localization of the tumor also favors secondary tumor involvement over a gastric primary. The morphological features specific to metastases from specific organ sites, their overlap with primary gastric carcinoma, and the role of ancillary immunohistochemical studies in arriving at a definite diagnosis are discussed in greater detail below.

BREAST CARCINOMA

Metastasis from breast cancer is not only one of the most common primary sites of origin but also one of the most challenging diagnostic scenarios. Invasive lobular carcinoma is the source of the majority (70%–75%) of metastatic breast cancer to the stomach.[14,19,20] The distinction between diffuse-type gastric cancer, which typically arises de novo, from metastatic lobular–type breast cancer is extremely difficult morphologically since both tumors show single cell infiltration and cytoplasmic lumen formation. Lack of a clinical history of breast cancer does not completely rule out the possibility of a metastatic carcinoma because rare cases of gastric metastasis as the first manifestation of an occult breast cancer have been reported.[21] Similarly, knowledge of a history of breast cancer is helpful but not sufficient for definite diagnosis because the gastric tumor may be a second primary. In a recent meta-analysis of 19,049 breast cancer survivors, 28 (0.15%) gastric malignancies were reported on follow-up. Eleven of these twenty-eight (39.3%) were primary gastric adenocarcinomas, and only 4/28 (14.3%) were metastases from the prior breast primary.[22] Tamoxifen use has been suggested to increase the risk of subsequent gastric cancer but a recent study failed to confirm this association. The authors did find, however, that the latency between the initial breast cancer and the second gastric primary appears to be significantly reduced in tamoxifen users as compared to those not exposed to tamoxifen. The reported latency was 4 years in tamoxifen users as compared to 13 years in nonusers in this study (Figs. 8-1–8-4).[23]

In metastatic breast cancer, more than half of the cases show diffuse infiltration of the stomach, mimicking the linitis plastica appearance of diffuse-type gastric cancer. Only a minor subset of metastases present as localized gastric lesions. There is a wide spectrum of nuclear features seen in these cases. Foci typical of lobular-type breast cancer with small, round nuclei and bland monomorphic nuclei are present in most cases. However, some cases show marked nuclear hyperchromasia, open chromatin with prominent nucleoli while retaining the single cell infiltration pattern of lobular carcinoma. The distinction between metastatic breast cancer and a second gastric primary can be particularly challenging in these latter instances.

The diagnostic dilemma is further compounded by reports in the literature of estrogen receptor (ER)-positive gastric carcinoma. The reported prevalence for this phenomenon was up to 50% in some studies and did not correlate with patient gender.[22–24] Fortunately, recent studies using more specific primary antibodies have consistently shown approximately 75% of metastatic breast cancers to be positive for ERα and gastric cancers to be consistently negative.[20,25] However, expression of ERβ has been reported recently in a subset of gastric carcinomas,[26] and surgical pathologists should be aware of the type and specificity of anti-ER antibody being used in their laboratory. Progesterone receptor expression is usually focal and variable in intensity and may not be useful in diagnostic workup. Complete loss of E-cadherin expression may be seen in diffuse type gastric cancer but is more common in metastatic breast cancer while expression of CDX-2 in the tumor cells favors a gastric primary. A useful immunohistochemical panel for distinguishing gastric carcinoma from metastatic breast cancer is listed in Table 8-1.

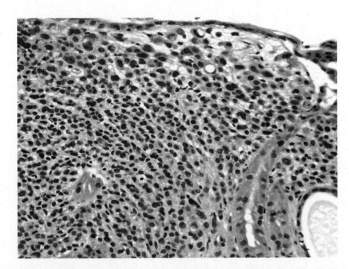

FIGURE 8-1 Gastric metastasis from lobular breast carcinoma can show morphological heterogeneity. Small, round, lymphoid-like tumor cells (bottom half) are admixed with larger more pleomorphic cells underneath the surface epithelium. Note tumor cells with lumen formation close to the top that resemble signet-ring cell carcinoma.

FIGURE 8-2 CK7 immunostain in metastatic breast cancer highlights single cell tumor infiltration in the mid gastric pit zone imparting a near perfect resemblance to diffuse-type gastric cancer (**A**). Diffuse nuclear positivity for ER in the tumor cells is diagnostic of metastatic breast cancer (**B**).

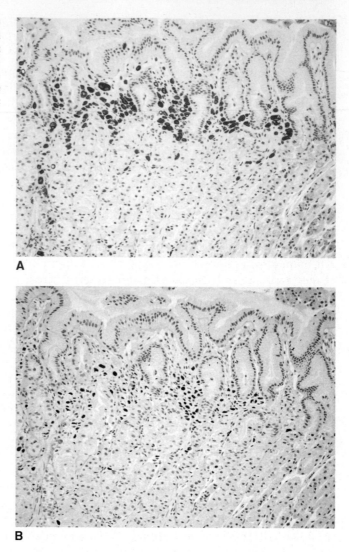

A

B

FIGURE 8-3 Immunoreactivity for PR is usually focal and variable in intensity and may not always be helpful in distinguishing metastatic breast cancer from a gastric primary.

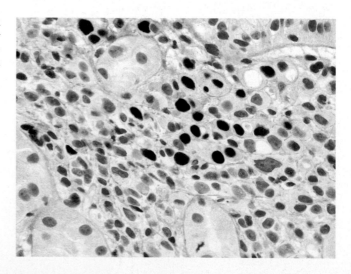

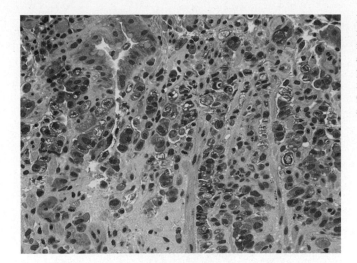

FIGURE 8-4 Diffuse-type gastric carcinoma in a patient with a prior history of invasive breast carcinoma. The tumor cells are pleomorphic, show vacuolated cytoplasm with prominent intracytoplasmic mucin. The tumor cells were positive for CDX-2 and intestinal-type mucin MUC-2 and were negative for ER and PR.

MALIGNANT MELANOMA

Malignant melanoma involving the gastrointestinal tract may be primary or secondary. The commonest sites for primary gastrointestinal melanomas include the esophagus and the anorectum. Even at these sites, metastatic melanoma is more common than primary tumors. The presence of a junctional mucosal melanocytic component is typically seen in primary malignant melanomas of the GI tract but may not be discernible in large tumors that have overrun the precursor lesion. Another problematic scenario is gastric metastasis from a primary cutaneous melanoma that has undergone spontaneous regression. The cutaneous lesion in these cases shows dermal lymphoid infiltrate with melanophages, vascular proliferation, and fibrosis. The presence of concurrent involvement of other visceral sites is helpful in these cases to establish the diagnosis of a metastatic melanoma. Finally, clear cell sarcoma of tendons and aponeurosis, also known as malignant melanoma of soft parts, may rarely occur as a primary tumor in the gastrointestinal tract, and examples of primary gastric clear cell sarcoma have also been reported.[27] Although the histological and immunohistochemical features of clear cell sarcoma overlap with those of malignant melanoma, the presence of t(12,22)(q13;q12) resulting in fusion transcripts *EWS-ATF1* or *EWS-CREB1* is diagnostic of clear cell sarcoma and has not been demonstrated in cutaneous malignant melanomas (Table 8-2). EWS rearrangement in these tumors can be demonstrated by FISH on paraffin sections and is extremely helpful in establishing the diagnosis (Fig. 8-5).

Table 8-1	Immunohistochemical panel useful in distinguishing metastatic breast cancer from primary gastric adenocarcinoma	
Antibody	Breast Carcinoma	Gastric Carcinoma
ER	+	−
PR	+	−
GCDFP-15	±	−
CDX2	−	+
Villin	−	+
Hepar-1	−	+

Table 8-2	Markers useful in differential diagnosis of malignant melanoma metastatic to the stomach			
Marker	**Malignant Melanoma**	**Clear Cell Sarcoma**	**GIST**	**Schwannoma**
S-100	Diffuse, strong	Diffuse, strong	Rare focal positivity	Diffuse, strong
HMB45	++	++	–	–
MART-1	++	++	–	–
KIT	++	++	+++	–
DOG1	–	–	+++	–
t(12,22)(q13;q12)	–	+	–	–

FIGURE 8-5 Malignant melanoma is known for gastrointestinal tropism and is one of the commonest metastatic tumors involving the stomach. Partially necrotic tumor cells (left) are present below surface foveolar epithelium (**A**) and show nuclear pleomorphism, prominent cherry red nucleoli, and abundant amphophilic cytoplasm with scattered melanin pigment (**B**).

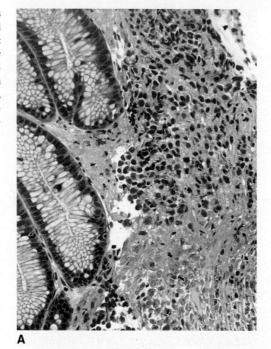

A

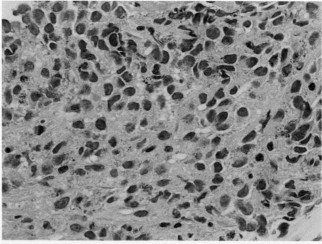

B

Malignant melanoma metastasizes to the stomach in approximately 20% to 25% of patients[5,28] and may be detected synchronously at the time of diagnosis of the primary lesion or years later as recurrent disease. Solitary or multiple lesions, often with ulceration and pigmentation are detected on endoscopy. The microscopic features are similar to those seen in cutaneous lesions. Round to oval- or spindle-shaped cells with large, smooth contoured nuclei with open chromatin and prominent nucleoli are present and the cytoplasm is abundant pale to amphophilic with or without melanin pigmentation. Metastatic melanomas to the stomach with a predominance of spindle cells can be mistaken for a gastrointestinal stromal tumor, an error that may be further compounded by the fact that both tumors may stain positively for KIT and S-100. Diffuse and strong immunoreactivity for S-100 and positive staining with markers of melanocytic differentiation such as HMB-45 and MART-1 is diagnostic of malignant melanoma. Gastric schwannomas also show strong S-100 positivity but are negative for melanocytic markers. The peripheral lymphoid cuff and lack of nucleolar prominence and mitotic activity in gastric schwannomas is distinctive enough that they seldom pose a challenge in distinction from metastatic melanoma.

PULMONARY CARCINOMA

In a large autopsy study of 423 primary lung cancer patients, gastrointestinal metastases were found in 58 (14%) cases. The esophagus was the most frequent sites of involvement and the commonest histologic type of metastasis was squamous cell carcinoma followed by large cell undifferentiated carcinoma and pulmonary small cell carcinoma.[29] However, contiguous spread to the esophagus was also included as metastatic disease in this autopsy study. Dysphagia is the commonest symptom when the metastasis involves the proximal stomach around the GE junction. The presence of a dysplastic precursor lesion in the gastric mucosa is the most definitive way of establishing the diagnosis of a gastric primary. Ancillary studies may be helpful if the metastatic lung tumor is an adenocarcinoma. Nearly 75% of pulmonary adenocarcinomas are positive for TTF-1 and over half for surfactant-A protein. Gastric adenocarcinomas are often positive for CDX-2 and CK20, but these markers are also expressed by a minor subset of pulmonary carcinomas with intestinal differentiation. Primary gastric small cell neuroendocrine carcinomas are rare, bulky tumors that are often high stage at presentation, usually arise in a preexisting adenoma, and may show an admixed glandular tubulo-papillary component. Unfortunately, the expression of TTF-1 is not helpful in this setting to diagnose metastasis from a lung primary since over 10% of primary gastric small cell carcinomas have also been shown to be TTF-1 positive.[30] We have also seen rare examples of metastatic Merkel cell carcinoma to the stomach that morphologically resembles primary or metastatic small cell carcinoma. As at other sites, the paranuclear, dot-like, CK20 positivity is diagnostic of Merkel cell carcinoma (Figs. 8-6 and 8-7).

GENITOURINARY TRACT CARCINOMAS

Renal cell carcinomas may involve the stomach due to local tumor recurrence or as a result of hematogenous spread. Not surprisingly, concurrent pulmonary metastasis is also present in most patients. Gastric metastasis from renal cell carcinoma is rare and occurs in only about 0.2% of patients, and almost all tumors are of the clear cell type.[13] The morphological features are those of large, clear cells in a nested or alveolar pattern with variable nuclear size and nucleolar prominence typical of clear cell carcinoma. Primary gastric carcinomas may also rarely show prominent clear cell cytoplasmic change that may be mistaken for a metastatic renal cell carcinoma. These tumors occur more commonly in the gastric cardia and GE junction area and show at least some areas of tubulo-papillary architecture typical of gastric adenocarcinomas.[31] Immunohistochemical staining may be helpful in small biopsy material, particularly if a prior history of renal cell carcinoma is unknown. Clear cell carcinomas of the kidney are PAX-8 positive and co-express EMA and vimentin, while gastric cancers with clear cell change typically stain with CEA and CDX-2 and express gastrointestinal mucins MUC5AC or MUC2 (Figs. 8-8–8-10).

FIGURE 8-6 Pulmonary carcinomas of all histologic types have been reported to metastasize to the stomach. A small focus of partially crushed tumor cells is present deep in a mucosal biopsy (**A**) obtained from a patient with a history of pulmonary small cell carcinoma. On higher power, the tumor cells show nuclear crush artifact and marked nuclear hyperchromasia (**B**). The tumor cells were also diffusely positive for synaptophysin.

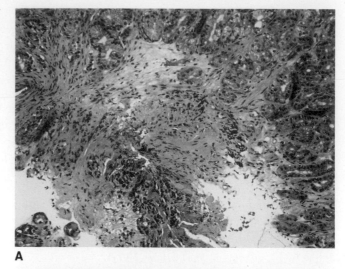

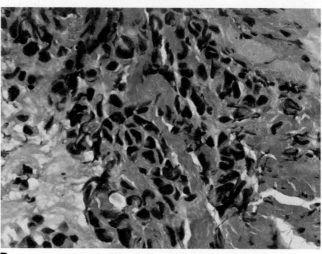

FIGURE 8-7 Merkel cell carcinoma metastatic to the stomach. Uniform, small round tumor cells with high nuclear-cytoplasmic ratio, pale powdery chromatin, and brisk mitotic activity (**A**).

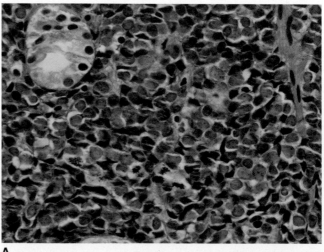

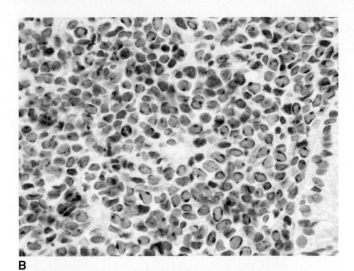

B

FIGURE 8-7 (*continued*) Diffuse dot-like paranuclear positivity for CK20 was diagnostic in this case. Note the portion of gastric glandular epithelium present at bottom right which is negative (**B**).

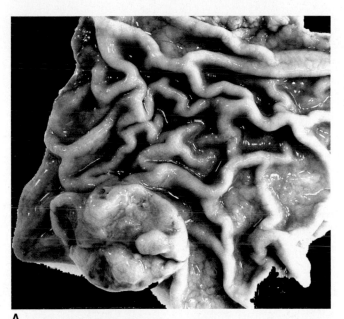

A

FIGURE 8-8 Partial gastrectomy specimen from a patient with metastatic renal cell carcinoma. The gastric mucosa overlying the tumor nodule is stretched but smooth with no ulceration (**A**). This appearance is common to submucosal-based primary gastric tumors such as carcinoids and GIST. On low-power examination, the metastatic tumor is located in the submucosa and shows nests of pale clear cells separated by a delicate vascular stroma (**B**).

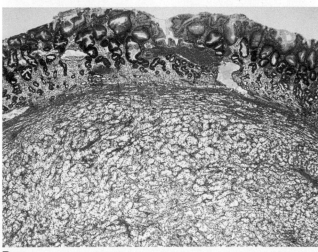

B

FIGURE 8-8 (*continued*) The tumor cells co-express EMA (**C**) and vimentin (**D**) consistent with clear cell carcinoma of the kidney.

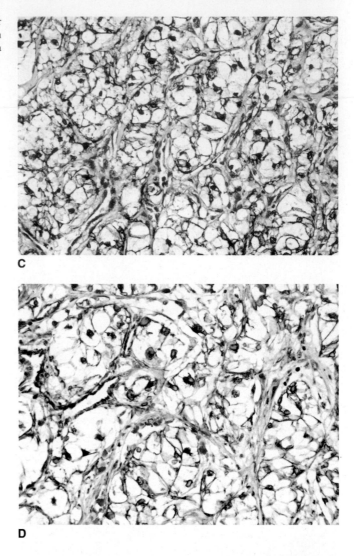

FIGURE 8-9 Primary gastric carcinoma may show prominent clear cell change but usually this is focal and not a diagnostic challenge. In the rare cases where this change is diffuse, it may mimic metastatic clear cell carcinoma (**A**).

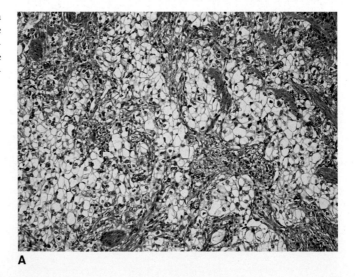

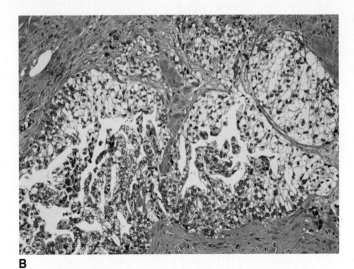

B

FIGURE 8-9 (*continued*) Tubulo-papillary glandular formations are almost always present in such cases and point to the diagnosis of primary gastric cancer with clear cell change (**B**).

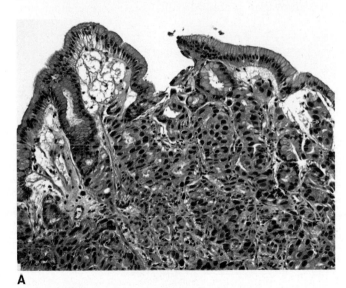

A

FIGURE 8-10 Metastatic prostate cancer involving the stomach. Small glands and nests of tumor cells with abundant cytoplasm infiltrate the gastric epithelium (**A**). The lack of a precursor lesion should raise suspicion for a metastatic tumor. Diffuse, strong positivity for PSA was diagnostic of metastatic prostate cancer in this case (**B**).

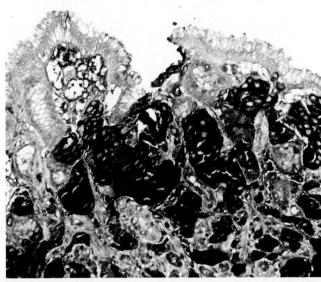

B

Clinically, symptomatic gastric metastases from prostate cancer are very rare.[32,33] However, autopsy studies in patients with metastatic prostate cancer have shown a 1% to 4% incidence of gastric metastasis.[2,3] The tumor cells infiltrate the gastric mucosa as small, tubular glands or solid nests and show prominent nucleoli, abundant amphophilic cytoplasm, and immunohistochemical positivity for prostate-specific antigen. Six cases of gastric metastasis were described in a large autopsy study of 367 patients with muscle-invasive bladder cancer,[34] and an extremely unusual case of metastatic bladder cancer with diffuse gastric infiltration mimicking linitis plastica was also reported recently.[35] Metastases from urothelial cancers co-express CK7 and CK20 and are also positive for p63 and CK34βE12 that is helpful in making the diagnosis. Extremely rare instances of testicular choriocarcinoma metastatic to the stomach have been described.[36]

GYNECOLOGIC CANCERS

Ovarian metastases from a gastric primary result in the well-recognized phenomenon of Krukenberg tumor. The reverse scenario of gastric metastasis from an ovarian primary is extremely rare. Nonetheless, in some instances, high-stage ovarian cancers may cause gastroduodenal obstruction. In a series of 438 women with ovarian cancer, 11 patients (2.5%) presented with

FIGURE 8-11 Serosal tumor deposit involving the stomach in a patient with high-grade ovarian papillary serous carcinoma (**A**). The tumor may involve the entire gastric wall in some cases and cause obstruction. The mural and mucosal components of the metastatic tumor in such cases may show a more nested architecture, and the papillary configuration may not be apparent (**B**).

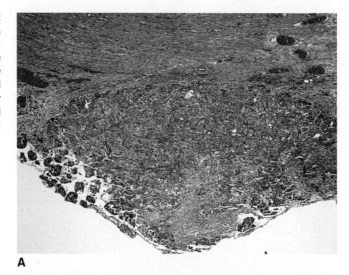

A

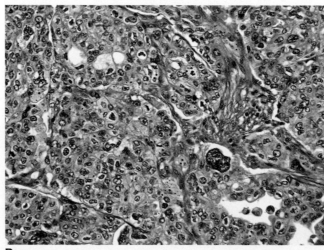

B

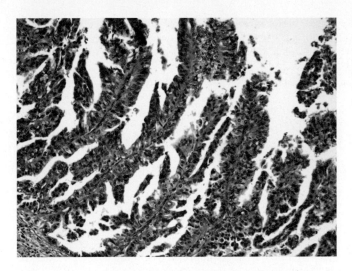

FIGURE 8-12 Primary papillary gastric carcinomas, as seen here, may resemble metastatic ovarian papillary serous carcinoma. These tumors typically arise in a background of gastritis and dysplasia, which helps in establishing the diagnosis of primary gastric cancer.

symptomatic gastroduodenal relapse, and six of these showed predominant involvement of the gastric body.[37] There are also reports of intramural gastric metastases from ovarian cancers presenting clinically with upper GI bleeding.[38,39] Histologically, high-grade serous papillary ovarian carcinoma is the most common subtype. The serosal deposits show high-grade nuclei with intense hyperchromasia typical of serous carcinomas. The mural deposits may cluster together in large nests and the papillary architecture may not be easily apparent. The tumor cells also tend to show a more bland morphology in the mural component, which may be mistaken for a primary gastric carcinoma. Primary papillary gastric carcinoma may mimic metastatic serous carcinomas but the nuclei are usually low grade and the cells have abundant cytoplasm in primary papillary gastric tumors. Numerous psammoma bodies, when present, favor metastatic serous carcinoma. Immunohistochemically, serous carcinomas stain positively with ER and PR and often show diffuse, strong positivity for p53, while primary gastric carcinomas are pCEA and CDX-2 positive. Rare examples of metastatic uterine endometrial stromal sarcoma presenting as gastric submucosal mass lesions have also been reported (Figs. 8-11 and 8-12).[40]

ESOPHAGEAL, HEPATOBILIARY, AND PANCREATIC CARCINOMA

Lymphatic emboli from squamous cell carcinomas of the mid or upper esophagus may involve the gastric cardia and can be detected at autopsy in about 15% of patients.[6–8] Pancreatico-biliary tumors spread to the stomach most often due to direct extension but may also present as isolated submucosal metastases either at presentation or at the time of tumor recurrence. Colon cancer metastatic to the stomach has been reported but is extraordinarily rare.[36] Retrograde hematogenous spread of hepatocellular carcinoma to the stomach[41] occurs rarely and needs to be distinguished from hepatoid gastric carcinoma. The latter shows true gland formation and mucin positivity in contrast to metastatic hepatocellular carcinoma that infiltrates in a nested or trabecular pattern with canalicular formations that may be highlighted with pCEA immunostain.

References

1. Menuck LS, Amberg JR. Metastatic disease involving the stomach. *Am J Dig Dis.* 1975;20(10):903–913.
2. Green, LK. Hematogenous metastases to the stomach. A review of 67 cases. *Cancer.* 1990;65(7): 1596–1600.

3. Oda I, Kondo H, Yamao T, et al. Metastatic tumors to the stomach: analysis of 54 patients diagnosed at endoscopy and 347 autopsy cases. *Endoscopy*. 2001;33(6):507–510.

4. Telerman A, Gerard B, Van den Heule B, et al. Gastrointestinal metastases from extra-abdominal tumors. *Endoscopy*. 1985;17(3):99–101.

5. Dasgupta TK, Brasfield RD. Metastatic melanoma of the gastrointestinal tract. *Arch Surg*. 1964;88: 969–973.

6. Saito T, Iizuka T, Kato H, et al. Esophageal carcinoma metastatic to the stomach. A clinicopathologic study of 35 cases. *Cancer*. 1985;56(9):2235–2241.

7. Anderson LL, Lad TE. Autopsy findings in squamous-cell carcinoma of the esophagus. *Cancer*. 1982;50(8):1587–1590.

8. Mandard AM, Chasle J, Marnay J, et al. Autopsy findings in 111 cases of esophageal cancer. *Cancer*. 1981;48(2):329–335.

9. Choi SH, Sheehan FR, Pickren JW. Metastatic involvement of the stomach by breast cancer. *Cancer*. 1964;17:791–797.

10. Asch MJ, Wiedel PD, Habif DV. Gastrointestinal metastases from carcinoma of the breast. Autopsy study and 18 cases requiring operative intervention. *Arch Surg*. 1968;96(5):840–843.

11. Kadakia SC, Parker A, Canales L. Metastatic tumors to the upper gastrointestinal tract: endoscopic experience. *Am J Gastroenterol*. 1992;87(10):1418–1423.

12. Hsu CC, Chen JJ, Changchien CS. Endoscopic features of metastatic tumors in the upper gastrointestinal tract. *Endoscopy*. 1996;28(2):249–253.

13. Pollheimer MJ, Hinterleitner TA, Pollheimer VS, et al. Renal cell carcinoma metastatic to the stomach: single-centre experience and literature review. *BJU Int*. 2008;102(3):315–319.

14. Taal BG, Peterse H, Boot H. Clinical presentation, endoscopic features, and treatment of gastric metastases from breast carcinoma. *Cancer*. 2000;89(11):2214–2221.

15. Christoph F, Grunbaum M, Wolkers F, et al. Prostate cancer metastatic to the stomach. *Urology*. 2004;63(4):778–779.

16. Hu ML, Tai WC, Chuah SK, et al. Gastric metastasis of hepatocellular carcinoma via a possible existing retrograde hematogenous pathway. *J Gastroenterol Hepatol*. 2010;25:408–412.

17. Campoli PM, Ejima FH, Cardoso DM, et al. Metastatic cancer to the stomach. *Gastric Cancer*. 2006;9(1):19–25.

18. Kobayashi O, Murakami H, Yoshida T, et al. Clinical diagnosis of metastatic gastric tumors: clinicopathologic findings and prognosis of nine patients in a single cancer center. *World J Surg*. 2004;28(6):548–551.

19. Pectasides D, Psyrri A, Pliarchopoulou K, et al. Gastric metastases originating from breast cancer: report of 8 cases and review of the literature. *Anticancer Res*. 2009;29(11):4759–4763.

20. O'Connell FP, Wang HH, Odze RD. Utility of immunohistochemistry in distinguishing primary adenocarcinomas from metastatic breast carcinomas in the gastrointestinal tract. *Arch Pathol Lab Med*. 2005;129(3):338–347.

21. Clavien PA, Laffer U, Torhost J, et al. Gastro-intestinal metastases as first clinical manifestation of the dissemination of a breast cancer. *Eur J Surg Oncol*. 1990;16(2):121–126.

22. Kojima O, Takahashi T, Kawakami S, et al. Localization of estrogen receptors in gastric cancer using immunohistochemical staining of monoclonal antibody. *Cancer*. 1991;67(9):2401–2406.

23. Wu CW, Tsay SH, Chang TJ, et al. Clinicopathologic comparisons between estrogen receptor-positive and -negative gastric cancers. *J Surg Oncol*. 1992;51(4):231–235.

24. Harrison JD, Jones JA, Ellis IO, et al. Oestrogen receptor D5 antibody is an independent negative prognostic factor in gastric cancer. *Br J Surg*. 1991;78(3):334–336.

25. van Velthuysen ML, Taal BG, van der Hoeven JJ, et al. Expression of oestrogen receptor and loss of E-cadherin are diagnostic for gastric metastasis of breast carcinoma. *Histopathology*. 2005;46(2):153–157.

26. Matsuyama S, Ohkura Y, Eguchi H, et al. Estrogen receptor beta is expressed in human stomach adenocarcinoma. *J Cancer Res Clin Oncol*. 2002;128(6):319–324.

27. Lagmay JP, Ranalli M, Arcila M, et al. Clear cell sarcoma of the stomach. *Pediatr Blood Cancer*. 2009;53(2):214–216.

28. Patel JK, Didolkar MS, Pickren JW, et al. Metastatic pattern of malignant melanoma. A study of 216 autopsy cases. *Am J Surg*. 1978;135(6):807–810.

29. Antler AS, Ough Y, Pitchumoni CS, et al. Gastrointestinal metastases from malignant tumors of the lung. *Cancer*. 1982;49(1):170–172.

30. Li AF, Li AC, Hsu CY, et al. Small cell carcinomas in gastrointestinal tract: immunohistochemical and clinicopathological features. *J Clin Pathol.* 2010;63(7):620–625.

31. Ghotli ZA, Serra S, Chetty R. Clear cell (glycogen rich) gastric adenocarcinoma: a distinct tubulo-papillary variant with a predilection for the cardia/gastro-oesophageal region. *Pathology.* 2007;39(5):466–469.

32. Hong KP, Lee SJ, Hong GS, et al. Prostate cancer metastasis to the stomach. *Korean J Urol.* 2010;51(6):431–433.

33. Onitilo AA, Engel JM, Resnick JM. Prostate carcinoma metastatic to the stomach: report of two cases and review of the literature. *Clin Med Res.* 2010;8(1):18–21.

34. Wallmeroth A, Wagner U, Moch H, et al. Patterns of metastasis in muscle-invasive bladder cancer (pT2-4): an autopsy study on 367 patients. *Urol Int.* 1999;62(2):69–75.

35. Hong WS, Chung DJ, Lee JM, et al. Metastatic gastric linitis plastica from bladder cancer mimicking a primary gastric carcinoma: a case report. *Korean J Radiol.* 2009;10(6):645–648.

36. Kanthan R, Sharanowski K, Senger JL, et al. Uncommon mucosal metastases to the stomach. *World J Surg Oncol.* 2009;7:62.

37. Spencer JA, Crosse BA, Mannion RA, et al. Gastroduodenal obstruction from ovarian cancer: imaging features and clinical outcome. *Clin Radiol.* 2000;55(4):264–272.

38. Taylor RR, Phillips WS, O'Connor DM, et al. Unusual intramural gastric metastasis of recurrent epithelial ovarian carcinoma. *Gynecol Oncol.* 1994;55(1):152–155.

39. Saunders NJ. Haematemesis due to gastric involvement by metastatic ovarian carcinoma 30 years after removal of the primary tumour. *Br J Clin Pract.* 1986;40(7):298–299.

40. Kethu SR, Zheng S, Eid R. Metastatic low-grade endometrial stromal sarcoma presented as a subepithelial mass in the stomach was diagnosed by EUS-guided FNA. *Gastrointest Endosc.* 2005;62(5):814–816.

41. Hu ML, Tai WC, Chuah SK, et al. Gastric metastasis of hepatocellular carcinoma via a possible existing retrograde hematogenous pathway. *J Gastroenterol Hepatol.* 2010;25(2):408–412.

9

Gastrointestinal Stromal Tumor

▶ Min En Nga

▶ Amitabh Srivastava

INTRODUCTION

The predominant mesenchymal tumor of the gastrointestinal tract, until recently, was believed to be of smooth muscle origin. However, it was well recognized that these gastrointestinal "smooth muscle tumors" were quite distinct from their soft tissue counterparts. In 1941, Stout and Golden recognized that in the gastrointestinal tract it was impossible to "be entirely certain that any leiomyoma is necessarily benign, except the small intramural tumors, which are chance findings at autopsy or operation."[1] In a later publication, focusing on the epithelioid variant of these tumors, Stout reported that most gastric tumors behaved in a benign fashion but that some displayed malignant behavior and even the ability to metastasize. The propensity for malignant behavior, he indicated, "cannot be recognized by any clinical or gross characteristics" but may be suspected if the tumor showed an "elevated mitotic count in 50 high power fields(hpf)."[2] This uncertainty in predicting malignant behavior led to the use of terms such as "malignant leiomyoma" and "leiomyoblastoma" to describe these tumors.

The purported smooth muscle origin of these tumors became questioned when immunohistochemistry came into widespread use. These tumors were found to be largely devoid of conventional markers of smooth muscle differentiation.[3,4] Moreover, a subset was also found to express neural markers. In 1983, Mazur and Clark proposed the term "stromal tumor" for these unique neoplasms, reflecting the uncertainty regarding their line of differentiation.[5] In the early 1990s, CD34 emerged as the first relatively specific marker for these stromal tumors and similarities between these tumors and the interstitial cells of Cajal were recognized soon thereafter by multiple groups.[6–8] This explained the mixed smooth muscle—neural phenotype of these lesions. The designation of "gastrointestinal pacemaker cell tumor,"[7] however, did not gain acceptance and the term "gastrointestinal stromal tumor (GIST)" came into widespread use. Tumors previously classified as gastrointestinal autonomic nerve tumors were also accepted as variants of GISTs.[9]

In their seminal discovery in 1998, Hirota et al. reported that the majority of GISTs had activating mutations in the *KIT* gene and also expressed the KIT protein on immunohistochemistry.[10] A subset of KIT-negative GISTs were later found to harbor mutations in platelet-derived growth factor receptor-alpha (PDGFR-α), another receptor tyrosine kinase closely related to KIT.[11] Treatment with tyrosine kinase inhibitors (TKIs) led to marked improvement in outcome of these previously treatment refractory tumors[12,13] and this heralded an era of unprecedented developments in molecular targeted therapy. GISTs have now become a model for molecular targeted therapy of solid tumors.

CLINICAL FEATURES

GISTs are the most common mesenchymal tumors of the gastrointestinal tract and affect both sexes equally. However, they constitute only about 2% of all neoplastic lesions involving the gastrointestinal tract. The age at presentation is variable but most patients are >50 years old (median age around 60 years).[14] GIST occurs rarely in children, most commonly in the second decade of life, but because of its unique clinicopathological characteristics, pediatric GIST is widely considered to be a distinct entity.[15,16] Recent population-based studies suggest an incidence of 11 to 14.5 cases per million and the estimated incidence of GIST in the United States is around 4,500 to 6,000 new cases per year.[17–19] The majority of GISTs are sporadic, but some are familial with inherited germline mutations and others occur in syndromic settings. Well-recognized examples of syndromic GISTs include those that occur in patients with neurofibromatosis type I, Carney's triad (GIST, paraganglioma, pulmonary chondroma), and the Carney-Stratakis syndrome (gastric GIST with paraganglioma). The syndromic GISTs are discussed in detail later in this chapter.

The stomach is the most common site of involvement (50%–60%) by GISTs, followed by the small intestine (25%) and the colorectum (~10%). In the small intestine, two thirds of the tumors arise in the jejunum and about one third in the ileum. The duodenum and esophagus are primary sites of involvement of about 5% of cases each and appendiceal involvement is extremely rare (<1%). GISTs may also arise outside the gastrointestinal wall in the mesentery, omentum, or the retroperitoneum and are then referred to as extragastrointestinal stromal tumors.[20–23]

The majority of GISTs (70%) are clinically symptomatic and the spectrum of presenting symptoms is wide and related to tumor size. Most patients present with bleeding, early satiety, or bloating[17] while chronic blood loss leading to fatigue or anemia may be the first manifestation in some patients. Approximately 20% of GISTs are asymptomatic and detected during clinical workup for unrelated reasons. Another 10% are found at autopsy or incidentally in gastric or esophageal resections performed for another primary tumor, which suggests that not all GISTs progress to clinically symptomatic tumors despite the presence of *KIT* gene mutations.[24–26]

The preoperative tissue diagnosis of GISTs is often challenging, owing to their submucosal location and relative inaccessibility to standard endoscopic biopsy techniques. In recent years, endoscopic ultrasound (EUS) coupled with fine needle aspiration (FNA) cytology has significantly improved the ability to image gastric intramural masses and to obtain representative tissue samples. Distinctive features of GIST on EUS have been described, and this coupled with FNA not only provides a means for preoperative diagnosis but also allows for ancillary immunohistochemical or molecular testing on cell block material.[27–29]

MORPHOLOGY

Macroscopic Features

GISTs are well-circumscribed tumors, most often centered in the wall of the stomach or small intestine. The size range is wide and tumors may range from 1 cm to over 30 cm with a median size of about 5 cm. Extension into mucosa with surface ulceration or into the serosa with perforation of the serosal surface may be present in large tumors. Most tumors are gray-white and fleshy in appearance. Hemorrhage, necrosis, and cystic degeneration may be present. The latter two features are often quite prominent in large tumors or in resections performed after neoadjuvant treatment (Figs. 9-1 to 9-3).

Microscopic Features

GISTs are divided microscopically into spindle, epithelioid, and mixed types. The spindle cell tumors are the most common (70%) type and show variable cellularity. The cells are arranged in a fascicular or storiform pattern and show pale, eosinophilic, fibrillary cytoplasm with ill-defined cell borders, which imparts a syncytial appearance to the tumor. The overwhelming majority of GISTs are monomorphic. They display oval, uniform nuclei with inconspicuous nucleoli. Paranuclear vacuoles, once thought to be a specific feature of true smooth muscle tumors, are particularly prominent in gastric GISTs. Striking nuclear palisading, reminiscent of neural tumors is present in about 50% of gastric and 70% of small intestinal GISTs. Approximately 20% of GISTs are composed exclusively of epithelioid tumor cells and the remaining 10% of tumors show a

FIGURE 9-1 GISTs appear as well-circumscribed submucosal mass lesions. The overlying mucosa is stretched over the lesion and may ulcerate in some cases.

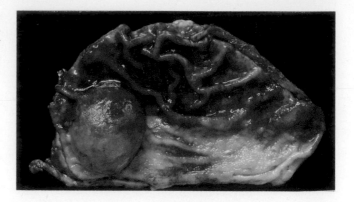

mixed spindle and epithelioid phenotype. Epithelioid GISTs occur more often in the stomach than in the small intestine. These tumors show round to polygonal cells arranged in a nested or sheetlike architecture. The tumor cells show a central or peripheral nucleus with abundant eosinophilic or clear cytoplasm and sharply defined cell borders. Epithelioid tumors with prominent paranuclear vacuoles may mimic signet ring cell carcinoma. Mitotic activity is variable and high mitotic counts may be seen in any subgroup.

Various degenerative changes can be seen. The stroma may be sclerotic and hyalinized or myxoid in appearance. Calcification may be present in some tumors and is usually a degenerative change seen in the center of large tumors. Small intestinal tumors often show peculiar bright eosinophilic hyaline or fibrillar structures composed of tangles of collagen fibers that stain positively with a periodic acid-Schiff stain. These are known as "skeinoid" fibers and are present

FIGURE 9-2 The cut surface, particulary in small tumors, is homogenenous, fleshy white in consistency.

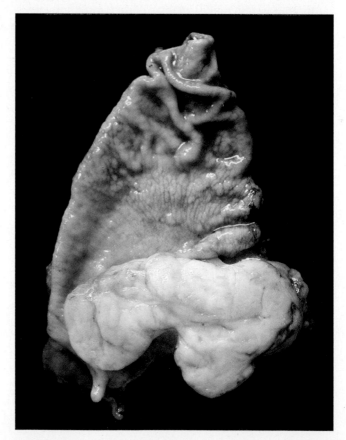

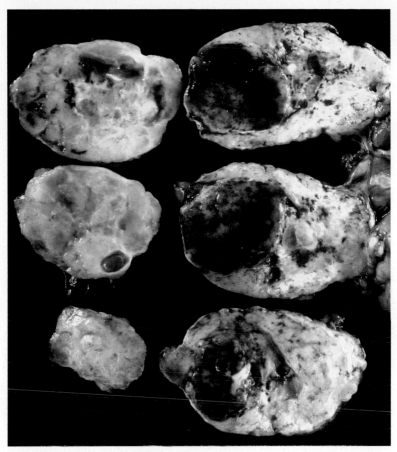

FIGURE 9-3 Large tumors show a more variegated appearance with cystic change, hemorrhage, and necrosis.

in up to 40% of small intestinal GISTs and have been reported to be associated with a better prognosis in some studies.[22]

As mentioned above, the majority of GISTs are monomorphic and presence of significant nuclear atypia should prompt consideration of an alternate diagnosis. However, about 2% of true GISTs may show marked nuclear atypia to a degree usually seen in pleomorphic sarcomas. Molecular analysis of *KIT* and *PDGFRA* gene mutations is extremely useful in these cases.

Neoadjuvant chemotherapy with TKIs may lead to a marked reduction in cellularity accompanied by a myxohyaline stroma. In most instances, the tumor morphology following TKI therapy is comparable to the primary untreated tumor. However, transformation of spindle cell tumors to an epithelioid morphology and pseudopapillary growth patterns due to residual cuffs of viable tumor clustering around blood vessels have also been described. In rare instances, GISTs may show dedifferentiation, either de novo or following TKI therapy, into a high-grade sarcoma. Rhabdomyosarcomatous dedifferentiation has been described in which the transformed rhabdomyosarcomatous and the typical GIST components both show similar mutations in either the *KIT* or *PDGFRA* genes (Figs. 9-4–9-17).[30–32]

IMMUNOHISTOCHEMICAL FEATURES

Immunoreactivity for KIT (CD117) is a sensitive and specific marker for GIST and is extremely useful in the differential diagnosis of mesenchymal lesions of the gastrointestinal tract. KIT is expressed in up to 95% of GISTs. CD34 is expressed in 60% to 70% of GISTs but is less sensitive

FIGURE 9-4 Spindle cell GISTs show a fascicular architecture. The tumor cells are monomorphic and show bland, elongated nuclei with prominent paranuclear vacuoles.

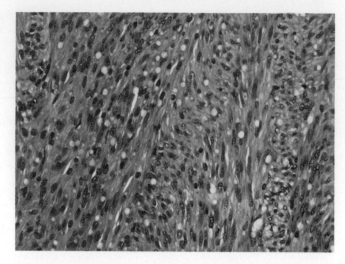

FIGURE 9-5 Epithelioid GISTs are also monomorphic and composed of round cells with central nuclei, abundant eosinophilic cytoplasm, and sharp cell borders.

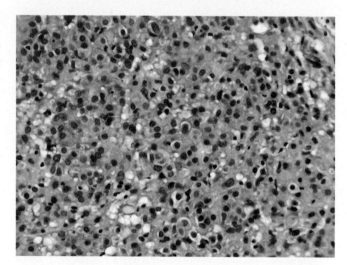

FIGURE 9-6 The degree of cellularity in GISTs is variable. Hypercellular tumors may resemble a monomorphic spindle cell sarcoma, such as synovial sarcoma, MPNST, or fibrosarcoma.

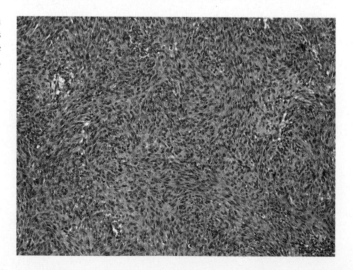

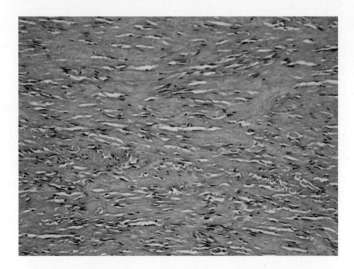

FIGURE 9-7 Hypocellular tumors show prominent collagenized stroma and resemble hypocellular areas of IMT. Unlike IMTs, plasma cell infiltration is not a conspicuous feature of GISTs.

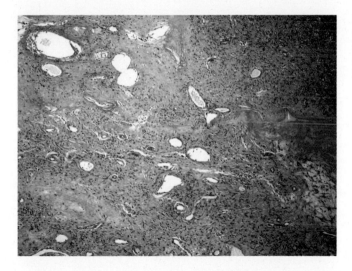

FIGURE 9-8 Central portions of large tumors may undergo infarction and necrosis. Ectatic vessels and hyalinized stroma impart a solitary fibrous tumor-like appearance to these areas.

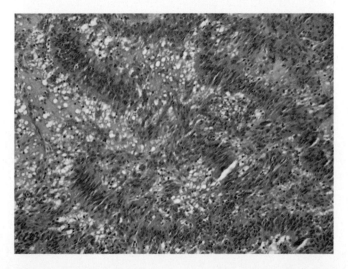

FIGURE 9-9 Nuclear palisading, reminiscent of neural tumors, is a common feature in GISTs and may be quite prominent, as in this example.

FIGURE 9-10 Diffuse presence of para-nuclear vacuoles in spindle cell GISTs can be mistaken for a clear cell epithelial or mesenchymal neoplasm, particularly in small biopsy specimens.

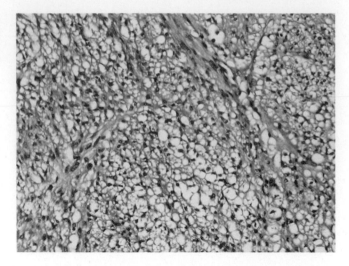

FIGURE 9-11 Epithelioid GISTs with prominent paranuclear vacuoles resemble a signet ring cell carcinoma. The background stroma is myxoid, unlike the desmoplastic stroma seen in infiltrating carcinomas.

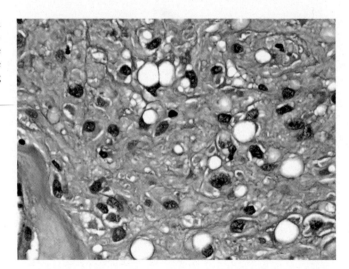

FIGURE 9-12 Bright, eosinophilic, hyaline or fibrillary tangles of collagen fibers, known as skeinoid fibers, are more commonly seen in small intestinal GISTs.

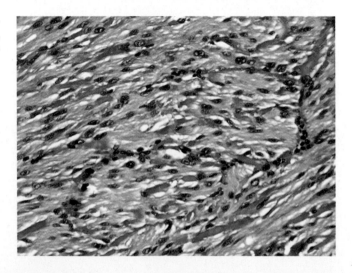

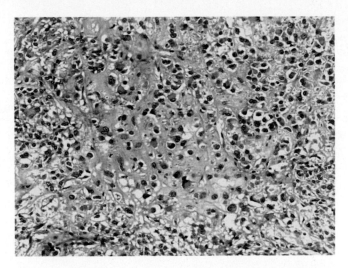

FIGURE 9-13 Some examples of epithelioid GISTs show eccentric nuclei and dense eosinophilic cytoplasm imparting a plasmacytoid appearance to the tumor cells. Although the majority of GISTs are monomorphic tumors, some cases may show binucleate cells and mild nuclear atypia.

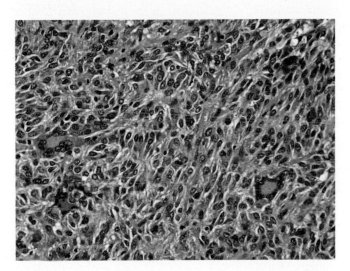

FIGURE 9-14 Multinucleated giant cells are rarely seen in some GISTs. Tumor giant cells with peripheral arrangement of nuclei resembling Touton type giant cells are present in this case. Osteoclastic giant cells have also been described.

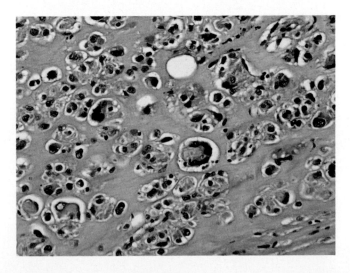

FIGURE 9-15 The presence of nuclear pleomorphism is rare in GISTs and occurs in <2% of tumors. Nuclear enlargement, hyperchromasia and multinucleated tumor giant cells are present in this epithelioid GIST.

FIGURE 9-16 Marked stromal sclerosis and pseudopapillary pattern are seen in GISTs resected following neoadjuvant chemotherapy. Viable cuffs of tumor cells remain around blood vessels imparting a pseudopapillary appearance.

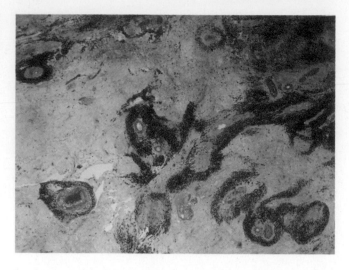

and specific than KIT.[14,33] Immunoreactivity for KIT is variable in intensity and pattern. Most cases show strong and diffuse cytoplasmic staining. Membranous or perinuclear dotlike (Golgi zone) staining may be present in some tumors, particularly in epithelioid GISTs. Focal weak staining may be present in some tumors that may be completely negative. Cases negative for KIT immunostain are more likely to be *KIT* wild type or *PDGFRA* mutant GISTs. Both KIT and CD34 may be negative in about 5% of GISTs[34] and these tumors are more likely to be of epithelioid morphology. The stomach is a preferred location for these KIT-negative, epithelioid or mixed spindle and epithelioid GISTs. Treatment with TKI may also lead to loss of expression of both KIT and CD34, coupled with a gain in desmin reactivity.[31,35]

Smooth muscle actin (SMA), desmin, and H-caldesmon show variable reactivity in GISTs. SMA positivity ranges from 10% to 45%[33] of cases, and is seen particularly in small intestinal GISTs. The largest series of gastric GISTs yielded SMA-positivity in only 19% of cases, and when positive, the staining was patchy.[14,33] Desmin reactivity is much less prevalent but in the stomach has been reported in up to 30% of cases.[14,36] H-caldesmon is reported to be positive in close to 80% of GISTs.[35] Thus, of the three markers of myoid differentiation, desmin is the most discriminatory in differential diagnostic workup, since diffuse strong reactivity is seldom seen in GISTs and favors a primary smooth muscle tumor instead.

FIGURE 9-17 Dedifferentiated GISTs are extremely rare and resemble an undifferentiated pleomorphic sarcoma. Foci of typical GIST were also present in this case of dedifferentiated GIST and both components showed an exon 11 mutation.

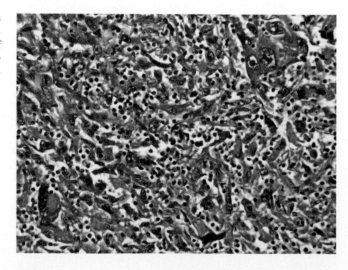

S-100 protein is positive in 1% to 5% of GISTs and is usually focal.[14,33] Cytokeratin positivity is rare and occurs in <1% of tumors and high molecular weight keratins are generally absent.[37–39] Keratin-positive epithelioid GISTs may be mistaken for a carcinoma involving the gut and peritoneum, particularly in small biopsy specimens and this pitfall should be kept in mind. Bcl-2 positivity has also been reported but is neither specific nor sensitive enough for diagnostic purposes.[14,40,41]

Recent markers reported to be highly sensitive for GISTs include DOG1 ("discovered on GIST"), protein kinase C-theta (PKC-θ), and nestin.[38,42–46] DOG1, also known as TMEM16A, is a highly sensitive marker for both *KIT* and *PDGFRA* mutated GISTs. DOG1 stains about a third of KIT-negative GISTs and its utility is greatest in tumors lacking *KIT/PDGFRA* mutations, such as GISTs in pediatric patients and in the setting of neurofibromatosis.[36,42] DOG1 reactivity has also been reported in germ cell tumors, melanomas, carcinomas, and normal gastric epithelium. PKC-θ is expressed on Western blots in nearly all GISTs. However, commercially available antibodies to this antigen show limited specificity and PKC-θ is not in widespread diagnostic use at present. PKC-θ is also positive in a significant proportion of schwannomas.[38,45] Similarly, immunostaining with PDGFRA may be helpful and has been proposed to be useful in KIT-negative GISTs with *PDGFRA* mutation, but currently available antibodies do not show reproducible results and the published data is contradictory.[34,47] Nestin, an intermediate filament protein, is expressed in GISTs but also highly expressed in neural tumors, including schwannomas, gliomas and primitive neuroectodermal tumors, and melanocytic and vascular tumors.[38] Carbonic anhydrase II (CA II) has been recently proposed as marker of GISTs and reported to be expressed in 95% of tumors regardless of mutational status. About 50% of KIT-negative GISTs have been reported to be CA II-positive. These results need to be validated in other studies before CA II immunostaining comes into routine use (Figs. 9-18–9-21).[48]

MOLECULAR FEATURES

GISTs harbor mutually exclusive mutations in either the *KIT* or *PDGFRA* genes.[10,11] In the physiologic state, these are activated by binding with their ligands, stem cell factor, and PDGF. Gain-of-function mutations result in constitutional phosphorylation of these receptors, causing activation of downstream effectors, which perpetuates proliferation signals and decreases apoptosis. The nature and loci of mutations correlate, to some extent, with clinicopathological features and clinical behavior. *KIT* mutations have been demonstrated in up to 85% of GISTs and occur preferentially in spindle cell GISTs. Most commonly (65%) these are in-frame deletions involving the juxtamembrane domain of exon 11, followed by exon 9 mutations in another 15%.[49] Exon 13 and

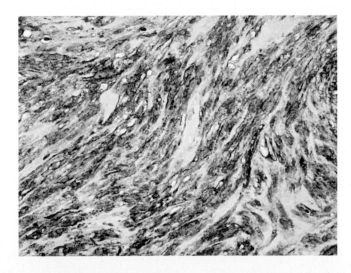

FIGURE 9-18 Immunohistochemical expression of KIT is a sensitive and specific marker of GISTs and is present in up to 95% of cases. Membranous and cytoplasmic positivity is present in this spindle cell GIST.

FIGURE 9-19 Membranous KIT positivity, with little cytoplasmic staining, is more commonly seen in epithelioid GISTs.

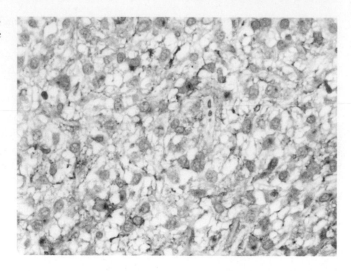

FIGURE 9-20 Perinuclear, dotlike, Golgi pattern of staining is prominent in some examples and is more commonly seen in *KIT* mutant GISTs.

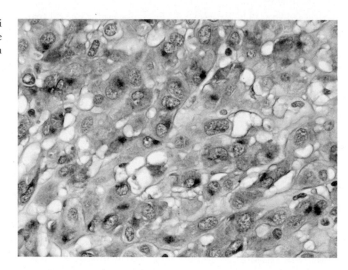

FIGURE 9-21 CD34 positivity is seen in 60% to 70% of GISTs but is less specific than KIT. CD34 positivity is also present in IFPs and solitary fibrous tumors involving the stomach.

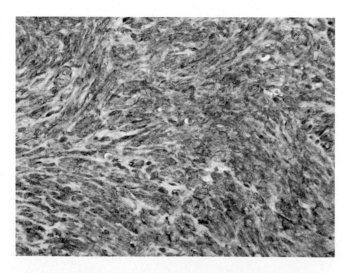

17 *KIT* mutations are rare.[47,50] Familial GISTs may additionally exhibit exon 8 *KIT* mutations.[51,52] *PDGFRA* mutations occur in 4% to 18% of GISTs, preferentially in gastric and omental tumors, and are more likely to be seen in epithelioid variants.[10,33,47,49] The D842V point mutation in exon 18 is the most frequently affected locus, followed by exons 12 and 14. GISTs developing in neurofibromatosis type I (NF-1) and in patients with Carney's triad tend to be negative for both *KIT* and *PDGFRA* mutations.[50,53,54]

Tumor progression in GISTs is the result of further mutations characterized by both chromosomal gains and losses. Loss of chromosome 14, 22q, 1p, 9p, or 11p and gains of 5p and 20q have been implicated in aggressive tumors.[55–58] Secondary mutations may occur in *KIT* and *PDGFRA* following treatment with TKI and confer resistance to chemotherapy.[59] However, tumors with unusual phenotypic changes following therapy may not show any secondary mutations while still exhibiting resistance to TKI treatment. *BRAF* mutations have been reported as another possible mechanism for chemoresistance.[60]

DIFFERENTIAL DIAGNOSIS

The differential diagnosis of spindle cell GISTs includes smooth muscle tumors, schwannomas, fibromatosis (desmoid tumors), inflammatory fibroid polyp (IFP), inflammatory myofibroblastic tumor (IMT), solitary fibrous tumor, monophasic synovial sarcoma, and the recently described plexiform angiomyxoid myofibroblastic tumor. All lesions to be considered in the differential diagnosis of spindle cell GISTs are typically negative for KIT.

Leiomyomas involving the gastrointestinal tract occur most commonly in the esophagus. The tumor cells show intense cytoplasmic eosinophilia and better defined cell boundaries in contrast to the syncytial appearance usually seen in GISTs. Diffuse and strong desmin expression is particularly helpful in the diagnosis of true smooth muscle tumors. SMA and caldesmon positivity are of limited value as both can be found in GISTs and in smooth muscle tumors. The presence of significant nuclear pleomorphism in a spindle cell tumor should prompt consideration of a leiomyosarcoma since the majority of GISTs are monomorphic tumors with little nuclear atypia. Leiomyomas and leiomyosarcomas are consistently negative for KIT.

Schwannomas of the gastrointestinal tract show a uniform cellularity and lack the Antoni A and Antoni B areas typically seen in their soft tissue counterparts. Schwannomas are surrounded by a distinctive cuff of lymphoid tissue and show diffuse and strong S-100 immunoreactivity. Glial fibrillary acidic protein is also expressed commonly in gastrointestinal schwannomas and is negative in GISTs.

Deep intra-abdominal fibromatosis is composed of long, sweeping fascicles of spindle cells in a collagenous or myxoid stroma. The nuclei may be pointed and buckled or stellate-shaped in fibromatosis and show cytoplasmic amphophilia consistent with myofibroblastic differentiation. Aberrant nuclear localization of beta-catenin is present in 75% to 80% of fibromatosis cases and is a useful feature for diagnosis. However, lack of nuclear expression of beta-catenin does not rule out a diagnosis of fibromatosis.

IMT typically presents in children and young adults and is composed of a fascicular myofibroblastic proliferation admixed with a prominent inflammatory infiltrate rich in plasma cells. Hypocellular, richly collagenized zones are often present in IMTs. These tumors are diffusely and strongly positive for SMA and about 50% to 60% are also positive for ALK. Rearrangement of the *ALK* gene may be demonstrated by FISH in approximately 45% of IMTs.

IFP is a distinctive polypoid lesion involving the stomach and small intestine, which is centered in the submucosa and often ulcerates the overlying mucosal surface. The lesion is composed of granulation tissuelike stroma with perivascular hyalinization and a prominent eosinophilic infiltrate. The spindle-shaped fibroblasts in the lesion show a perivascular onion skin–like proliferation and are CD34-positive.

Solitary fibrous tumors may also occur in the gastrointestinal tract and are composed of a branching, ectatic, hemangiopericytoma-like vasculature with spindle cells proliferating in a "patternless pattern." The cellularity is variable within the same tumor and thick collagen bundles are usually present in the hypocellular zones. The tumor cells express CD34 and CD99.

Monophasic synovial sarcoma rarely involves the gastrointestinal tract. These tumors are highly cellular and positivity for cytokeratin and EMA is helpful in making the diagnosis. Demonstration of the t(X;18)(p11;q11) translocation by FISH or PCR is diagnostic of monophasic synovial sarcomas.

Plexiform angiomyxoid myofibroblastic tumor is a recently described entity in the stomach. The tumor exhibits a plexiform architecture with bland spindle cells present in an abundant myxoid matrix. The tumor cells are positive for smooth muscle and muscle specific actin, consistent with myofibroblastic differentiation, while S-100, KIT, and CD34 are negative. No mutations in *KIT* or *PDFRA* have been identified.[61,62]

Epithelioid GISTs may be mistaken for glomus tumors, neuroendocrine tumors, epithelioid leiomyosarcomas, metastatic malignant melanomas, epithelioid malignant peripheral nerve sheath tumors (MPNSTs), and clear cell sarcomas.

Glomus tumors almost exclusively involve the stomach when they occur in the gastrointestinal tract. The perivascular accentuation of epithelioid cells, bland nuclear morphology, and SMA positivity are diagnostic of glomus tumors. Immunostains for desmin, S-100, and KIT are negative.

The nested pattern of epithelioid GISTs may be confused for a neuroendocrine tumor. However, the latter are KIT-negative, keratin-positive and show reactivity for markers of neuroendocrine differentiation, such as chromogranin and synaptophysin.

Epithelioid leiomyosarcomas are more pleomorphic than GISTs and show positivity for desmin, SMA, and caldesmon and are negative for KIT. Although KIT-negative GISTs may be positive for desmin, reactivity is usually focal and weak. Molecular analysis for *KIT* or *PDGFRA* mutations may be necessary in some cases for definite diagnosis.

Metastatic malignant melanomas show nuclear pleomorphism, diffuse S-100 expression, and positivity for melanocytic markers HMB-45 and MART-1. A prior clinical history of malignant melanoma can be elicited in most instances. Epithelioid MPNSTs are also strongly S-100 positive but are negative for other markers of melanocytic differentiation.

Clear cell sarcomas of the gastrointestinal tract also express S-100 and may lack melanocytic differentiation. However, just like their soft tissue counterparts, rearrangements of *EWSR1* (22q12) gene has been demonstrated in most reported instances of primary clear cell sarcomas of the gastrointestinal tract.

PREDICTORS OF AGGRESSIVE BEHAVIOR AND PROGNOSIS

GISTs may recur or metastasize even after complete surgical resection and common sites of metastasis include the liver, omentum, and the peritoneal cavity. Metastatic spread to bones and lungs is less common.[33,39] Rather than classify GISTs into definite benign or malignant categories, the current approach employs tumor site, size, and mitotic activity to stratify tumors into groups varying from very low to high risk of aggressive behavior. This conceptual shift was proposed by Fletcher and colleagues at The National Institute of Health (NIH) Consensus meeting in April 2001 and initially incorporated only size and mitotic count, regardless of tumor site.[63] However, the proposed scheme appeared to overestimate the risk of gastric GISTs and based on additional data from larger case series, tumor site was incorporated into the risk stratification scheme. This forms the basis of the current National Comprehensive Cancer Network (NCCN) guidelines for evaluating risk of aggressive behavior in GISTs (Table 9-1).[14,33,64]

There is some data to support that "sarcomatous" appearing spindle or epithelioid GISTs behave in an aggressive manner.[14] However, traditional morphologic parameters of adverse outcome such as nuclear atypia or necrosis are not currently used in assessing risk in GISTs. This is largely because the presence of significant atypia or necrosis correlates very closely with large tumor size and a high mitotic count. Within the stomach, GISTs involving the gastric cardia or

Table 9-1	Risk stratification of gastric gist using tumor size and mitotic activity		
Group	**Tumor Characteristics**		**Number of Patients With Progressive Disease (%)**
	Size (cm)	**Mitotic rate (per 50 hpf)**	
Very low	≤2	≤5	0
Low	≤2	≥5	0*
	>2 to ≤5	≤5	1.9
	>5 to ≤10	≤5	3.6
Intermediate	>10	≤5	12
	>2 to ≤5	>5	16
High	>5 to ≤10	>5	55
	>10	>5	86

*Very few cases analyzed to be certain of the clinical outcome.
Source: Modified from Miettinen M, Sobin LH, Lasota J. Gastrointestinal stromal tumors of the stomach: a clinicopathologic, immunohistochemical, and molecular genetic study of 1765 cases with long-term follow-up. *Am J Surg Pathol.* 2005;29(1):52–68.

fundus appear to exhibit a greater tendency toward aggressive behavior as compared to antral GISTs.[14]

Several immunohistochemical markers of adverse outcome have been studied but none has gained acceptance thus far. Down-regulation of cell cycle inhibitors p16 and p27 has been associated with malignant behavior.[65–68] Tumors classified as low risk by current morphologic criteria but with p16 down-regulation have been shown to behave aggressively. However, more recent data has shown contradictory findings.[69] High-risk GISTs have also been shown to upregulate cell cycle regulatory proteins such as cyclins D, E, and B1, as well as CDK2, CDK4, and CDK6. Increased expression of cyclin A, p53, and RB has also been reported[40,69,70] and the expression of vascular endothelial growth factor has been recently proposed as a marker of poor response to imatinib therapy.[71]

The genetic profile of GISTs is rapidly emerging as an important tool in predicting clinical behavior and response to specific agents. The type of receptor tyrosine kinase mutation correlates with response to therapy and a molecular classification of GISTs has been proposed.[50,72] The response rates following therapy vary from 72% to 86% for patients with exon 11 mutations, to 38% to 48% for those with exon 9 mutations, to only around 28% for wild type GISTs. The commonest *PDGFRA* mutation (D842V) seen in GISTs confers complete resistance to imatinib. More recent data suggest that patients with *KIT* exon 9 mutation may benefit from a higher starting dose of imatinib (800 mg instead of 400 mg) and sunitinib may be a better first-line drug choice for patients with exon 9 mutant or *KIT* wild type GISTs.[73–76] The type of mutation in the *KIT* gene may also have some bearing on prognosis. In general, patients with deletions in exon 11 fare worse than those with point mutations.[49,50]

TREATMENT AND OUTCOME

In patients with low- to intermediate-risk primary GISTs, surgical resection can be curative, with 5-year survival rates ranging from 50% to 80%. However, despite complete tumor resection, postoperative recurrence or metastasis occurs in a substantial proportion of patients.[77,78] The KIT TKI imatinib mesylate has become the standard first-line pharmacologic therapy for unresectable or metastatic GIST.[20,79] In patients with recurrent or metastatic GIST, treatment with imatinib results in an overall response rate of 68%. The median time to progression is about 24 months and the median overall survival around 57 months.[80–83] In patients with locally advanced primary GISTs, the neoadjuvant (preoperative) use of imatinib may be beneficial since tumor shrinkage after therapy often leads to a less extensive surgical resection and improved patient outcome.[84] In patients with inoperable or metastatic GIST, surgical intervention is not generally recommended. However, response following neoadjuvant imatinib treatment may lead to consideration of surgery even in this setting if there is evidence of significant disease response.

PEDIATRIC, FAMILIAL, AND SYNDROMIC GISTs

Pediatric GISTs

Only about 1% to 2% of GISTs occur in the pediatric age group, the standard accepted definition being tumors occurring in patients up to 18 years of age. Pediatric GISTs show unique clinico-pathological characteristics and are generally regarded as a distinct entity. A marked female predominance is observed in pediatric GISTs, the tumors occur preferentially in the stomach, and an epithelioid morphology is quite common. Although pediatric GISTs consistently express the KIT protein, they lack mutations in *KIT* and *PDGFRA* genes. These tumors often spread to regional lymph nodes, a phenomenon seldom seen in adult GISTs. About 10% of pediatric GISTs may be syndromic, and an attempt should be made during initial workup of these patients to look for any evidence of familial predisposition and for manifestations of any of the clinical syndromes associated with GISTs, which are discussed below.

The tumor size and mitotic rate-based risk stratification system used in adult tumors do not predict behavior in pediatric GISTs. Multifocal tumors occur in about 23% of cases, which explains the high incidence of local recurrences. However, despite multiple recurrences, pediatric GISTs follow an indolent course and the few patients who succumb to their disease do so after a protracted clinical course. Progression to malignancy occurs in pediatric GISTs even in the absence of large-scale chromosomal aberrations that characterize their adult counterparts. On gene expression profiling studies, pediatric GISTs cluster separately from adult GISTs, further supporting a unique phenotype.[15,16,85]

Familial GIST Syndrome

About 20 families have been described in literature, thus far, with germline mutations in either *KIT* or *PDGFRA* genes. The inheritance is autosomal dominant with high penetrance and most affected family members go on to develop one or more tumors. Familial GISTs occur at a younger mean age (around 45 years) than sporadic tumors. Both sexes are affected equally and the tumors are morphologically similar to their sporadic counterparts. The small intestine is involved more often than the stomach. Diffuse hyperplasia of the myenteric plexus in association with multiple GISTs is present in some cases.[86] Patients with germline *KIT* mutations in exon 13 or 17 develop multiple GISTs. Cutaneous manifestations such as hyperpigmentation, urticaria pigmentosa, or increased numbers of nevi and mast cell disease have been described in patients with germline *KIT* mutations in exon 11. The majority of familial GISTs follow a benign clinical course.[87–90]

GIST in Neurofibromatosis Type I

Neurofibromatosis type I (NF1; von Recklinghausen disease) occurs in 1:3,000 live births due to a germline mutation in the *NF1* gene, which encodes the GTPase activating protein neurofibromin. It is inherited in an autosomal dominant manner. The most characteristic features are café au lait spots, freckles in the axilla and groin, and multiple dermal neurofibromas and ocular hamartomas known as Lisch nodules.

Gastrointestinal manifestations of NF1 include myenteric plexus hyperplasia and GISTs. The clinical features of GISTs in NF1 resemble those of GISTs in familial GIST syndrome patients. There is a slight female predominance, and the tumors are often small and multiple and occur more frequently in the small intestine. *KIT* or *PDGFRA* mutations are not prevalent in NF1-associated GISTs, suggesting a *KIT*-independent pathway for tumor development.[91,92]

Carney's Triad and Carney-Stratakis Syndrome

The triad of gastric epithelioid GIST, pulmonary chondroma, and extra-adrenal paraganglioma is known as Carney's triad. Most reported cases have been in women (85%) and occur at a median age of around 30 years. Although these are sporadic tumors with no known heritable predisposition, GISTs in the setting of Carney's triad do not harbor *KIT* or *PDGFRA* mutations. The tumors are often multifocal, show frequent nodal metastasis and multiple recurrences. The risk of aggressive behavior cannot be predicted using the criteria proposed for the typical adult GISTs.[93] The Carney-Stratakis syndrome consists of the paraganglioma/gastric GIST dyad and appears to be an autosomal dominant condition with incomplete penetrance and variable expressivity. Mutations in succinic dehydrogenase subunits SDHB, SDHC, and SDHD have recently been described in Carney-Stratakis syndrome.[94]

SUMMARY

In the short span of a little more than a decade, the understanding of these once enigmatic tumors has been rapidly consolidated into a vast archive of clinical, morphologic, immunophenotypic, and genotypic data that is helpful in diagnosis, in prognosis, and in guiding therapy. EUS-guided FNA has made preoperative diagnosis and ancillary testing possible. Additional molecular insights in the coming years are likely to enhance the repertoire of targeted therapeutic agents available for treatment and will hopefully help in improving patient outcomes in GISTs.

References

1. Golden T, Stout AP. Smooth muscle tumors of the gastrointestinal tract and retroperitoneal tissues. *Surg Gynecol Obstet.* 1941;73:784–810.
2. Stout AP. Bizarre smooth muscle tumors of the stomach. *Cancer.* 1962;15:400–409.
3. Appelman HD. Smooth muscle tumors of the gastrointestinal tract. What we know now that Stout didn't know. *Am J Surg Pathol.* 1986;10(Suppl 1).83–99.
4. Welsh RA, Meyer AT. Ultrastructure of gastric leiomyoma. *Arch Pathol.* 1969;87(1):1–81.
5. Mazur MT, Clark HB. Gastric stromal tumors. Reappraisal of histogenesis. *Am J Surg Pathol.* 1983;7(6):507–519.
6. Huizinga JD, Thuneberg L, Klüppel M, et al. W/kit gene required for interstitial cells of Cajal and for intestinal pacemaker activity. *Nature.* 1995;373(6512):347–349.
7. Kindblom LG, Remotti HE, Aldenborg F, et al. Gastrointestinal pacemaker cell tumor (GIPACT). Gastrointestinal stromal tumors show phenotypic characteristics of the interstitial cells of Cajal. *Am J Pathol.* 1998;152(5):1259–1269.
8. Robinson TL, Sircar K, Hewlett BR, et al. Gastrointestinal stromal tumors may originate from a subset of CD34-positive interstitial cells of Cajal. *Am J Pathol.* 2000;156(4):1157–1163.
9. Miettinen M, Lasota J. Gastrointestinal stromal tumors—definition, clinical, histological, immunohistochemical, and molecular genetic features and differential diagnosis. *Virchows Arch.* 2001;438(1):1–12.
10. Hirota S, Isozaki K, Moriyama Y, et al. Gain-of-function mutations of c-kit in human GISTs. *Science.* 1998;279(5350):577–580.
11. Heinrich MC, Corless CL, Duensing A, et al. PDGFRA activating mutations in gastrointestinal stromal tumors. *Science.* 2003;299(5607):708–710.
12. Joensuu H, Roberts PJ, Sarlomo-Rikala, et al. Effect of the tyrosine kinase inhibitor STI571 in a patient wit a metastatic gastrointestinal stromal tumor. *N Eng J Med.* 2001;344(14);1052–1056.
13. Heinrich MC, Maki RG, Corless CL, et al. Sunitinib (SU) response in imatinib-resistant (IM-R) GIST correlates with KIT and PDGFRA mutation status. 2006 ASCO Annual Meeting Proceedings Part I. *J Clin Onc.* 2006;24(18S)(June 20 Suppl):9502.

14. Miettinen M, Sobin LH, Lasota J. Gastrointestinal stromal tumors of the stomach: a clinicopathologic, immunohistochemical, and molecular genetic study of 1765 cases with long-term follow-up. *Am J Surg Pathol.* 2005;29(1):52–68.

15. Prakash S, Sarran L, Socci N, et al. Gastrointestinal stromal tumors in children and young adults: a clinicopathologic, molecular, and genomic study of 15 cases and review of the literature. *J Pediatr Hematol Oncol.* 2005;27(4):179–187.

16. Janeway KA, Liegl B, Harlow A, et al. Pediatric KIT wild-type and platelet-derived growth factor receptor alpha- wild-type gastrointestinal stromal tumors share KIT activation but not mechanisms of genetic progression with adult gastrointestinal stromal tumors. *Cancer Res.* 2007;67(19):9084–9088.

17. Nilsson B, Bumming P, Meis-Kindblom JM, et al. Gastrointestinal stromal tumors: the incidence, prevalence, clinical course, and prognostication in the preimatinib mesylate era—a population-based study in western Sweden. *Cancer.* 2005;103(4):821–829.

18. Goettsch WG, Bos SD, Breekveldt-Postma N, et al. Incidence of gastrointestinal stromal tumours is underestimated: results of a nation-wide study. *Eur J Cancer.* 2005;41(18):2868–2872.

19. Tryggvason G, Gislason HG, Magnusson MK, et al. Gastrointestinal stromal tumors in Iceland, 1990–2003: the Icelandic GISTstudy, a population-based incidence and pathologic risk stratification study. *Int J Cancer.* 2005;117(2):289–293.

20. DeMatteo RP, Lewis JJ, Leung D, et al. Two hundred gastrointestinal stromal tumors: recurrence patterns and prognostic factors for survival. *Ann Surg.* 2000;231(1):51–58.

21. Miettinen M, Monihan JM, Sarlomo-Rikala M, et al. Gastrointestinal stromal tumors/smooth muscle tumors (GISTs) primary in the omentum and mesentery: clinicopathologic and immunohistochemical study of 26 cases. *Am J Surg Pathol.* 1999;23(9):1109–1118.

22. Miettinen M, Makhlouf H, Sobin LH, et al. Gastrointestinal stromal tumors of the jejunum and ileum: a clinicopathologic, immunohistochemical, and molecular genetic study of 906 cases before imatinib with long-term follow-up. *Am J Surg Pathol.* 2006;30(4):477–489.

23. Reith JD, Goldblum JR, Lyles RH, et al. Extragastrointestinal (soft tissue) stromal tumors: an analysis of 48 cases with emphasis on histologic predictors of outcome. *Mod Pathol.* 2000;13(5):577–585.

24. Abraham SC, Krasinskas AM, Hofstetter WL, et al. "Seedling" mesenchymal tumors (gastrointestinal stromal tumors and leiomyomas) are common incidental tumors of the esophagogastric junction. *Am J Surg Pathol.* 2007;31(11):1629–1635.

25. Kawanowa K, Sakuma Y, Sakurai S, et al. High incidence of microscopic gastrointestinal stromal tumors in the stomach. *Hum Pathol.* 2006;37(12):1527–1535.

26. Agaimy A, Wunsch PH, Dirnhofer S, et al. Microscopic gastrointestinal stromal tumors in esophageal and intestinal surgical resection specimens: a clinicopathologic, immunohistochemical, and molecular study of 19 lesions. *Am J Surg Pathol.* 2008;32(6):867–873.

27. Boggino HE, Fernandez MP, Logroño R. Cytomorphology of gastrointestinal stromal tumors: diagnostic role of aspiration cytology, core biopsy, and immunochemistry. *Diagn Cytopathol.* 2000;23(3):156–160.

28. Gomes AL, Bardales RH, Milanezi F, et al. Molecular analysis of c-Kit and PDGFRA in GISTs diagnosed by EUS. *Am J Clin Pathol.* 2007;127(1);89–96.

29. Pang NK, Chin SY, Nga ME, et al. Comparative validation of c-kit exon 11 mutation analysis on cytology samples and corresponding surgical resections of gastrointestinal stromal tumours. *Cytopathology.* 2009;20(5):297–303.

30. Abdulkader I, Cameselle-Teijeiro J, Forteza J. Pathological changes related to Imatinib treatment in a patient with a metastatic gastrointestinal stromal tumour. *Histopathology.* 2005;46(4):470–472.

31. Pauwels P, Debiec-Rychter M, Stul M, et al. Changing phenotype of gastrointestinal stromal tumours under imatinib mesylate treatment: a potential diagnostic pitfall. *Histopathology.* 2005;47(1):41–47.

32. Liegl B, Hornick JL, Antonescu C, et al. Rhabdomyosarcomatous differentiation in gastrointestinal stromal tumors after tyrosine kinase inhibitor therapy: a novel form of tumor progression. *Am J Surg Pathol.* 2009;33(2):218–226.

33. Rubin BP. Gastrointestinal stromal tumors: an update. *Histopathology.* 2006;48(1):83–96.

34. Rossi G, Valli R, Marchioni A, et al. PDGFR expression in differential diagnosis between KIT-negative gastrointestinal stromal tumors and other primary soft-tissue tumors of the gastrointestinal tract. *Histopathology.* 2005;46(5):522–531.

35. Yamaguchi U, Hasegawa T, Masuda T, et al. Differential diagnosis of gastrointestinal stromal tumor and other spindle cell tumors in the gastrointestinal tract based on immunohistochemical analysis. *Virch Arch.* 2004:445(2);142–150.

36. Liegl B, Hornick JL, Corless C, et al. Monoclonal antibody DOG 1.1 shows higher sensitivity than KIT in the diagnosis of Gastrointestinal stromal tumors, including unusual subtypes. *Am J Surg Pathol.* 2009;33(3):437–446.

37. Nga ME, Wong AS, Wee A, et al. Cytokeratin expression in gastrointestinal stromal tumors: A word of caution. *Histopathology.* 2002;40(5):480–481.

38. Sarlomo-Rikala M, Tsujimura T, Lendahl U, et al. Patterns of nestin and other intermediate filament expression distinguish between gastrointestinal stromal tumors, leiomyomas and schwannomas. *APMIS.* 2002;110(6):499–507.

39. Miettinen M, Lasota J. Gastrointestinal stromal tumors: review on morphology, molecular pathology, prognosis, and differential diagnosis. *Arch Pathol Lab Med.* 2006;130(10):1466–1478.

40. Feakins RM. The expression of p53 and bcl-2 in gastrointestinal stromal tumors is associated with anatomical site, and p53 expression is associated with grade and clinical outcome. *Histopathology.* 2005;46(3):270–279.

41. Steinert DM, Oyarzo M, Wang X, et al. Expression of bcl-2 in gastrointestinal stromal tumors. Correlation with progression-free survival in 81 patients treated with imatinib mesylate. *Cancer.* 2006;106(7): 1617–1623.

42. Espinosa I, Lee CH, Kim MK, et al. A novel monoclonal antibody against DOG1 is a sensitive and specific marker for gastrointestinal stromal tumours. *Am J Surg Pathol.* 2008;32(2):210–218.

43. West RB, Corless CL, Chen X, et al. The novel marker, DOG1, is expressed ubiquitously in gastrointestinal stromal tumors irrespective of KIT or PDGFRA mutation status. *Am J Pathol.* 2004;165(1):107–113.

44. Lee HE, Kim MA, Lee HS, et al. Characteristics of KIT-negative gastrointestinal stromal tumours and diagnostic utility of protein kinase C theta immunostaining. *J Clin Pathol.* 2008;61(6):722–729.

45. Kim KM, Kang DW, Moon WS, et al. PKCh expression in gastrointestinal stromal tumor. Gastrointestinal Stromal Tumor Committee, The Korean Gastrointestinal Pathology Study Group. *Mod Pathol.* 2006;19(11):1480–1486.

46. Blay P, Astudillo A, Buesa JM, et al. Protein kinase c theta is highly expressed in gastrointestinal stromal tumors but not in other mesenchymal neoplasms. *Clin Canc Res.* 2004;10(12 Pt 1):4089–4095.

47. Pauls K, Merkelbach-Bruse S, Thal D, et al. PDGFR alpha- and c-kit-mutated GISTs are characterised by distinctive histological and immunohistochemical features. *Histopathology.* 2005;46(2):166–175.

48. Parkkila S, Lasota J, Fletcher JA, et al. Carbonic anhydrase II. A novel biomarker for gastrointestinal stromal tumors. *Mod Pathol.* 2010;2(5)3:743–750.

49. Lasota J, Miettinen M. Clinical significance of oncogenic KIT and PDGFRA mutations in gastrointestinal stromal tumors. *Histopathology.* 2008;53(3):245–266.

50. Corless CL, Fletcher JA, Heinrich MC. Biology of Gastrointestinal Tumours. *J Clin Oncol.* 2004;22(18):3813–3825.

51. Hirota S, Nishida T, Izosaki K, et al. Familial gastrointestinal stromal tumors associated with dysphagia and novel type germline mutation of KIT gene. *Gastroenterology.* 2002;122(5):1493–1499.

52. Hartmann K, Wardelmann E, Yongsheng MA, et al. Novel germline mutation of KIT associated with familial gastrointestinal stromal tumors and mastocytosis. *Gastroenterology.* 2005;129(3):1042–1046.

53. Diment J, Tamborini E, Casali P, et al. Carney triad: case report and molecular analysis of gastric tumor. *Hum Pathol.* 2005;36(1):112–116.

54. Yantis RK, Rosenberg AE, Sarran L, et al. Multiple gastrointestinal stromal tumors in type 1 neurofibromatosis: a pathologic and molecular study. *Mod Pathol.* 2005;18(4):475–484.

55. Heinrich MC, Rubin BP, Longley BJ, et al. Biology and genetic aspects of gastrointestinal stromal tumors: KIT activation and cytogenetic alterations. *Hum Pathol.* 2002;33(5):484–495.

56. Bermann F, Gunawan B, Hermnns B, et al. Cytogenetic and morphologic characteristics of gastrointestinal stromal tumors. Recurrent rearrangement of chromosome 1 and losses of chromosomes 14 and 22 are common anomalies. *Verh Dtsch Ges Pathol.* 1998;82:275–278.

57. Debiec-Rychter M, Lasota J, Sarlomo-Rikala M, et al. Chromosomal aberrations in malignant gastrointesintal sromal tumors: correlation with c-KIT gene mutation. *Cancer Genet Cytogenet.* 2001;12(1)8:24–30.

58. El-Rifai W, Sarlomo-Rikala M, Andersson LC, et al. High-resolution deletion mapping of chromosome 14 in stromal tumors of the gastrointestinal tract suggests two distinct tumor supressor loci. *Genes Chromosomes Cancer.* 2000;27(4):387–391.

59. Antonescu CR, Besmer P, Guo T, et al. Acquired resistance to imatinib in gastrointestinal stromal tumors occurs through secondary gene mutation. *Clin Canc Res.* 2005;11(11):4182–4190.

60. Agaram NP, Wong GC, Guo T, et al. Novel V600E BRAF mutations in imatinib-naive and imatinib-resistant gastrointestinal stromal tumors. *Genes Chromosomes Cancer.* 2008;47(10):853–859.

61. Takahashi Y, Shimizu S, Ishida T, et al. Plexiform angiomyxoid myofibroblastic tumor of the stomach. *Am J Surg Pathol.* 2007;31(5):724–728.

62. Miettinen M, Makhlouf H, Sobin L, et al. Plexiform fibromyxoma: a distinctive benign gastric antral neoplasm not to be confused with a myxoid GIST. *Am J Surg Pathol.* 2009;33(11):1624–1632.

63. Fletcher CD, Berman JJ, Corless C, et al. Diagnosis of gastrointestinal stromal tumors: a consensus approach. *Hum Pathol.* 2002;33(5):459–465.

64. Miettinen M, el-Rifai W, Sobin L, et al. Evaluation of malignancy and prognosis of gastrointestinal stromal tumors: a review. *Hum Pathol.* 2002;33(5):478–483.

65. Sabah M, Cummins R, Leader M, et al. Loss of heterozygosity of chromosome 9p and loss of p16INK4A expression are associated with malignant gastrointestinal stromal tumors. *Mod Pathol.* 2004;17(11):1364–1371.

66. Schneider-Stock R, Boltze C, Lasota J, et al. High prognostic value of p16INK4 alterations in gastrointestinal stromal tumors. *J Clin Oncol.* 2003;21(9):1688–1697.

67. Schneider-Stock R, Boltze C, Lasota J, et al. Loss of p16 protein defines high risk patients with gastrointestinal stromal tumors: a tissue microarray study. *Clin Cancer Res.* 2005;11(2 Pt 1):638–645.

68. Nemoto Y, Mikami T, Hana K, et al. Correlation of enhanced cell turnover with prognosis of gastrointestinal stromal tumors of the stomach: relevance of cellularity and p27kip1. *Pathol Int.* 2006;56(12):724–731.

69. Steigen SE, Bjerkehagen B, Haugland HK, et al. Diagnostic and prognostic markers for gastrointestinal stromal tumors in Norway. *Mod Pathol.* 2008;21(1):46–53.

70. Pruneri G, Mazzarol G, Fabris S, et al. Cyclin D3 immunoreactivity in gastrointestinal stromal tumors is independent of cyclin D3 gene amplification and is associated with nuclear p27 accumulation. *Mod Pathol.* 2003;16(9):886–892.

71. McAuliffe JC, Lazar AJ, Yang D, et al. Association of intratumoral vascular endothelial growth factor expression and clinical outcome for patients with gastrointestinal stromal tumors treated with imatinib mesylate. *Clin Cancer Res.* 2007;13(22 Pt 1):6727–6734.

72. Corless CL, Heinrich MC. Molecular pathobiology of gastrointestinal stromal sarcomas. *Annu Rev Pathol.* 2008;3:557–586.

73. Debiec-Rychter M, Sciot R, Le Cesne A, et al. KIT mutations and dose selection for imatinib in patients with advanced gastrointestinal stromal tumours. *Eur J Cancer.* 2006;42(8):1093–1103.

74. Heinrich MC, Corless CL, Blanke CD, et al. Molecular correlates of imatinib resistance in gastrointestinal stromal tumors. *J Clin Oncol.* 2006;24(29):4764–4774.

75. Blanke CD, Demetri GD, von Mehren M, et al. Long-term results from a randomized phase II trial of standard- versus higher-dose imatinib mesylate for patients with unresectable or metastatic gastrointestinal stromal tumors expressing KIT. *J Clin Oncol.* 2008;26(4):620–625.

76. Hirota S, Ohashi A, Nishida T, et al. Gain-of-function mutations of platelet derived growth factor receptor alpha gene in gastrointestinal stromal tumors. *Gastroenterology.* 2003;125(3):660–667.

77. Hassan I, You YN, Shyyan R, et al. Surgically managed gastrointestinal stromal tumors: a comparative and prognostic analysis. *Ann Surg Oncol.* 2008;15(1):52–59.

78. Langer C, Gunawan B, Schuler P, et al. Prognostic factors influencing surgical management and outcome of gastrointestinal stromal tumours. *Br J Surg.* 2003;90(3):332–339.

79. Dagher R, Cohen M, Williams G, et al. Approval summary: imatinib mesylate in the treatment of metastatic and/or unresectable malignant gastrointestinal stromal tumors. *Clin Cancer Res.* 2002;8(10):3034–3038.

80. Blanke CD, Rankin C, Demetri GD, et al. Phase III randomized, intergroup trial assessing imatinib mesylate at two dose levels in patients with unresectable or metastatic gastrointestinal stromal tumors expressing the kit receptor tyrosine kinase: S0033. *J Clin Oncol.* 2008;26(4):626–632.

81. Demetri GD, von Mehren M, Blanke CD, et al. Efficacy and safety of imatinib mesylate in advanced gastrointestinal stromal tumors. *N Engl J Med.* 2002;347(7):472–480.

82. Andtbacka RH, Ng CS, Scaife CL, et al. Surgical resection of gastrointestinal stromal tumors after treatment with imatinib. *Ann Surg Oncol.* 2007;14(1):14–24.

83. Eisenberg BL, Harris J, Blanke CD, et al. Phase II trial of neoadjuvant/adjuvant imatinib mesylate (IM) for advanced primary and metastatic/recurrent operable gastrointestinal stromal tumor (GIST): early results of RTOG 0132/ACRIN 6665. *J Surg Oncol.* 2009;99(1):42–47.

84. DeMatteo RP, Maki RG, Singer S, et al. Results of tyrosine kinase inhibitor therapy followed by surgical resection for metastatic gastrointestinal stromal tumor. *Ann Surg.* 2007;245(3):347–352.

85. Miettinen M, Lasota J, Sobin LH. Gastrointestinal stromal tumors of the stomach in children and young adults: a clinicopathologic, immunohistochemical, and molecular genetic study of 44 cases with long-term follow-up and review of the literature. *Am J Surg Pathol.* 2005;29(10):1373–1381.

86. O'Brien P, Kapusta L, Dardick I, et al. Multiple familial gastrointestinal autonomic nerve tumors and small intestinal neuronal dysplasia. *Am J Surg Pathol.* 1999;23(2):198–204.

87. Beghini A, Tibiletti MG, Roversi G, et al. Germline mutation in the juxtamembrane domain of the kit gene in a family with gastrointestinal stromal tumors and urticaria pigmentosa. *Cancer.* 2001;92(3): 657–662.

88. Isozaki K, Terris B, Belghiti J, et al. Germline-activating mutation in the kinase domain of KIT gene in familial gastrointestinal stromal tumors. *Am J Pathol.* 2000;57(5):1581–1585.

89. Maeyama H, Hidaka E, Ota H, et al. Familial gastrointestinal stromal tumor with hyperpigmentation: association with a germline mutation of the c-kit gene. *Gastroenterology.* 2001;120(1):210–215.

90. Nishida T, Hirota S, Taniguchi M, et al. Familial gastrointestinal stromal tumours with germline mutation of the KIT gene. *Nat Genet.* 1998;19(4):323–324.

91. Miettinen M, Fetsch JF, Sobin LH, et al. Gastrointestinal stromal tumors in patients with neurofibromatosis 1: a clinicopathologic and molecular genetic study of 45 cases. *Am J Surg Pathol.* 2006;30(1):90–96.

92. Takazawa Y, Sakurai S, Sakuma Y, et al. Gastrointestinal stromal tumors of neurofibromatosis type I (von Recklinghausen's disease). *Am J Surg Pathol.* 2005;29(6):755–763.

93. Zhang L, Smyrk TC, Young WF Jr, et al. Gastric stromal tumors in Carney triad are different clinically, pathologically, and behaviorally from sporadic gastric gastrointestinal stromal tumors: findings in 104 cases. *Am J Surg Pathol.* 2010;34(1):53–64.

94. Pasini B, McWhinney SR, Bei T, et al. Clinical and molecular genetics of patients with the Carney-Stratakis syndrome and germline mutations of the genes coding for the succinate dehydrogenase subunits SDHB, SDHC, and SDHD. *Eur J Hum Genet.* 2008;16(1):79–88.

10 Primary Gastric Lymphoma

▶ X. Frank Zhao

▶ Sanford A. Stass

INTRODUCTION

The gastrointestinal tract (GI) is the most common site of extranodal malignant lymphomas, accounting for 30% to 50% of cases.[1] Within the GI organs, the stomach is the most commonly involved followed by the ileocecal region, small and large bowel. Since primary nodal lymphoma can also involve secondarily the stomach, it may be difficult to define primary gastric lymphoma (PGL). Gastric non-Hodgkin lymphomas (NHLs) have been defined as lymphomas that uniquely involve the stomach or for which the involvement represents >75% of total tumor volume.[2] More strictly, PGL may be defined as the stomach being the only organ involved by lymphoma. Since there were no consensus criteria for the origin of PGL in the past, some cases previously reported in the literature may have included lymphomas of nongastric origin.

PATHOGENESIS OF PRIMARY GASTRIC LYMPHOMA

The pathogenesis of extronodal marginal zone B-cell lymphoma of mucosa-associated lymphoid tissue (MALT), also called MALT lymphoma, serves as a classical mechanism for gastric lymphomas. This type of lymphoma originates from MALT, which represents the accumulation of extranodal lymphoid tissue (characterized by follicular hyperplasia) in the setting of chronic inflammation.[3] Although there is normally no organized lymphoid tissue in the stomach, MALT forms in response to chronic inflammation or bacterial infection.[4] *Helicobacter pylori* has been confirmed as the pathogen responsible for some chronic gastritis and PGL.[5] If chronic stimulation persists, *H. pylori*–specific T cells will promote the proliferation of polyclonal B cells in the MALT. Over time one clone may become dominant,[6] by either activation of an oncogene (such as BCL10) or inactivation of a tumor suppressor gene (such as p53), and gain an advantage in proliferation over the other B-cell clones. This dominant B-cell clone eventually develops into a MALT lymphoma.

EPIDEMIOLOGY OF PRIMARY GASTRIC LYMPHOMA

PGL comprises approximately 2% of all NHLs. A British study of 153 PGL reported an annual incidence of 1.2% of all gastric malignancies, with most (97%) being NHL.[7] A more recent Danish study revealed an incidence of approximately 7% for PGL.[2] Significant geographic disparities have been noted. Comparing the incidence of PGL in northern Italy to UK communities, Doglioni et al. reported 13 times more cases of PGL in the Italian community (66 vs. 5 per 100,000 per 5 years).[8] Notably, a much higher incidence of gastric carcinoma and *H. pylori* chronic gastritis was also found in the same Italian community,[8] supporting the role of *H. pylori* in the pathogenesis of PGL as well as gastric carcinoma.

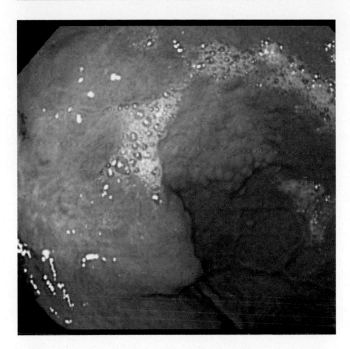

FIGURE 10-1 Endoscopic appearance of MALT lymphoma. MALT lymphoma can have protean presentation from thickened gastric folds and polypoid projection (like in this example) or be flat or ulcerated.

MACROSCOPIC MORPHOLOGY OF PRIMARY GASTRIC LYMPHOMA

The appearance of PGL at endoscopy or on gross examination can be diverse and similar to other malignant tumors of the stomach (Fig. 10-1). They may present as a polypoid nodular growth, as a large fungating mass, or thickened mucosal folds or perforating ulceration. PGL may involve a portion of the stomach, but may also be diffuse or multifocal. Therefore, malignant lymphoma should always be on the list of differential diagnoses of gastric cancers.

CLASSIFICATION OF PRIMARY GASTRIC LYMPHOMA

Currently, the WHO classification is used for PGL. Except for the unique gastric MALT lymphoma, almost all the nodal counterparts of lymphomas can be found in the stomach. Like lymphomas in other organs, PGLs are largely divided into Hodgkin and NHLs. Primary gastric Hodgkin lymphomas are extremely rare. Based on the histology, primary gastric NHLs can be seen as either small cell type or large cell type. Immunophenotyping further divides the lymphomas into B-cell and T-cell types. The distribution of PGL histologic types differs among several studies.[9–11] However, the most cited are the data of a 2005 German multicenter study (GIT NHL 02/96) of 747 patients[11] that indicated that the most common PGL is diffuse large B-cell lymphoma (DLBCL), accounting for more than half of all the 398 PGLs (Table 10-1).

GASTRIC MALT LYMPHOMA

MALT lymphoma is the most common PGL in Western countries.[9] The stomach is also the most common organ involved by MALT lymphoma (Table 10-2). The concept of MALT lymphoma was first proposed by Isaacson and Wright in 1983.[12] Its connection with *H. pylori* infection was later demonstrated by Wotherspoon et al.[13] Since the progression of chronic gastritis to MALT lymphoma is a continuous process, morphological overlap exists between gastritis and early MALT lymphoma.[13] Although there is no consensus on the morphologic criteria for differentiating

Table 10-1	Histological types of the localized PGL
Histological Types	**Frequency (%)**
Diffuse large B-cell lymphoma	59.5
With small cell component (18.1%)	
Without small cell component (81.9%)	
MALT lymphoma	37.9
T-cell lymphoma	1.3
Mantle cell lymphoma	0.8
Follicular lymphoma	0.5

Source: From Koch P, Probst A, Berdel WE, et al. Treatment results in localized primary gastric lymphoma: data of patients registered within the German multicenter study (GIT NHL 02/96). *J Clin Oncol*. 2005;23:7050–7059.

gastritis and MALT lymphoma, Wotherspoon et al.[14] have proposed a scoring system for this purpose (Table 10-3). Generally speaking, expansion of the marginal zone of the hyperplastic lymphoid follicles (Fig. 10-2), dense lymphoid infiltrate composed of predominantly small B cells (Fig. 10-3), increase in plasmacytoid lymphocytes, dropping out of gastric glands (Fig. 10-4), and conspicuous lymphoepithelial lesions (LELs) (Fig. 10-5) are all morphological features that favor MALT lymphoma. However, these features also can be seen in rare cases of severe gastritis. When in doubt, molecular study to detect VDJ rearrangement should be performed to rule out a B-cell clonal process.[15]

Microscopically, MALT lymphoma is morphologically heterogenous. The characteristic lymphoma cells are small to medium in size and have a bland appearance with relatively increased cytoplasm, slightly irregular nuclei, moderately dispersed chromatin, and inconspicuous nucleoli, resembling centrocytes. The relative abundant, pale cytoplasm allows the cells to exhibit a "monocytoid" morphology[16] (Fig. 10-6). The neoplastic cells can also infiltrate the gastric glands and form clusters within the glandular epithelium, fostering "lymphoepithelial lesions" (Fig. 10-5A). The characteristic LELs can be highlighted by staining for pancytokeratin (Fig. 10-5B).

Table 10-2	Organ distribution of MALT lymphoma	
Lymphoma (Other Names)	**Organ**	**Frequency (%)**
Primary gastric MALT lymphoma	Stomach	70
Extranodal marginal zone B-cell lymphoma of bronchus-associated lymphoid tissue (BALT lymphoma)	Lung	14
Ocular MALT lymphoma	Ocular adnexa (conjunctiva; eye socket; lacrimal glands)	12
Thyroid MALT lymphoma	Thyroid	4
Immunoproliferative small intestinal disease	Small intestine	1

Table 10-3	Scoring system for the diagnosis of MALT lymphoma	
Grade	**Description**	**Histological Features**
0	Normal	Scattered plasma cells in lamina propria. No lymphoid follicles.
1	Chronic active gastritis	Small clusters of lymphocytes in lamina propria. No lymphoid follicles. No LELs
2	Chronic active gastritis with florid lymphoid follicle formation	Prominent lymphoid follicles with surrounding mantle zone and plasma cells. No LELs.
3	Suspicious lymphoid infiltrate in lamina propria, probably reactive	Lymphoid follicles surrounded by small lymphocytes that infiltrate diffusely in lamina propria and occasionally into epithelium
4	Suspicious lymphoid infiltrate in lamina propria, probably lymphoma	Lymphoid follicles surrounded by CCL that infiltrate diffusely in lamina propria and into epithelium in small groups
5	Low-grade B-cell lymphoma of MALT	Presence of dense diffuse infiltrate of CCL cells in lamina propria with prominent LELs

CCL, centrocyte-like; LEL, lymphoepithelial lesion.
Source: From Wotherspoon AC, Doglioni C, Diss TC, et al. Regression of primary low-grade B-cell gastric lymphoma of mucosa-associated lymphoid tissue type after eradication of *Helicobacter pylori*. *Lancet*. 1993;342:575–577.

The cells are almost always positive for CD19, CD20 (Fig. 10-7), CD22, and CD79a and show surface immunoglobulin light chain kappa or lambda restriction. They are frequently positive for CD43. Typically negative for CD5 and CD10, an immunophenotype differs from those of most other small B-cell lymphomas (chronic lymphocytic leukemia/small lymphocytic lymphoma, follicular lymphoma, and mantle cell lymphoma [MCL]). The neoplastic B cells often are accompanied by plasmacytic differentiation as well as monoclonal plasma cells. Although primary lymphoplasmacytic lymphoma in the stomach is much rarer than MALT lymphoma, it has been reported.[17] Because of the overlapping features, differentiating between these two diseases is extremely difficult. In addition to Waldenstrom macroglobulinemia, which is often

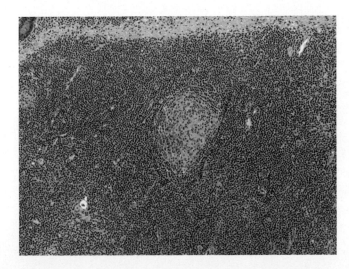

FIGURE 10-2 Histology of MALT lymphoma (medium power). Marginal zone expansion of a monotonous population of small bland lymphoid cells is one of the characteristic histology.

FIGURE 10-3 MALT lymphoma (low power). Gastric glands with dense lymphoid infiltration of small lymphoid cells in the lamina propria with occasional dropping out of gastric glands.

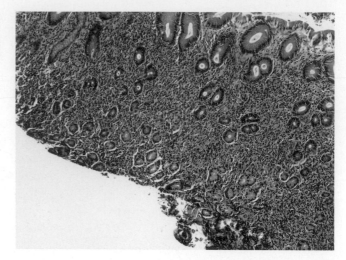

FIGURE 10-4 MALT lymphoma (low power). Dropping out of atrophic gastric glands with intestinal metaplasia in an otherwise lamina propria crowded with Lymphoma cells.

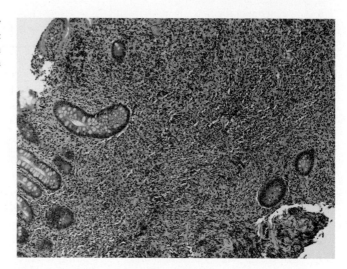

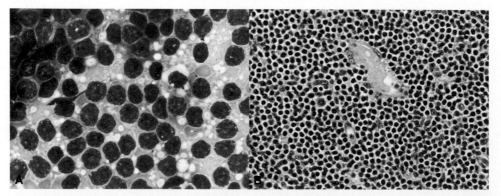

FIGURE 10-5 MALT lymphoma (high power). **A:** On the touch prep, the lymphoma cells are bland with small amount of basophilic cytoplasm, round or occasionally cleaved nuclei, clumped chromatin and inconspicuous nucleoli. Mitotic figures are not present. **B:** A monotonous population of monocytoid lymphoid cells with relatively more abundant cytoplasm provide ample clear space between the nuclei of the adjacent lymphoma cells.

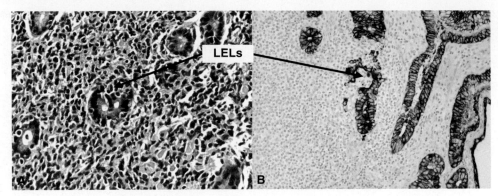

FIGURE 10-6 LELs of MALT lymphoma (high power). **A:** Characteristic LELs in the gastric glands (*arrows*). **B:** LELs can be easily demonstrated by immunostaining for pancytokeratin.

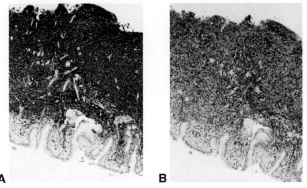

FIGURE 10-7 Immunophenotype of MALT lymphoma (low power). Immunohistochemistry for CD20 (**A**) and CD3 (**B**) reveals that the majority of the infiltrate cells are positive for CD20.

associated with lymphoplasmacytic lymphoma, cytogenetic analysis is helpful in differentiating these two lymphomas.[18]

Typically, the immunoglobulin heavy chain (IgH) and light chain (IgL) genes of MALT lymphoma cells are rearranged with somatic *hyper*mutations. Multiple genetic abnormalities have been identified in MALT lymphoma (Table 10-4). In approximately 30% of gastric cases, MALT lymphoma cells can obtain a recurrent t(11;18)(q21;q21) genetic abnormality,[19] which results in the fusion of *API2* to *MALT1* genes[20]. This translocation has been associated with resistance to *H. pylori* eradication therapy (see below). *MALT1* can also be activated by a t(14;18)(q32;q21) in ocular MALT lymphoma.[21] A recurrent t(1;14)(p22;q32) occurs in approximately 5% of gastric MALT lymphomas, together with several other genetic abnormalities, such as +3, +12, and +18.[22] This recurrent translocation brings BCL10 under the control of *IGH* enhancer (Fig. 10-8) and activates NFκB pathway,[23,24] which in turn promotes B-cell proliferation.[5] Cases with this translocation unlikely respond to *H. pylori* eradication either. Finally, the majority of MALT lymphomas (65% of cases) acquire deletion of p53 gene[25] or inactivation of *CDKN2A* (p16) gene,[26,27] which plays important roles in the large B-cell transformation of MALT lymphoma.

Most MALT lymphomas follow an indolent clinical course and thus conservative treatment is highly advisable. Eradication of *H. pylori* infection can lead to regression of the lymphoma at an early stage in many patients[13,28,29] (Table 10-5). Therefore, it is necessary to rule out active *H. pylori* infection whenever MALT lymphoma is diagnosed. Giemsa or immunohistochemical

Table 10-4	Common genetic abnormalities in PGL		
Lymphoma	Chromosomal Abnormality	Genes Involved	Reference
Gastric MALT lymphoma	t(11;18)(q21;q21)	*API2-MALT1*	19,20
	t(1;14)(p22;q32)	*IGH-BCL10*	47
	t(1;2)(p22;p12)	*IGκ-BCL10*	48
	t(14;18)(q32;q21)	*IGH-MALT1*	43
	+3, +12, +18	?	47
Primary gastric large B-cell lymphoma	3q27 rearrangement	*BCL6*	49,50
	t(8;14)(q24;q32)	c-*MYC*	51
	6q23 rearrangement	?	51
Primary gastric MCL	t(11;14)(q13;q32)	*IGH-CCND1*	40
Primary gastric follicular lymphoma	t(14;18)(q21;q21)	*IGH-BCL2*	42

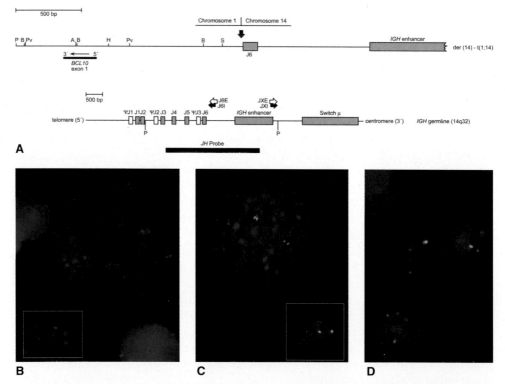

FIGURE 10-8 The t(1;14)(p22;q32) and its molecular detection. **A:** Schematic of t(1;14)(p22;q32). The breakpoint is indicated by an *arrow*. **B:** FISH assigns BCL10 gene to chromosome 1p22. **C,D:** The t(1;14)(p22;q32) is detected by FISH in two patients with MALT lymphoma (Reproduced from Ott G, Katzenberger T, Greiner A, et al. The t(11;18)(q21;q21) chromosome translocation is a frequent and specific aberration in low-grade but not high-grade malignant non-Hodgkin lymphomas of the mucosa-associated lymphoid tissue (MALT-) type. *Cancer Res.* 1997;57:3944–3948.)

Table 10-5	Treatment of MALT lymphomas	
Treatment	**Indication**
Eradication of *H. pylori*	Stage IE, *H. pylori* (+), low grade (or with focal large cell transformation), no t(11;18)(q21;q21)
Local radiation	Stage IE, failed *H. pylori* treatment in *H. pylori* (+) cases, or *H. pylori* (−), t(11;18)(q21;q21)
Combination therapy (rituximab alone, or in combination with chemotherapeutic agents)	Stage IIE/IV, failed local therapy, recurrent disease

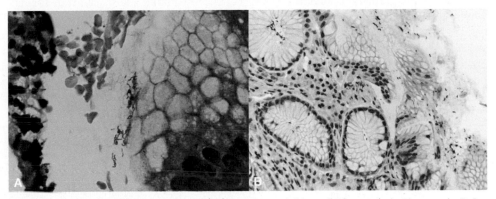

FIGURE 10-9 Identification of active *H. pylori* infection in the gastric biopsy (high power). **A:** Giemsa stain. **B:** Immunohistochemical stain.

stain often can identify the bacteria in the gastric glands (Fig. 10-9). Because of the resistance to *H. pylori* eradication that they confer, all diagnosed MALT lymphomas should be analyzed for t(11;18)(q21;q21) and t(1;14)(p22;q32) by FISH studies.[30] In cases with no *H. pylori* infection and cases with the t(11;18)(q21;q21) or t(1;14)(p22;q32) rearrangements, local low-dose radiation can be an effective treatment in the majority of MALT lymphomas. Although early stage low-grade MALT lymphoma can be cured by surgical resection, because of the morbidity caused by surgery and almost equally effective response rate to radiation (95%), surgical resection is not usually recommended for MALT lymphoma.[11] Gastric MALT lymphomas are slow to disseminate; even extragastric and bone marrow involvements do not appear to confer a worse prognosis. For advanced diseases, rituximab (a monoclonal CD20 antibody) alone or in combination with other chemotherapeutic agents may be warranted.[31,32] Although the data may vary from one report to another, if the patients are properly treated (Table 10-5), the 5-year and 10-year overall survival can reach >90% and >80%.[33]

PRIMARY GASTRIC DIFFUSE LARGE B-CELL LYMPHOMA

DLBCL remains the most common PGL diagnosed in the world and could account for more than half of the cases.[27] However, since many DLBCLs found in the stomach do not originate from the stomach, a complete workup should be carried out to exclude other primary locations. Primary gastric DLBCLs are morphologically similar to nodal DLBCL and that of other organs. The lymphoma cells diffusely infiltrate or completely destroy the gastric glands (Fig. 10-10). The cells are large with abundant cytoplasm, vesicular nuclei, and occasionally prominent nucleoli (Fig. 10-11). Since DLBCL is a heterogeneous group of neoplasms, variations in morphology are present (Figs. 10-12–10-14). The centroblastic DLBCL cells have vesicular nuclei with multiple nuclear membrane–associated small nucleoli (Fig. 10-11), whereas the immunoblastic variants display a single centrally located prominent nucleolus in most of the cells (Fig. 10-13). The anaplastic variant morphologically can be confused with a poorly differentiated carcinoma.

DLBCL arising (*transformation*) from MALT has been reported.[34,35] Most such cases were based on the coexistence of both low-grade MALT lymphoma and DLBCL.[36] Since primary gastric DLBCL can arise from preexisting MALT lymphoma (and can overgrow the underlying low grade component), it is not known how many of these are actually de novo or are the result of transformation. Although the clinical behaviors of these two lymphomas are similar, differentiating de novo DLBCL from large B-cell transformation of MALT lymphoma is important, since there are reports that large B-cell lymphoma transformed from-low grade MALT lymphoma can benefit from treatment of *H. pylori* infection.[28,29] Practically, if there is a coexisting low-grade component, DLBCL may be considered a large cell transformation of MALT lymphoma.[36] However, it remains unresolved whether a de novo DLBCL and a low-grade MALT lymphoma can coexist. The presence of LELs has been used to differentiate high-grade MALT lymphoma from de novo DLBCL.[37] However, this approach may be limited in practice by the small amount of biopsied tissue. While CD10- and BCL2-positivity favor de novo DLBCL,[38] CD10- and BCL2-negativity, commonly seen in large B-cell transformation

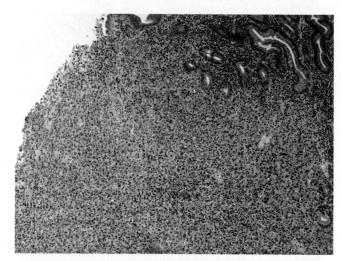

FIGURE 10-10 Primary gastric diffuse large B-cell lymphoma (medium power). The lamina propria is diffusely infiltrated by a population of large atypical lymphoid cells with destruction of gastric glands. Since lymphoma cells have more abundant cytoplasm, the infiltrate appears less dense than MALT lymphoma.

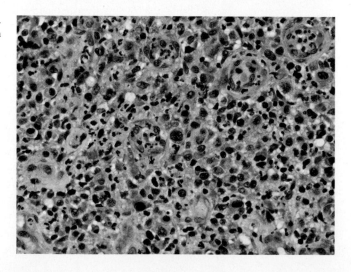

FIGURE 10-11 DLBCL (high power). Scattered large atypical lymphoid cells in a background of severe inflammation.

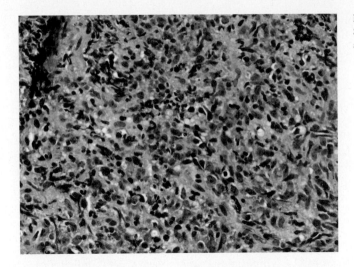

FIGURE 10-12 DLBCL (high power). Sheets of large atypical cells with occasional eosinophils.

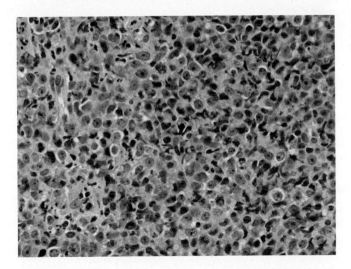

FIGURE 10-13 DLBCL (high power). Sheets of large lymphoid cells with immunoblastic morphology.

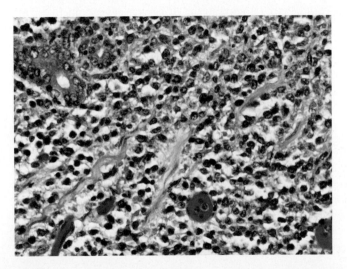

FIGURE 10-14 DLBCL (high power). Because of processing artifact, infiltrating large B cells may occasionally appear small. However, abundant cytoplasm (clear space) and vesicular nuclei feature them as large cells.

of MALT lymphoma, cannot completely exclude de novo DLBCL. Presence of the same *IGH* rearrangement in both the large B cells and the coexisting low-grade component is the most convincing evidence that the large B-cell lymphoma results from the progression of the MALT lymphoma.[36]

PRIMARY GASTRIC MANTLE CELL LYMPHOMA

Although MCL often presents in the lower GI as "lymphomatous polyposis,"[39] primary gastric MCL can be seen. The cells of MCL are small or medium-sized and usually have an irregular nuclear contour. Compared to MALT lymphoma cells, these cells are more monotonous in morphology, with rare or absent plasma cells. Larger cells (centroblast-like or immunoblast-like) are absent. Mitotic figures are often seen, which is almost always absent in MALT lymphoma. The cells of MCL are typically CD19+ and CD20+ and aberrantly express CD5 and cyclin D1. They also can be CD43+ and CD5−.[40] Cyclin D1 positivity and t(11;14)(q13;q32) (which results in overexpression of *CCND1* mRNA/protein) are required for the diagnosis, as well as the differential diagnosis from MALT lymphoma. Primary gastric MCL may follow a similar clinical course as the nodal MCL, which has a median survival of 3 to 5 years and mostly is incurable.

PRIMARY GASTRIC FOLLICULAR LYMPHOMA

Follicular lymphoma is a neoplasm of follicular center B cells (centrocytes and centroblasts). Primary gastric follicular lymphoma is very rare and most follicular lymphomas diagnosed in stomach represent secondary involvement. When the lymphoid follicles in the MALT increase in number and become crowded, a neoplasm should be suspected. The neoplastic follicles typically lose polarity and have ill-defined mantle zones or a lack of tingible-body macrophages. Immunostaining for BCL2 is most helpful in distinguishing follicular lymphoma from hyperplasia. The neoplastic cells are heterogeneous, with mixed small centrocytes and large centroblasts. The nuclei of most cells characteristically are cleaved. The cells are CD19+, CD20+, CD10+, BCL6+, and BCL2+ and are negative for CD5, CD43, and cyclin D1.[41] When the neoplastic cells diffusely infiltrate the interfollicular regions, follicular lymphoma can mimic MALT lymphoma, with parafollicular monocytoid B cells and remarkable LELs.[42] When it occurs, CD10- and BCL6-positivity help to distinguish follicular lymphoma from MALT lymphoma. The translocation t(14;18) (q32;q21), which is considered specific for nodal follicular lymphoma, has also been detected in 38% of ocular adnexal MALT lymphoma.[43] However, the chromosomal breakpoint at 18q21 in MALT lymphoma involves the *MALT1* gene,[43] rather than the *BCL2* gene, as in follicular lymphoma. Interestingly, to date the t(14;18)(q32;q21) (involving either *BCL2* or *MALT1*) has not been identified in either primary gastric follicular lymphoma or gastric MALT lymphoma. Due to the rarity of primary gastric follicular lymphoma, there are sparse data on its natural history and patient survival. Its natural history may be similar to that of the nodal follicular lymphoma, with low-grade cases being indolent but high-grade cases having a more aggressive clinical course.

PRIMARY GASTRIC T-CELL LYMPHOMAS

Primary gastric T-cell lymphoma (PGTCL) is a rare condition with only five examples recognized in a series of 398 PGLs.[11] Yet, it ought to be considered in the differential diagnosis of all PGLs, in particular MALT lymphoma.[44] Since T-cell lymphoma cells are small and often have clear cytoplasm, PGTCL can mimic MALT lymphoma morphologically (Fig. 10-15A). Although LELs are considered relatively specific for MALT lymphoma,[37] they can be seen in T-cell lymphoma as well (Fig. 10-15B). Occasional large cell transformation can be observed as well

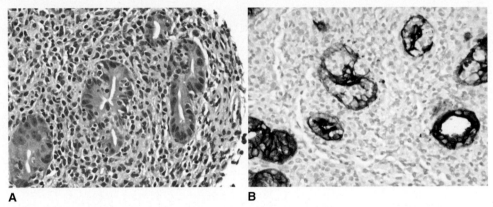

FIGURE 10-15 Primary gastric T-cell lymphoma with LELs (high power). **A:** H&E stain. **B:** Immunoperoxidase stain for pancytokeratin.

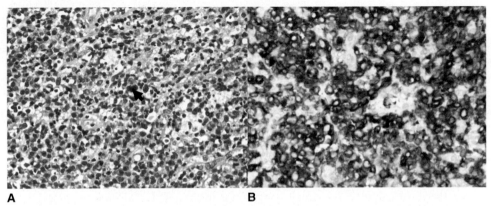

FIGURE 10-16 Primary gastric T-cell lymphoma (high power). **A:** Large neoplastic cell (indicated by an *arrow*) in a background of small neoplastic T cells and scattered eosinophils (H&E stain). **B:** Immunoperoxidase stain for CD3.

(Fig. 10-16A). A T-cell immunophenotype (Fig. 10-16B) can easily distinguish this entity from MALT lymphoma. Based on the immunophenotypes, PGTCL has been classified into two major subtypes: (1) helper/inducer T-cell subtype and (2) cytotoxic/suppressor T-cell subtype (Table 10-6). The latter may have originated from the CD103+ intraepithelial lymphocytes that also give rise to the enteropathy-associated T-cell lymphoma.[44] PGTCL is an aggressive peripheral T-cell lymphoma usually requiring systemic chemotherapy with or without radiotherapy, followed by stem cell transplantation. Based on one study of five patients with localized gastric T-cell lymphoma,[45] the median progression-free survival and median overall survival are 53 months and 123 months, respectively.

IMMUNODEFICIENCY-ASSOCIATED LYMPHOMA

Immunodeficiency-associated lymphoma has become a distinct entity in recent years. This group of lymphomas is mostly found in patients with acquired immunodeficiency syndrome (AIDS), status post organ transplantation, iatrogenic or congenital immunodeficiency. The majority of these cases are driven by Epstein-Barr virus as a consequence of compromised immunosurveillance. They are almost exclusively aggressive B-cell lymphomas: DLBCL and Burkitt lymphoma.[46] The lymphoma cells frequently appear monotonous and have high proliferation indices (numerous mitotic figures) and associated tumor necrosis. The atypical morphology may cause difficulty in accurate classification of these lymphomas. FISH analysis for c-*MYC* rearrangement

Table 10-6	Classification of PGTCLs	
Subtypes	Helper/Inducer	Cytotoxic/Suppressor
CD3	+	+
CD4	+	−
CD8	−	±
CD56	−	±
CD103	−	+
Granzyme B	−	+
TIA-1	±	+

TIA-1, T-cell intracellular antigen 1.

is helpful in identifying atypical Burkitt lymphoma. Some lymphomas in transplant patients can regress if immunosuppressants are withdrawn, whereas Burkitt lymphoma and aggressive large B-cell lymphoma usually require aggressive clinical management. However, withdrawal of immunosuppressants can lead to remission of lymphoma in posttransplant patients, whereas HAART therapy can improve the overall survival of HIV-infected patients. Since this group of diseases is quite heterogeneous, the clinical courses vary from only limited in the low-grade MALT lymphoma to rapidly progressive in Burkitt lymphoma.

SUMMARY

PGLs are the most common malignant lymphomas in the GI tract. Diagnosis of gastric cancers should always include PGL in the differential diagnosis. The most common PGLs are MALT lymphoma and gastric DLBCL, which comprise >95% of all the PGLs. Although LELs are the most characteristic morphologic feature of MALT lymphoma, occasional mimics of MALT lymphoma are seen. Since *H. pylori* infection plays an important role in the development of PGLs, its eradication by antibiotics could lead to protracted remission of *H. pylori*–associated gastric MALT lymphoma. However, multiple genetic abnormalities have been identified in MALT lymphomas, and the t(11;18)(q21;q21) is particularly associated with the resistance to *H. pylori* therapy. Radiotherapy is preferred for the localized low-grade lymphomas that are resistant to eradication of *H. pylori*. For cases of de novo DLBCL, large B-cell lymphoma transformed from MALT lymphoma, and rarely peripheral T-cell lymphoma, combination therapy is warranted.

References

1. Ferrucci PF, Zucca E. Primary gastric lymphoma pathogenesis and treatment: what has changed over the past 10 years? *Br J Haematol.* 2007;136:521–538.
2. d'Amore F, Brincker H, Grønbaek K, et al. Non-Hodgkin's lymphoma of the gastrointestinal tract: a population-based analysis of incidence, geographic distribution, clinicopathologic presentation features, and prognosis. Danish Lymphoma Study Group. *J Clin Oncol.* 1994;12:1673–1684.
3. Isaacson PG, Du MQ. MALT lymphoma: from morphology to molecules. *Nat Rev Cancer.* 2004;4: 644–653.
4. Isaacson PG, Du MQ. Gastrointestinal lymphoma: where morphology meets molecular biology. *J Pathol.* 2005;205:255–274.

5. Li Z, Wang H, Xue L, et al. Emu-BCL10 mice exhibit constitutive activation of both canonical and noncanonical NF-kappaB pathways generating marginal zone (MZ) B-cell expansion as a precursor to splenic MZ lymphoma. *Blood.* 2009;114:4158–4168.

6. Nakamura S, Aoyagi K, Furuse M, et al. B-cell monoclonality precedes the development of gastric MALT lymphoma in *Helicobacter pylori*-associated chronic gastritis. *Am J Pathol.* 1998;152:1271–1279.

7. Hockey MS, Powell J, Crocker J, et al. Primary gastric lymphoma. *Br J Surg.* 1987;74:483–487.

8. Doglioni C, Wotherspoon AC, Moschini A, et al. High incidence of primary gastric lymphoma in northeastern Italy. *Lancet.* 1992;339:834–835.

9. Liu C, Crawford JM. The gastrointestinal tract. In: Kumar, et al. eds. *Robbins and Cotran pathologic basis of disease.* 7th ed. Philadelphia, PA: Elsevier; 2005:797.

10. Ferreri AJ, Montalbán C. Primary diffuse large B-cell lymphoma of the stomach. *Crit Rev Oncol Hematol.* 2007;63:65–71.

11. Koch P, Probst A, Berdel WE, et al. Treatment results in localized primary gastric lymphoma: data of patients registered within the German multicenter study (GIT NHL 02/96). *J Clin Oncol.* 2005;23:7050–7059.

12. Isaacson P, Wright DH. Malignant lymphoma of mucosa-associated lymphoid tissue. A distinctive type of B-cell lymphoma. *Cancer.* 1983;52:1410–1416.

13. Wotherspoon AC, Ortiz-Hidalgo C, Falzon MR, et al. *Helicobacter pylori*-associated gastritis and primary B-cell gastric lymphoma. *Lancet.* 1991;338:1175–1176.

14. Wotherspoon AC, Doglioni C, Diss TC, et al. Regression of primary low-grade B-cell gastric lymphoma of mucosa-associated lymphoid tissue type after eradication of *Helicobacter pylori*. *Lancet.* 1993;342:575–577.

15. Hummel M, Oeschger S, Barth TF, et al. Wotherspoon criteria combined with B cell clonality analysis by advanced polymerase chain reaction technology discriminates covert gastric marginal zone lymphoma from chronic gastritis. *Gut.* 2006;55:782–787.

16. Piris MA, Rivas C, Morente M, et al. Monocytoid B-cell lymphoma, a tumour related to the marginal zone. *Histopathology.* 1988;12:383–392.

17. Okada Y, Mori H, Maeda T, et al. Autopsy case of lymphoplasmacytic lymphoma with a large submucosal tumor in the stomach. *Pathol Int.* 2001;51:802–806.

18. Ye H, Chuang SS, Dogan A, et al. t(1;14) and t(11;18) in the differential diagnosis of Waldenström's macroglobulinemia. *Mod Pathol.* 2004;17:1150–1154.

19. Levine EG, Arthur DC, Machnicki J, et al. Four new recurring translocations in non-Hodgkin lymphoma. *Blood.* 1989;74:1796–1800.

20. Dierlamm J, Baens M, Wlodarska I, et al. The apoptosis inhibitor gene API2 and a novel 18q gene, MLT, are recurrently rearranged in the t(11;18)(q21;q21) associated with mucosa-associated lymphoid tissue lymphomas. *Blood.* 1999;93:3601–3609.

21. Auer IA, Gascoyne RD, Connors JM, et al. t(11;18)(q21;q21) is the most common translocation in MALT lymphomas. *Ann Oncol.* 1997;8:979–985.

22. Wotherspoon AC, Soosay GN, Diss TC, et al. Low-grade primary B-cell lymphoma of the lung. An immunohistochemical, molecular, and cytogenetic study of a single case. *Am J Clin Pathol.* 1990;94:655–660.

23. Willis TG, Jadayel DM, Du MQ, et al. Bcl10 is involved in t(1;14)(p22;q32) of MALT B cell lymphoma and mutated in multiple tumor types. *Cell.* 1999;96:35–45.

24. Zhang Q, Siebert R, Yan M, et al. Inactivating mutations and overexpression of BCL10, a caspase recruitment domain-containing gene, in MALT lymphoma with t(1;14)(p22;q32). *Nat Genet.* 1999;22:63–68.

25. Du M, Peng H, Singh N, et al. The accumulation of p53 abnormalities is associated with progression of mucosa-associated lymphoid tissue lymphoma. *Blood.* 1995;86:4587–4593.

26. Neumeister P. Deletion analysis of the p16 tumor suppressor gene in gastrointestinal mucosa-associated lymphoid tissue lymphomas. *Gastroenterology.* 1997;112:1871–1875.

27. Huang Q, Ai L, Zhang ZY, et al. Promoter hypermethylation and protein expression of the p16 gene: analysis of 43 cases of B-cell primary gastric lymphomas from China. *Mod Pathol.* 2004;17:416–422.

28. Bayerdörffer E, Neubauer A, Rudolph B, et al. Regression of primary gastric lymphoma of mucosa-associated lymphoid tissue type after cure of *Helicobacter pylori* infection. MALT Lymphoma Study Group. *Lancet.* 1995;345:1591–1594.

29. Montalban C, Santon A, Boixeda D, et al. Regression of gastric high grade mucosa associated lymphoid tissue (MALT) lymphoma after *Helicobacter pylori* eradication. *Gut.* 2001;49:584–587.

30. Liu H, Ruskon-Fourmestraux A, Lavergne-Slove A, et al. Resistance of t(11;18) positive gastric mucosa-associated lymphoid tissue lymphoma to *Helicobacter pylori* eradication therapy. *Lancet.* 2001;357(9249):39–40.

31. Montalban C, Norman F. Treatment of gastric mucosa-associated lymphoid tissue lymphoma: *Helicobacter pylori* eradication and beyond. *Expert Rev Anticancer Ther.* 2006;6:361–371.

32. Martinelli G, Laszlo D, Ferreri AJ, et al. Clinical activity of rituximab in gastric marginal zone non-Hodgkin's lymphoma resistant to or not eligible for anti-*Helicobacter pylori* therapy. *J Clin Oncol.* 2005;23:1979–1983.

33. Stathis A, Chini C, Bertoni F, et al. Long-term outcome following *Helicobacter pylori* eradication in a retrospective study of 105 patients with localized gastric marginal zone B-cell lymphoma of MALT type. *Ann Oncol.* 2009;20:1086–1093.

34. Chan JK, Ng CS, Isaacson PG. Relationship between high-grade lymphoma and low-grade B-cell mucosa-associated lymphoid tissue lymphoma (MALT lymphoma) of the stomach. *Am J Pathol.* 1990;136:1153–1164.

35. Montalban C, Manzanal A, Castrillo JM, et al. low-grade gastric B-cell MALT lymphoma progressing into high-grade lymphoma. Clonal identity of the two stages of the tumour, unusual bone involvement and leukemic dissemination. *Histopathology.* 1995;27:89–91.

36. Chan JK, Ng CS, Isaacson PG. Relationship between high-grade lymphoma and low-grade B-cell mucosa-associated lymphoid tissue lymphoma (MALToma) of the stomach. *Am J Pathol.* 1990;136:1153–1164.

37. Hsi ED, Eisbruch A, Greenson JK, et al. Classification of primary gastric lymphomas according to histologic features. *Am J Surg Pathol.* 1998;22:17–27.

38. Villuendas R, Piris MA, Orradre JL, et al. Different bcl-2 protein expression in high-grade B-cell lymphomas derived from lymph node or mucosa-associated lymphoid tissue. *Am J Pathol.* 1991;139:989–993.

39. Cornes JS. Multiple lymphomatous polyposis of the gastrointestinal tract. *Cancer.* 1961;14:249–257.

40. Raderer M, Püspök A, Birkner T, et al. Primary gastric mantle cell lymphoma in a patient with long standing history of Crohn's disease. *Leuk Lymphoma.* 2004;45:1459–1462.

41. Goodlad JR, MacPherson S, Jackson R, et al. Extranodal follicular lymphoma: a clinicopathological and genetic analysis of 15 cases arising at non-cutaneous extranodal sites. *Histopathology.* 2004;44:268–276.

42. Tzankov A, Hittmair A, Müller-Hermelink HK, et al. Primary gastric follicular lymphoma with parafollicular monocytoid B-cells and lymphoepithelial lesions, mimicking extranodal marginal zone lymphoma of MALT. *Virchows Arch.* 2002;441:614–617.

43. Streubel B, Lamprecht A, Dierlamm J, et al. T(14;18)(q32;q21) involving IGH and MALT1 is a frequent chromosomal aberration in MALT lymphoma. *Blood.* 2003;101:2335–2339.

44. Holanda D, Zhao MY, Rapoport AP, et al. Primary gastric T cell lymphoma mimicking marginal zone B cell lymphoma of mucosa-associated lymphoid tissue. *J Hematop.* 2008;1:29–35.

45. Park YH, Kim WS, Bang S-M, et al. Primary gastric T-cell lymphoma: clinicopathologic features and treatment outcome. *Blood (ASH Annual Meeting Abstracts).* 2005;106: Abstract 3355.

46. Ho-Yen C, Chang F, van der Walt J, et al. Gastrointestinal malignancies in HIV-infected or immunosuppressed patients: pathologic features and review of the literature. *Adv Anat Pathol.* 2007;14:431–443.

47. Willis TG, Jadayel DM, Du MQ, et al. BCL10 is involved in t(1; 14)(p22; q32) of MALT B-cell lymphoma and mutated in multiple tumour types. *Cell.* 1999;96:35–45.

48. Achuthan R, Bell SM, Carr IM, et al. BCL10 in malignant lymphomas–an evaluation using fluorescence in situ hybridization. *J Pathol.* 2002;196:59–66.

49. Liang R, Chan WP, Kwong YL, et al. High incidence of BCL-6 gene rearrangement in diffuse large B-cell lymphoma of primary gastric origin. *Cancer Genet Cytogenet.* 1997;97:114–118.

50. Chen YW, Liang AC, Au WY, et al. Multiple BCL6 translocation partners in individual cases of gastric lymphoma. *Blood.* 2003;102(5):1931–1932; author reply 1932.

51. Ott G, Katzenberger T, Greiner A, et al. The t(11;18)(q21;q21) chromosome translocation is a frequent and specific aberration in low-grade but not high-grade malignant non-Hodgkin's lymphomas of the mucosa-associated lymphoid tissue (MALT-) type. *Cancer Res.* 1997;57:3944–3948.

52. Zhang Q, Siebert R, Yan M, et al. Inactivating mutations and overexpression of BCL10, a caspase recruitment domain-containing gene, in MALT lymphoma with t(1;14)(p22;q32). *Nat Genet.* 1999;22(1):63–68.

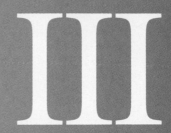

III

Endoscopy and Emerging Techniques

Correlation of Endoscopy with Histopathology in Gastric Neoplasm

11

▶ Michio Shimizu

▶ Hiroto Kita

▶ Koji Nagata

INTRODUCTION

Conventional (white light) endoscopy and endoscopically directed biopsies of the upper gastrointestinal tract are routinely performed in gastroenterology units. In practice, the biopsy sampling is obtained on the basis of gross morphological changes, so that the pathological diagnosis is directed by the endoscopic findings. Generally speaking, gastric lesions are endoscopically divided into two broad types: elevated and depressed. The differential diagnosis of elevated lesions is broad and includes polyps (fundic gland and hyperplastic), polypoid dysplasia (i.e., adenoma), adenocarcinoma, and protruding submucosal tumor (e.g., carcinoid). Depressed lesions encompass benign erosion, ulcer, and scar (from previous ulceration) and malignant processes (e.g., adenocarcinoma and malignant lymphoma).

The endoscopic appearance of early gastric cancer is variable: poorly differentiated type adenocarcinoma (the so-called undifferentiated type) tends to present as a depressed lesion, but the well to moderately differentiated type (the so-called differentiated-type adenocarcinoma) can present as either a protruding lesion or a depressed lesion.[1,2] Further evaluation of the lesions includes assessment of shape, color, contour, margin, and size, all characteristics that help define the diagnosis. However, conventional endoscopy is limited by the detection of lesions on the basis of gross findings under direct vision; for example, the margin of depressed lesions is sometimes difficult to identify. Instead, chromoendoscopy, that is, the use of stains or dyes such as indigo carmine, improves the visualization and characterization of lesions.[3,4] In particular, it highlights and improves identification of 0-II type (depressed type) lesions that may not be otherwise discernible.[5–7] However, Western endoscopists rarely appreciate the routine use of chromoendoscopy.

Magnification endoscopy (or "magnifying endoscopy") and NBI play an especially important role in the diagnosis of gastric lesions.[8–10] These methods in particular allow precise evaluation of the microsurface structure and microvascular architecture of the mucosa that are closely related to pathological findings. Therefore, understanding the pathological findings becomes even more important for endoscopic diagnosis of gastric lesions.

Recent technical progress has expanded the use of endoscopy as not only a diagnosis modality but also a therapeutic modality. EMR and ESD are now performed as alternatives to surgery for the treatment of both premalignant lesions and carcinomas limited to the mucosa.[11,12] This chapter focuses on these new endoscopic techniques and the correlation between endoscopic and pathologic findings in commonly diagnosed gastric neoplasms. The readers are referred to each individual chapter for in-depth pathologic review of the various entities covered herein.

NEW ENDOSCOPIC TECHNIQUES

Magnification Endoscopy and Narrow-Band Imaging

Magnification endoscopy is very useful for detecting subtle mucosal lesions, including early stage gastric neoplasm. Practically, however, the best strategy is first to perform conventional endoscopy to detect any mucosal lesion. When an abnormality is found, visualization of the lesion is zoomed up to maximal magnification. Magnification endoscopy will enable the determination of whether the lesion is neoplastic, and its extent.

The findings of magnification endoscopy are based mainly on the evolution of microsurface structure and microvascular architecture. By white light alone, only the microvascular architecture can be identified, but with NBI, both the microsurface and microvascular architectures can be observed. NBI takes advantage of an intrinsic contrast agent, hemoglobin, to highlight the superficial microvascular anatomy. In recently developed endoscopes, it is easy to change the level of structure enhancement, and the light source can be changed from white light imaging to NBI by using switches on the scope.[13,14]

Magnification endoscopic findings in the normal stomach differ by location. The body mucosa reveals a honeycomb-like subepithelial capillary network pattern with collecting venules, while normal antral mucosa demonstrates a coil-shaped subepithelial capillary network pattern without any collecting venules. The microsurface structure also is variable; the openings of crypts in the body mucosa are round or oval, whereas the openings of crypts in the antrum display a linear or reticular pattern (Figs. 11-1 and 11-2).[15,16] Magnification endoscopy can identify *Helicobacter pylori*–associated gastritis and intestinal metaplasia. A regular pattern of collecting venules indicates the absence of *H. pylori* infection.[17–20] Using NBI, a fine, bluish-white line that appears on the crests of the epithelial surface/gyri is a good indicator of intestinal metaplasia.[20] The patterns of various neoplasms under magnification endoscopy with NBI are described separately below.

Endoscopic Mucosal Resection and Endoscopic Submucosal Dissection

Pioneered in Japan for treatment of superficial gastric cancers, EMR is now widely used in the West for treatment of Barrett esophagus-related neoplasms as well as uncommon early gastric neoplasms.[21,22] EMR is one of the most recommended procedures for therapy of early gastric cancer because it is noninvasive. In addition, in contrast to other endoluminal techniques (laser, plasma coagulation), EMR does not destroy the epithelium and thus allows collection of the complete specimen for pathological evaluation.[23,24] In EMR, however, mucosa sampling cut using a snare poses a high risk of piecemeal resection for lesions measuring 10 mm or more.[25]

ESD is a more recent technique that uses electrosurgical knives instead of a snare, extending the plane of resection in the deep submucosa. ESD provides more accurate resections of superficial neoplasms than EMR. It is a reliable technique for an *en bloc* resection regardless of the size and location of the lesion. It is also more effective therapeutically.[25]

Whether specimens are obtained through EMR or ESD, the handling is very important for providing optimal pathologic diagnosis. The histological type, the presence or absence of lymphatic and vascular invasion, the depth of invasion, and the status of vertical and lateral margins should be reported precisely.[26] If complete resection is not obtained, additional endoscopic resection or surgical treatment will be needed. The precise procedure of EMR and ESD has been described elsewhere.[25]

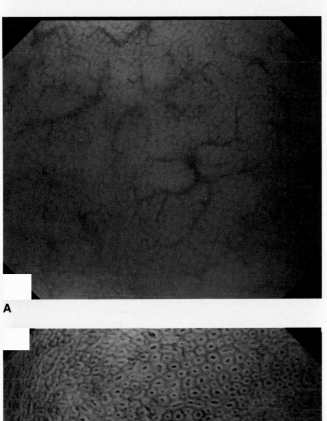

FIGURE 11-1 Magnification endoscopy in normal gastric mucosa. The body shows a honeycomb-like subepithelial capillary network pattern with the collecting venules (**A**). Magnification endoscopy combined with NBI also reveals a round or oval crypt-opening pattern (**B**).

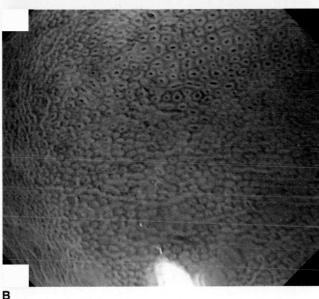

ENDOSCOPIC AND PATHOLOGIC FINDINGS IN REPRESENTATIVE GASTRIC NEOPLASMS

Adenoma

Adenomas account for 7% to 10% of all gastric polyps in most large series.[27] Most are sessile, and pure pedunculated lesions are rare. Under endoscopy, adenoma and carcinoma can produce 0-IIa type gastric lesion (superficial elevated or slightly elevated type).[9] However, a white opaque substance (WOS) noted during magnification endoscopy with NBI is detected more frequently in adenomas than in carcinoma (Fig. 11-3).[9] In addition, WOS shows a regular distribution (*regular* WOS) in adenomas, while it tends to be irregularly distributed (*irregular* WOS) in carcinomas.

FIGURE 11-2 Magnification endoscopy in normal gastric mucosa. The antrum shows a coil-shaped subepithelial capillary network without collecting venules (A). Magnification endoscopy combined with NBI also reveals a linear or reticular crypt-opening pattern (B).

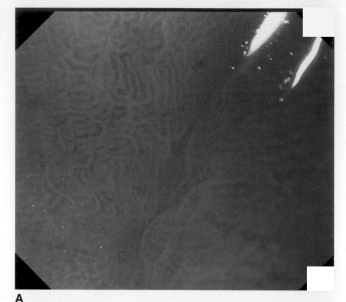

A

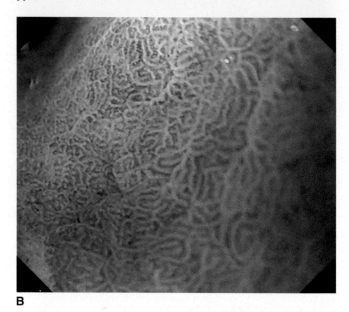

B

Microscopically, two phenotypes are recognized: intestinal type and gastric type.[27] Intestinal type adenomas resemble colorectal adenoma. They are composed of mostly tubular structures that typically reveal a double-layered structure in which the basal half of the mucosa contains cystic tubules (Fig. 11-4). They are characterized by the presence of goblet cells and Paneth cells. Adenomas are considered to be benign; however, malignant transformation occurs in about 2% of lesions measuring under 2 cm, and approximately 50% of lesions larger than 2 cm.[28] Gastric type or foveolar dysplasia is characterized by cuboidal to columnar cells with pale, clear to light eosinophilic cytoplasm and round to oval nuclei. Architecturally, the glands tend to be smaller than in adenomatous dysplasia.

Early Carcinoma

Early gastric cancer is defined as any carcinoma confined to the mucosa (intramucosal carcinoma) and the submucosa, regardless of the presence of lymph node metastasis. Superficial gastric cancers

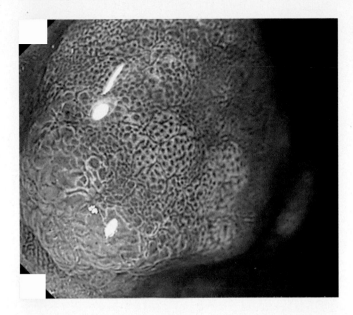

FIGURE 11-3 Magnification endoscopic findings with NBI within an adenoma of superficial elevated type. WOS with a regular distribution is observed.

are curable, with a 5-year survival rate surpassing 90%.[29] Although most early gastric cancers are <2 cm in diameter, larger cases have been described; therefore, the term "early" is not indicative of the size of the lesion.[30] Early gastric carcinomas are categorized into polypoid, superficial, ulcerated, and mixed forms.[31] The Japanese classification of gastric carcinoma organizes early gastric cancer into protruded type (Type I), superficial elevated type (Type IIa), flat type (Type IIb), superficial depressed type (Type IIc) (Figs. 11-5 and 11-6), and excavated type (Type III).[32] This terminology is useful for endoscopic as well as macroscopic findings, which often reveal subtle mucosal features.

By magnification endoscopy, the mucosa of gastric cancer shows an irregular microvascular architecture and/or an irregular microsurface structure distinguishable from chronic gastritis.[13] According to Nakayoshi et al., microvascular patterns of early gastric carcinoma can be classified into three groups: (a) a fine meshlike network pattern, (b) a corkscrew pattern, and (c) an unclassified pattern (Figs. 11-7 and 11-8). In depressed type lesions, differentiated-type carcinomas are more likely to show a fine meshwork pattern, while undifferentiated type carcinomas are more

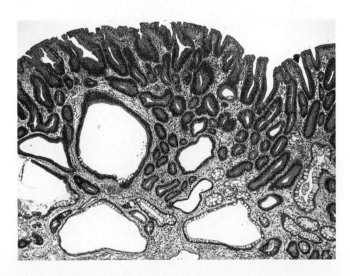

FIGURE 11-4 Histopathology of adenoma. A double-layered structure is observed. The upper half reveals dark staining intraepithelial neoplasia and the lower half shows cystic tubules.

FIGURE 11-5 Conventional endoscopic findings of early gastric cancer (Type IIc). A superficial depressed lesion is observed. Note the irregular border.

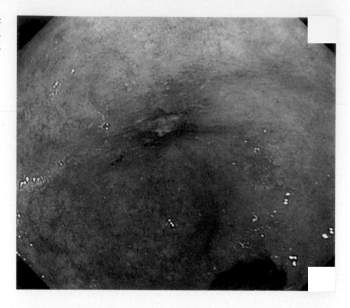

likely to exhibit a corkscrew pattern.[8] Furthermore, the surface pattern of the gastric mucosa can be classified into five types: type I, small round pits of uniform size and shape; type II, slitlike pits; type III, gyrus and villous patterns; type IV, of irregular arrangement and size; and type V, a destructive pattern. According to Tanaka, types IV and V are strongly correlated with a diagnosis of early gastric cancer.[33] Abnormal microvascular or microstructural findings are clinically helpful to distinguish gastritis from superficial cancer and to help determine tumor margins before endoscopy. In one study, Yao et al.[34] reported a diagnostic accuracy of 98.7% using irregular microvascular pattern to distinguish early cancer from gastritis.

Early gastric carcinomas show the same histopathologic patterns as advanced carcinomas (Figs. 11-9 and 11-10). However, mucinous adenocarcinomas are rarely seen among early gastric adenocarcinomas.

FIGURE 11-6 Chromoendoscopy of early gastric cancer (Type IIc). A superficial depressed lesion (unstained area) is clearly visualized by the use of indigo carmine.

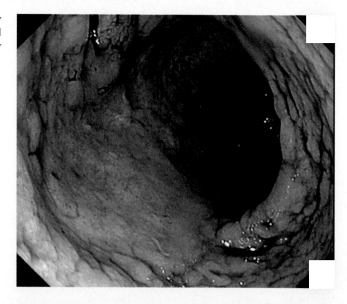

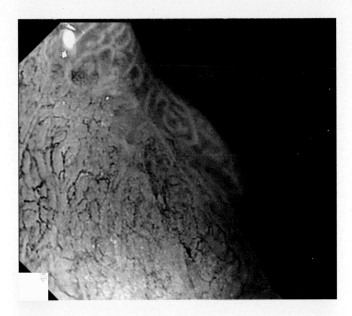

FIGURE 11-7 Microvascular patterns of well-differentiated early gastric carcinoma by magnified endoscopy combined with NBI. A fine meshlike network pattern is noted.

Advanced Carcinoma

Advanced adenocarcinomas penetrate into or beyond the muscularis propria. Macroscopically, they may be divided into an expanding growth pattern and an infiltrating growth pattern. In addition, according to the Japanese classification of gastric carcinoma, they can fall into Type 1 (polypoid tumors, sharply demarcated from the surrounding mucosa, usually resting on a wide base), Type 2 (ulcerated carcinomas with sharply demarcated and raised margins) (Fig. 11-11), Type 3 (ulcerated carcinomas without definite limits, infiltrating into the surrounding wall), Type 4 (diffusely infiltrating carcinomas in which ulceration is usually not a marked feature) (Fig. 11-12), and Type 5 (carcinomas that cannot be classified into any of the above types).[32]

The WHO classification lists microscopic subtypes based on the predominant morphologic component of the carcinoma. These include tubular adenocarcinoma, papillary adenocarcinoma,

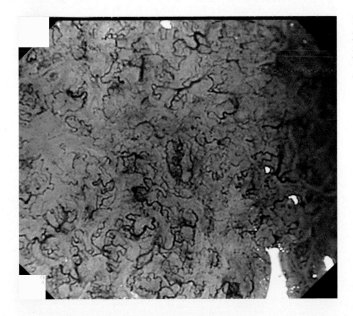

FIGURE 11-8 Microvascular pattern in poorly differentiated early gastric carcinoma using magnified endoscopy combined with NBI. A corkscrew pattern is seen.

FIGURE 11-9 Histopathology of early gastric carcinomas. A well to moderately differentiated tubular adenocarcinoma shows closely packed and cribriform structures (**A**) that invade into the lamina propria (**B**).

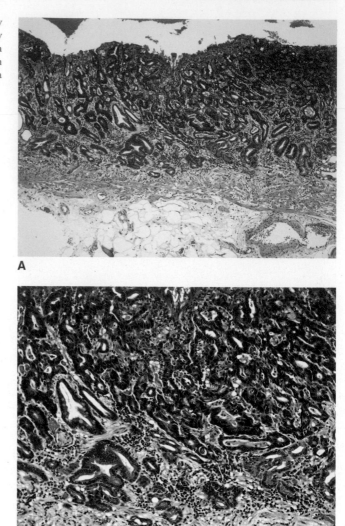

FIGURE 11-10 Histopathology of early gastric carcinomas. A poorly differentiated adenocarcinoma reveals irregular tubular structures and single cells.

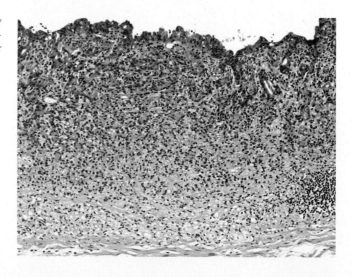

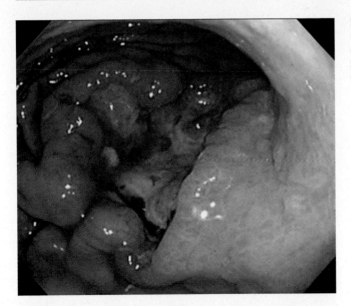

FIGURE 11-11 Advanced gastric cancer (Type 2). Conventional endoscopy shows a tumor with central ulceration. The margin of the tumor is sharply demarcated and raised.

mucinous adenocarcinoma, signet-ring cell carcinoma, adenosquamous carcinoma, squamous cell carcinoma, and undifferentiated carcinoma.[28]

Metastatic Carcinoma

Metastatic carcinomas are rare in the stomach and are found in <2% of autopsied cancer patients.[35] In general, metastatic tumors appear endoscopically as submucosal masses or raised (volcano) ulcerated masses, and multiple lesions can be observed (Fig. 11-13). They can appear as polypoid lesions or ulcerative lesions. Small black mucosal lesions can signify a metastatic melanoma. Breast carcinomas are the most common primary site, followed by malignant melanoma and lung cancer.[36] Breast carcinoma can be especially confusing in biopsy specimens, particularly when it is lobular rather than ductal type.[37,38] In an appropriate clinical setting, a panel of immunohistochemical markers, such as gross cystic disease fluid protein-15, estrogen receptor, and progesterone receptor, is very important to help rule out a primary breast carcinoma.[36–38]

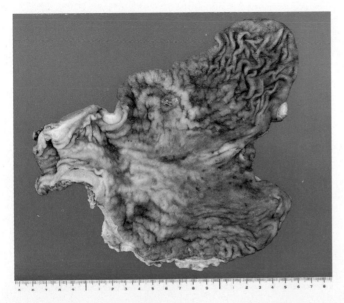

FIGURE 11-12 Resection specimen of advanced gastric cancer (Type 4). Marked thickening of the wall, which suggests the so-called linitis plastica (diffuse infiltrating carcinoma), is observed.

FIGURE 11-13 Metastatic carcinoma. Chromoendoscopy shows multiple submucosal tumors. Microscopically, metastatic mammary carcinoma was confirmed.

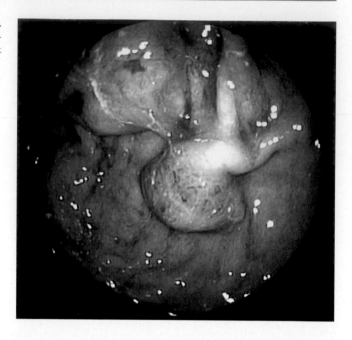

Carcinoid Tumor

The term "carcinoid tumor" recently has been replaced in the WHO classification by "neuroendocrine tumor" or "endocrine tumor."[28,39] Endoscopically, these lesions appear as polypoid or submucosal tumors (Fig. 11-14).[40] They commonly are multiple and can appear as multiple small polypoid lesions studding the body fundic mucosa. Histologically, endocrine tumors of the stomach are classified into (a) carcinoid (well-differentiated endocrine neoplasm), (b) small cell carcinoma (poorly differentiated endocrine neoplasm), and tumorlike lesions (hyperplasia and dysplasia). Typical carcinoids (the most common) show a ribbon or trabecular pattern and are argentaffin-negative but argyrophil-positive (Fig. 11-15).

MALT Lymphoma

Most primary gastric lymphomas are of B-cell origin, and the majority of cases formerly described as pseudolymphoma are now recognized as mucosa-associated lymphoma tissue (MALT)

FIGURE 11-14 Carcinoid tumor. Conventional endoscopy shows a tumor with central ulceration accompanied by a bridging fold.

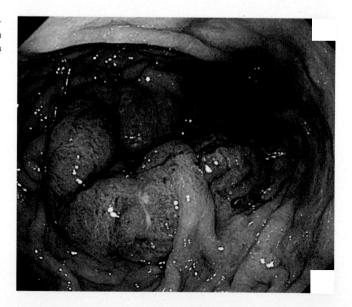

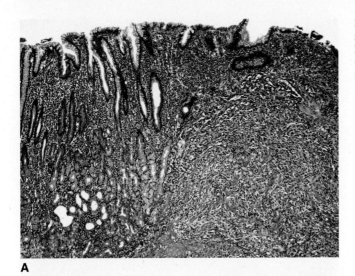

A

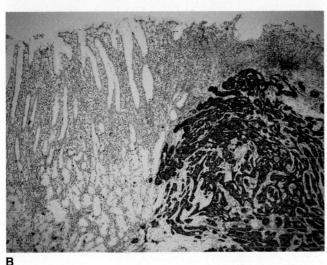

B

FIGURE 11-15 Histopathology of carcinoid tumor. Tumor cells with a trabecular pattern are observed at the right side of the photo (**A**). The tumor cells are immunopositive for chromogranin A (**B**).

lymphoma, which is a low-grade lymphoma. They arise in a background of *H. pylori* infection and may transform to diffuse large B-cell lymphoma.[41]

Endoscopically, MALT lymphoma may present either as an area of erythema, hemorrhage, or nodularity, or as a flat or ulcerated lesion. It also may appear as thickened gastric folds mimicking linitis plastica. Differential diagnoses include erosion, ulcer, gastritis, and carcinoma. In such cases, biopsy is essential, and it is important to take a large number of biopsies in order to reach the correct diagnosis. According to Nonaka et al., one unique finding suggestive of gastric MALT lymphoma is a treelike appearance of the abnormal blood vessels, clearly observed by magnification endoscopy with NBI (Fig. 11-16).[42,43] Recently, findings of gastric mantle cell lymphoma using magnification endoscopy with NBI also have been reported to show disappearance of the surface structure and a treelike appearance of abnormal blood vessels.[44]

Histologically, MALT lymphoma reveals an infiltrate of centrocyte-like cells, follicular colonization, destructive lymphoepithelial lesions, and plasma cell differentiation, including Dutcher bodies (Fig. 11-17).[45] In addition, biopsy specimens from patients with primary gastric lymphoma may show intestinal metaplasia, atrophy, and dysplasia.[46] About 10% of gastric MALT lymphomas are unresponsive to *H. pylori* eradication treatment. In addition, most of these cases contain an API2-MALT1 chimeric transcript mediated by t(11,18)(q21;q21) translocation.[41]

FIGURE 11-16 MALT lymphoma. Magnification endoscopy with NBI shows a treelike appearance of the abnormal blood vessels.

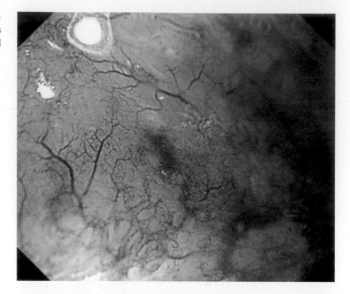

FIGURE 11-17 Histopathology of MALT lymphoma. Atypical lymphoid cells are diffusely infiltrated (**A**). Destructive lymphoepithelial lesions are highlighted by immunohistochemistry with CAM5.2 (**B**).

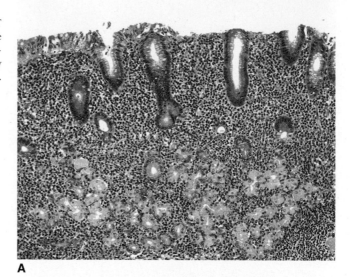

A

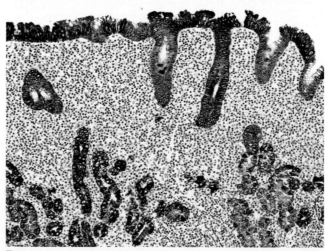

B

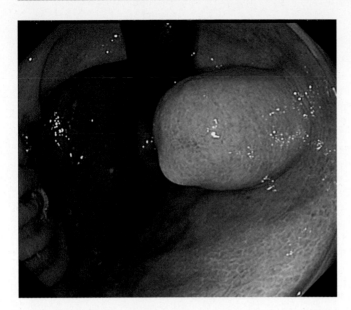

FIGURE 11-18 Gastrointestinal stromal tumor. Conventional endoscopy reveals a submucosal tumor.

Gastrointestinal Stromal Tumor

Gastrointestinal stromal tumors (GISTs) represent the most common gastric mesenchymal neoplasm. Microscopically, most GISTs are spindle cell tumors, and an epithelioid or perinuclear vacuolization pattern may be observed. Mitotic counts and the size of the lesion are important histological markers of malignancy.[47] Most GISTs have gained function mutations of the *KIT* gene and are positive for CD117. The most common mutations are the regulatory juxtamembrane domain (exon 11) of the *c-kit* gene. Less than 10% of GISTs have mutations of the platelet-derived growth factor alpha (PDGFRA) gene, which may be associated with a favorable clinical behavior.[48,49]

Endoscopically, GISTs commonly present as submucosal tumors (Fig. 11-18), and involve the muscularis propria and submucosa. Serosal and intraluminal extension (with mucosal erosion) may occur with large tumors. Luminal polypoid lesions with central mucosal ulceration can be seen. Therefore, differential diagnoses include most of the submucosal tumors. Endoscopic ultrasound (EUS) is a useful adjunct diagnostic tool; however, since it does not evaluate the degree of malignancy, an EUS-guided fine-needle aspiration is frequently conducted.[50,51] Recently, cooperative laparoscopic and endoscopic surgery has been reported for dissection of GIST.[52] In such cases, accurate preoperative EUS and computed tomography staging is cardinal.

SUMMARY

The introduction of magnification endoscopy with NBI has improved the detection of early neoplastic lesions. Using these methods, the microsurface structure and microvascular architecture of the gastric mucosa can be observed easily. In addition, EMR and ESD can be performed as alternatives to surgery for the treatment of early gastric cancers. We have focused on these new endoscopic techniques and discussed the correlation between endoscopic and pathologic findings in representative gastric neoplasms including adenoma, early and advanced gastric cancers, metastatic carcinoma, carcinoid tumor, MALT lymphoma, and GIST. Special attention was paid to the endoscopic findings of magnification endoscopy with NBI. With the recent rapid increase in articles on NBI, we can anticipate further progress in this field.

References

1. Takekoshi T, Baba Y, Ota H, et al. Endoscopic resection of early gastric carcinoma: results of a retrospective analysis of 308 cases. *Endoscopy*. 1994;296:352–358.

2. Maehara Y, Okuyama T, Oshiro T, et al. Early carcinoma of the stomach. *Surg Gynecol Obstet*. 1993;177:593–597.

3. Davila RE. Chromoendoscopy. *Gastrointest Endosc Clin N Am*. 2009;19:193–208.

4. Sakai Y, Eto R, Kasanuki J, et al. Chromoendoscopy with indigo carmine dye added to acetic acid in the diagnosis of gastric neoplasia: a prospective comparative study. *Gastrointest Endosc*. 2008;68:635–641.

5. The Paris endoscopic classification of superficial neoplastic lesions: esophagus, stomach, and colon: November 30 to December 1, 2002. *Gastrointest Endosc*. 2003;58:S3–S43.

6. Endoscopic Classification Review Group. Update on the Paris classification of superficial neoplastic lesions in the digestive tract. *Endoscopy*. 2005;37:570–578.

7. Dinis-Ribeiro M. Chromoendoscopy for early diagnosis of gastric cancer. *Eur J Gastroenterol Hepatol*. 2006;18:831–838.

8. Nakayoshi T, Tajiri H, Matsuda k, et al. Magnifying endoscopy combined with narrow band imaging system for early gastric cancer: correlation of vascular pattern with histopathology. *Endoscopy*. 2004;36:1080–1084.

9. Yao K, Iwashita A, Tanabe H, et al. White opaque substance within superficial elevated gastric neoplasia as visualized by magnification endoscopy with narrow-band imaging: a new optical sign for differentiating between adenoma and carcinoma. *Gastrointest Endosc*. 2008;68:574–580.

10. Gheorghe C. Narrow-band imaging endoscopy for diagnosis of malignant and premalignant gastrointestinal tract. *J Gastrointest Liver Dis*. 2006;15:77–82.

11. Larghi A, Waxman I. Endoscopic mucosal resection: treatment of neoplasia. *Gastrointest Endosc Clin N Am*. 2005;15:431–454.

12. Larghi A, Waxman I. State of the art on endoscopic mucosal resection and endoscopic submucosal dissection. *Gastrointest Endosc Clin N Am*. 2007;17:441–469.

13. Yao K, Takaki Y, Matsui T, et al. Clinical application of magnification endoscopy and narrow-band imaging in the upper gastrointestinal tract: new imaging techniques for detecting and characterizing gastrointestinal neoplasia. *Gastrointest Endoscopy Clin N Am*. 2008;15:415–433.

14. Guelrud M, Ehrlich EE. Enhanced magnification endoscopy in the upper gastrointestinal tract. *Gastrointest Endoscopy Clin N Am*. 2004;14:461–473.

15. Yao K. Gastric microvascular architecture as visualized by magnifying endoscopy: body and antral mucosa without pathologic change demonstrate two different patterns of microvascular architecture. *Gastrointest Endosc*. 2004;59:596–597.

16. Bansal A, Ulusarac O, Mathur S, et al. Correlation between narrow band imaging and nonneoplastic gastric pathology: a pilot feasibility trial. *Gastrointest Endosc*. 2008;67:210–216.

17. Nakagawa S, Kato M, Shimizu Y, et al. Relationship between histopathologic gastritis and mucosal microvascularity: observations with magnifying endoscopy. *Gastrointest Endosc*. 2003;58:71–75.

18. Anagnostopoulos GK, Yao K, Kaye P, et al. High-resolution magnification endoscopy can reliably identify normal gastric mucosa, *Helicobacter pylori*-associated gastritis, and gastric atrophy. *Endoscopy*. 2007;39:202–207.

19. Yagi K, Nakamura A, Sekine A. Comparison between magnifying endoscopy and histological, culture and urease test findings from the gastric mucosa of the corpus. *Endoscopy*. 2002;34:376–381.

20. Uedo N, Ishihara R, Iishi H, et al. A new method of diagnosing gastric intestinal metaplasia: narrow-band imaging with magnifying endoscopy. *Endoscopy*. 2006;38:819–824.

21. Mino-Kenudson M, Hull MJ, Brown I, et al. EMR for Barrett's esophagus-related superficial neoplasms offers better prognostic reproducibility than mucosal biopsy. *Gastrointest Endosc*. 2007;66:660–666.

22. Soetikno R, Kaltenbach T, Yeh R, et al. Endoscopic mucosal resection for early cancers of the upper gastrointestinal tract. *J Clin Oncol*. 2005;23:4490–4498.

23. Ponchon T. Endoscopic mucosal resection. *J Clin Gastroenterol*. 2001;32:6–10.

24. Conio M, Ponchon T, Blanchi S, et al. Endoscopic mucosal resection. *Am J Gastroenterology*. 2006;101:653–663.

25. Yamamoto H, Kita H. Endoscopic therapy of early gastric cancer. *Best Pract Res Clin Gastroenterol*. 2005;19:909–926.

26. Lauwers GY, Ban S, Mino M, et al. Endoscopic mucosal resection for gastric epithelial neoplasms: as study of 39 cases with emphasis on the evaluation of specimens and recommendations for optimal pathologic analysis. *Mod Pathol.* 2004;17:2–8.

27. Abraham SC, Montgomery EA, Singh VK, et al. Gastric adenomas: intestinal-type and gastric-type adenomas differ in the risk of adenocarcinoma and presence of background mucosal pathology. *Am J Surg Pathol.* 2002;26:1276–1285.

28. Stanley R, Hamilton R, Aaltonen LA. *World Health Organization Classification of Tumours, Pathology & Genetics, Tumours of the Digestive System.* Lyon, France: IARC press; 2000.

29. Green PH, O'Toole KM, Slonim D, et al. Increasing incidence and excellent survival of patients with early gastric cancer: experience in a United States medical center. *Am J Med.* 1988;85:658–661.

30. Bogomoletz WV. Early gastric cancer. *Am J Surg Pathol.* 1984;8:381–391.

31. Green PH, O'Toole KM, Weinberg LM, et al. Early gastric cancer. *Gastroenterlogy.* 1981;81:247–256.

32. Japanese Gastric Cancer Association. Japanese classification of gastric carcinoma, 2nd English edition. *Gastric Cancer.* 1998;1:10–24.

33. Tanaka K, Toyoda H, Kadowaki S, et al. Surface pattern classification by enhanced-magnification endoscopy for identifying early gastric cancers. *Gastrointest Endosc.* 2008;67:430–437.

34. Yao K, Iwashita A, Tanabe H, et al. Novel zoom endoscopy technique for diagnosis of small flat gastric cancer: a prospective, blind study. *Clin Gastroenterol Hepatol.* 2007;7:869–878.

35. Kanthan R, Sharanowski K, Senger JL, et al. Uncommon mucosal metastases to the stomach. *World J Surg Oncol.* 2009;7:62.

36. Jones GE, Strauss DC, Forshaw MJ, et al. Breast cancer metastasis to the stomach may mimic primary gastric cancer: report of two cases and review of literature. *World J Surg Oncol.* 2007;5:75.

37. Shimizu M, Matsumoto T, Hirokawa M, et al. Gastric metastasis from breast cancer: a pitfall in gastric biopsy specimens. *Pathol Int.* 1998;48:240–241.

38. Taal BG, den Hartog Jager FC, Steinmetz R, et al. The spectrum of gastrointestinal metastases of breast carcinoma: I. Stomach. *Gastrointest Endosc.* 1992;38:130–135.

39. Rindi G, Capella C, Solcia E. Introduction to a revised clinicopathological classification of neuroendocrine tumors of the gastroenteropancreatic tract. *Q J Nucl Med.* 2000;44:13–21.

40. Chuah SK, Hu TH, Kuo CM, et al. Upper gastrointestional carcinoid tumors incidentally found by endoscopic examinations. *World J Gastroenterol.* 2005;11:7028–7032.

41. Nakamura T, Inagaki H, Seto M, et al. Gastric low-grade B-cell MALT lymphoma: treatment, response, and genetic alteration. *J Gastroenterol.* 2003;38:921–929.

42. Nonaka K, Ishikawa K, Shimizu M, et al. Education and imaging. Gastrointestinal: gastric mucosa-associated lymphoma presented with unique vascular features on magnified endoscopy combined with narrow-band imaging. *J Gastroenterol Hepatol.* 2009;24:1697.

43. Isomoto H, Shikuwa S, Yamaguchi N, et al. Magnified endoscopic findings of gastric low-grade mucosa-associated lymphoid tissue lymphoma. *Endoscopy.* 2008;40:225–228.

44. Nonaka K, Ishikawa K, Arai S, et al. Magnifying endoscopic observation of mantle cell lymphoma in the stomach using the narrow-band imaging system. *Endoscopy.* 2010:42(Suppl 2):E94–E95.

45. Chan JK. Gastrointestinal lymphomas: an overview with emphasis on new findings and diagnostic problems. *Semin Diagn Pathol.* 1996;13:260–296.

46. Arista-Nasr J, Herrera-Goepfert R, Lazos-Ochoa M, et al. Histologic changes of the gastric mucosa associated with primary gastric lymphoma in endoscopic biopsy specimens. *Arch Pathol Lab Med.* 2000;124:1628–1631.

47. Fletcher CD, Berman JJ, Corless C, et al. Diagnosis of gastrointestinal stromal tumors: a consensus approach. *Hum Pathol.* 2002;33:459–465.

48. Kwon JE, Kang HJ, Kim SH, et al. Pathological characteristics of gastrointestinal stromal tumours with PDGFRA mutations. *Pathology.* 2009;41:544–554.

49. Braconi C, Bracci R, Bearzi I, et al. KIT and PDGFRalpha mutations in 104 patients with gastrointestinal stromal tumors (GISTs): a population-based study. *Ann Oncol.* 2008;19:706–710.

50. Okubo K, Yamao K, Nakamura T, et al. Endoscopic ultrasound-guided fine-needle aspiration biopsy for the diagnosis of gastrointestinal stromal tumors in the stomach. *J Gastroenterol.* 2004;39:747–753.

51. Sepe PS, Moparty B, Pitman MB, et al. EUS-guided FNA for the diagnosis of GI stromal cell tumors: sensitivity and cytologic yield. *Gastrointest Endosc.* 2009;70:254–261.

52. Hiki N, Yamamoto Y, Fukunaga T, et al. Laparoscopic and endoscopic cooperative surgery for gastrointestinal stromal tumor dissection. *Surg Endosc.* 2008;22:1729–1735.

New Imaging Techniques for the Diagnosis of Early Gastric Cancer and Premalignant Lesions

12

▶ Thomas Paulraj Thamboo

▶ Zhiwei Huang

▶ Ming Teh

INTRODUCTION

The advent of the flexible endoscope has revolutionized gross examination of the stomach and allowed real-time examination of subtle mucosal changes in situ. In practice, this enables directed biopsies of gastric mucosa for early premalignant changes and malignant lesions. Naturally, this has tremendous implications for screening surveillance programs for gastric cancers, as well as for patients on follow-up for conditions predisposing them to the development of gastric malignancies. Also, in endoscopic mucosal resection (EMR) and endoscopic submucosal dissection (ESD)— increasingly the definitive treatment for many early intestinal-type gastric cancers and high-grade dysplasias––careful endoscopic visualization is indispensable in ensuring the lesion is completely excised.

We hope that this chapter's images and descriptions of the different endoscopic modalities can serve as a useful introduction for the practicing GI pathologist to the tremendous advances in endoscopic imaging. Except for Raman spectroscopy, which could conceivably gain greater acceptance in the future, these techniques use conventional images, either "gross" or "microscopic." Notwithstanding the universal acknowledgement that histological analysis remains the diagnostic gold standard and is likely to continue to do so for a very long time, a basic understanding of these endoscopic images, easily accessible from most hospital information systems, can be helpful to the practicing GI pathologist and might just provide the gross-histological or light microscopic-endoscopic correlation that is so necessary in difficult diagnostic situations.

WHITE LIGHT REFLECTANCE ENDOSCOPY (CONVENTIONAL ENDOSCOPY)

White light reflectance forms the basis of conventional endoscopic examination and imaging and continues to be the modality used in most gastroscopic procedures, either on its own or in combination with newer techniques (image-enhanced endoscopy, see below). In white light reflectance endoscopy, white light is channeled to the tip of the endoscope via optical fibers and illuminates the gastric mucosa. Light reflected from the mucosa is received by a lens in the endoscope tip and channeled to a video CCD. This enables real-time video imaging of the mucosa with the ability to obtain a video recording of the procedure, as well as still images of selected fields. More recently, endoscopic magnification techniques have allowed the acquisition of magnified images of the mucosa under white light. Magnifying endoscopy has been shown to be able to identify gastric carcinoma on the basis of changes in the pattern of the gastric pits and mucosal microvasculature.[1-3] Magnifying endoscopy has also been used in conjunction with other techniques that enhance contrast (see below), for detection of intestinal metaplasia and dysplasia.[4-6]

IMAGE ENHANCED ENDOSCOPY

"Image enhanced endoscopy" is a term proposed by the American Gastroenterological Association to describe various means of enhancing contrast during endoscopy, using dye, optical, or electronic methods.[7] These techniques include chromoendoscopy, autofluorescence imaging (AFI) endoscopy, and narrow-band imaging (NBI). Confocal laser endomicroscopy is another technique that allows improved visualization of the mucosa during endoscopy, but this relies on increasing magnification rather than contrast. Other techniques are currently under study as well.

CHROMOENDOSCOPY

Chromoendoscopy, probably the oldest method of image enhancement in endoscopy, involves the application of dyes or stains to the mucosal surface during endoscopy in order to enhance the appearance of mucosal lesions and better differentiate them from surrounding normal mucosa under conventional white light. Staining is performed during the endoscopy procedure, and the stain may be applied to a wide area of the mucosa or targeted on a visible lesion. Contrast stains, such as indigo carmine, tend to concentrate in depressions and crevices in the mucosa, and in so doing, highlight the mucosal surface architecture and topography. Absorptive stains, such as methylene blue, are preferentially taken up by intestinal absorptive cells, which are then highlighted against the rest of the mucosa. Reactive stains, such as Congo red, react chemically with certain substances within cells, giving rise to a color change.

Indigo carmine is the most commonly used contrast stain in gastric chromoendoscopy. It has been used for over 30 years and continues to be shown to improve the endoscopic visualization of gastric neoplasia as compared to white light examination alone.[8] The dye allows visualization of the disordered gross architecture of the mucosa associated with gastric dysplasia and carcinoma (Fig. 12-1). Recently, indigo carmine combined with acetic acid has shown potential to be even more effective than indigo carmine alone in highlighting areas with gastric neoplasia.[8-10]

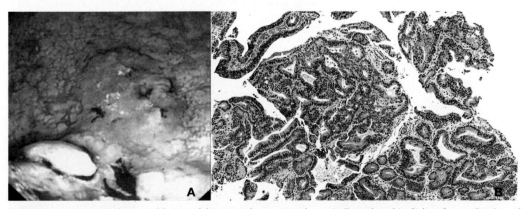

FIGURE 12-1 A: A raised mucosal lesion of the stomach as seen endoscopically under white light, after application of indigo carmine dye. The dye highlights the irregular topography of the lesion. **B:** A biopsy from the lesion showing high-grade dysplasia with areas suspicious for intramucosal carcinoma.

Methylene blue staining has been shown to improve the detection of intestinal metaplasia in the stomach.[4,5,11,12] The dye is applied to the mucosa, followed by irrigation with water. Areas of intestinal metaplasia show persistent blue staining with this technique, while normal non-metaplastic mucosa is not stained. Magnification chromoendoscopy using methylene blue has been shown to be able to detect intestinal metaplasia and dysplasia with an accuracy of 84% and 83%, respectively.[4] Areas of intestinal metaplasia stained blue but maintained a regular mucosal pattern. Areas of dysplasia showed no clear color change but showed loss of the regular mucosal pattern. A more recent study has shown this technique to be reproducible with high specificity (99%) for detection of dysplasia.[13]

AUTOFLUORESCENCE

AFI endoscopy involves illumination of the gastric mucosa with blue (short-wavelength) light that stimulates endogenous substances to fluoresce, that is, to emit visible light of a longer wavelength. These fluorescent substances, also known as fluorophores, vary in their distribution and concentration in different tissue types. Thus, under endoscopy, metaplastic and neoplastic tissue can be identified, as it has different autofluorescent colors compared to normal tissue. These differences can be enhanced by AFI systems to produce real-time images (Fig. 12-2).

AFI endoscopy has been shown to be able to identify gastric neoplasms, including early gastric cancers.[14,15] However, study results are mixed. One study found that for detection of early gastric neoplasia, AFI was less sensitive (68.1%) and specific (23.5%) than white light imaging (sensitivity 76.6%; specificity 84.3%).[16] Another study similarly found AFI to be of limited utility for the diagnosis of gastric neoplasia, with a sensitivity of 96.4% but a specificity of 49.1%.[14] Nonetheless, one study has shown that autofluorescence may be better than white light imaging at detecting the lateral extent of early gastric cancers, especially when these lateral extensions are flat or isochromatic, but was still not as good as chromoendoscopy.[15] AFI in combination with other modalities will likely prove more useful, and a combination of AFI, white light imaging, and NBI (trimodal imaging endoscopy) has been shown to be more sensitive and specific than AFI or white light imaging alone.[16]

NARROW-BAND IMAGING

NBI consists of illuminating the mucosa with selected narrow bands of wavelengths of light. White light from a conventional white light source is passed through narrow band filters to produce narrow bands of blue (centered on 415 nm) and green (centered on 540 nm) light that illuminate the mucosa. These bands of light are reflected by the mucosal surface but are maximally absorbed by hemoglobin within blood vessels. The reflected light from the bands is captured, either sequentially or simultaneously, and analyzed and displayed as an image. The images obtained with NBI

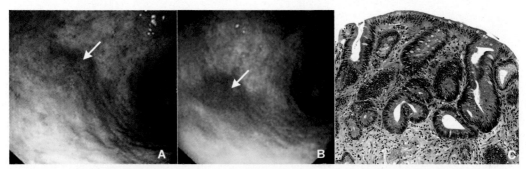

FIGURE 12-2 **A:** White light gastroscopy showing a slightly raised reddish mucosal lesion (*arrow*). **B:** The same lesion seen with autofluorescence imaging (*arrow*). **C:** A biopsy from the lesion showing low-grade dysplasia.

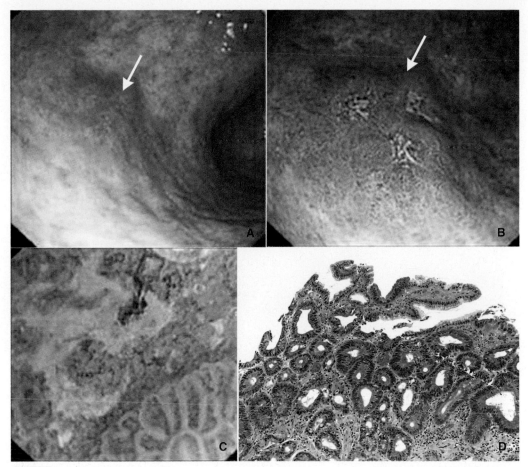

FIGURE 12-3 **A:** A raised mucosal lesion seen on white light gastroscopy (*arrow*). Not much detail of the surface of the lesion is discernible. **B:** With narrow-band imaging (NBI), the lesion appears more clearly defined (*arrow*) and some surface details are seen. **C:** A zoom magnification NBI image of the lesion, showing abnormal mucosal architecture. **D:** A biopsy from the lesion showing low-grade dysplasia.

thus show the mucosa and its vascular network with enhanced contrast. As disease processes alter the mucosal structure and vascular network, these changes allow the identification of preneo-plastic and neoplastic changes (Figs. 12-3 and 12-4). Under NBI, areas with intestinal metaplasia appear to have a light blue crest (blue-white lines on the epithelial surface) (Fig. 12-5).[17] Uedo et al. showed that NBI can demonstrate intestinal metaplasia in the gastric mucosa with a sensitivity and specificity of 89% and 93%, respectively.[17]

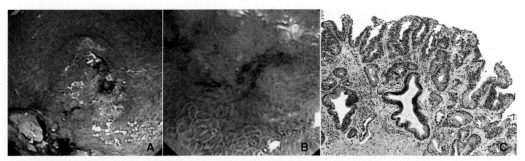

FIGURE 12-4 A raised mucosal lesion seen on NBI endoscopy without magnification (**A**) and with zoom magnification (**B**). The mucosal architecture is clearly abnormal. **C:** A biopsy from the lesion showing high-grade dysplasia.

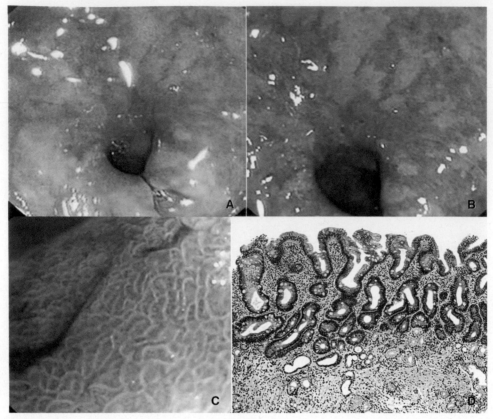

FIGURE 12-5 Areas of intestinal metaplasia in the stomach appearing as poorly defined slightly irregular areas under white light endoscopy (**A**) and as better-defined paler areas with NBI (**B**). Under zoom magnification, areas of intestinal metaplasia show anastomosing crestlike structures with a light blue appearance (*light blue crest*) (**C**). **D:** A biopsy from the lesion showing intestinal metaplasia.

With NBI, superficial gastric cancer shows an irregular microvascular pattern[6,18] and an irregular pattern of the mucosal surface. Three microvascular patterns (fine network; corkscrew and unclassified) are recognized in early gastric cancers with the first two more common in differentiated (tubular) and undifferentiated (discohesive), respectively.[18] However, there is currently no evidence that NBI is superior to magnified white light imaging for the detection of early gastric neoplasms, and prospective controlled trials are lacking.[19,20] Nonetheless, NBI with magnification has been shown to be effective in identifying the lateral extent of superficial gastric cancer,[6] which is useful in guiding EMR or ESD of these lesions.

CONFOCAL LASER ENDOMICROSCOPY

Confocal laser endomicroscopy (CLE) is a technique that enables in vivo visualization of the gastric mucosa at a microscopic level, providing real-time "virtual histology" images. A low-powered laser is transmitted through an optical fiber and focused through a lens onto a point on the mucosa. Light reflected from the illuminated point is focused by the same lens to converge back into the optical fiber (Fig. 12-6). In this way, the illuminating (incident) light and the reflected light detected by the system are in the same focal plane, hence the term "confocal." Light that is reflected back (or scattered) from other points and from other focal planes is rejected. This provides for a sharp, high-resolution optical image representing the tissue in one focal plane only.

Intravenous and topical fluorescence contrast agents that fluoresce under the incident laser light[21] are used in order to achieve high contrast at high resolution. The most commonly used

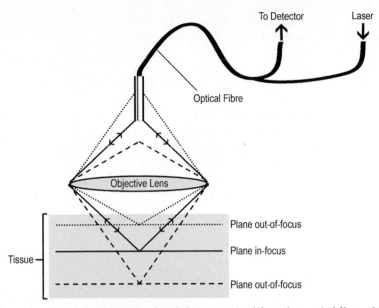

FIGURE 12-6 In confocal laser endomicroscopy, a laser light is transmitted through an optical fiber and focused through a lens on to a point on the mucosa (plane in-focus). Light reflected from the illuminated point is focused by the same lens to converge back into the optical fiber. Light that is reflected back from other planes that are out-of-focus is rejected.

contrast agents are intravenous fluorescein sodium and topically applied acriflavine. Fluorescein binds to albumin in the serum. Unbound fluorescein diffuses into the extracellular fluid and binds to the extracellular matrix. Cell nuclei and mucin are not stained by fluorescein and appear relatively dark.[22] Topical acriflavine stains the nuclei and acidic constituents of mucosal cells to a depth of 100 μm.[22]

At our institution, the Pentax EG-3870CIK (Pentax, Tokyo, Japan) is used. This system comprises a conventional endoscope with a confocal microscope at the tip and uses an incident

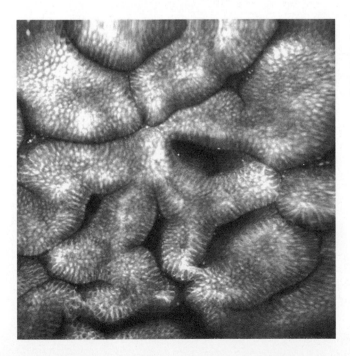

FIGURE 12-7 A confocal laser endomicroscopy image of normal gastric antral mucosa in a superficial plane (near the surface) showing the gastric foveolar pattern. Individual foveolar epithelial cells can be discerned in this image.

488 nm wavelength laser. Images of the mucosa can be obtained by focusing through the mucosa ("virtual sectioning") at 7-μm increments down to a depth of 250 μm. The images obtained by CLE, especially after contrast agents are used, are of a resolution roughly equivalent to a low-power image seen by a pathologist on a conventional microscope. On these images, structures such as foveolae or villi are apparent (Fig. 12-7). The obvious differences from conventional H&E microscopy are that the "sections" of mucosa in CLE are imaged in a horizontal plane (as opposed to vertical H&E sections) and that the images are in gray scale.

CLE imaging of normal gastric mucosa shows small irregular invaginations on the mucosal surface corresponding to the gastric pits, with the surface epithelial cells giving a cobblestone appearance.[23] These images correlate well with the histologic appearance of gastric mucosal biopsies (Fig. 12-8). In a study by Zhang et al.,[24] CLE images of fundic mucosa showed round gastric pits of approximately uniform size and shape, while those of pyloric mucosa showed continuous short rodlike pits with slitlike openings. These appearances were altered in a characteristic way with chronic inflammation. Intestinal metaplasia gives rise to a villuslike appearance on CLE, with interspersed goblet cells appearing as dark cells against the background of gastric foveolar cells[24–26] (Fig. 12-9). CLE has been shown in one study to be able to diagnose gastric intestinal metaplasia with a sensitivity of 98% and a specificity of 95%.[26] CLE has also been shown to be able to identify gastric adenocarcinoma, with CLE images showing a foveolar and glandular pattern that is either disorganized or indiscernible.[24,25,27,28] In the study by Yeoh et al.,[25] the diagnosis of gastric carcinoma could be made with good interobserver agreement by observing architectural atypia, vascular

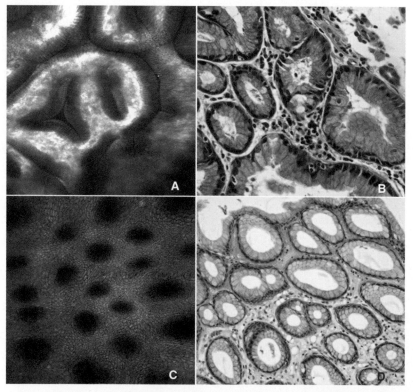

FIGURE 12-8 **A:** A confocal laser endomicroscopy (CLE) image of gastric antral mucosa, at a deeper plane than the image in Figure 12-7. The lamina propria structures are highlighted by intravenous fluorescein sodium used as a contrast agent. The corresponding biopsy (**B**) showed mild chronic gastritis, but no intestinal metaplasia or dysplasia. **C:** A CLE image of gastric fundic mucosa with the foveolae clearly visible and foveolar and surface epithelial cells identifiable, showing good morphologic correlation with the corresponding biopsy (**D**).

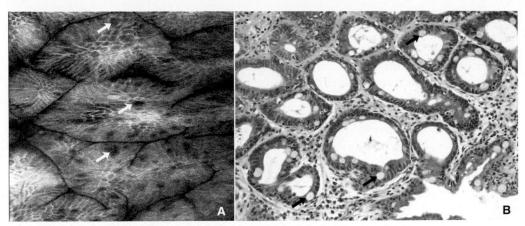

FIGURE 12-9 **A:** A confocal laser endomicroscopy image of gastric mucosa with intestinal metaplasia. The goblet cells appear as scattered dark cells (*arrows*). There is good morphologic correlation with the corresponding mucosal biopsy (**B**).

pattern derangement, increased nuclear-cytoplasmic ratio, chromatin condensation, and the presence of atypical "dark cells." (Fig. 12-10). In the study by Zhang et al.,[24] the normal gastric pit pattern was seen to disappear in cases of gastric carcinoma, with the appearance of atypical glands or cells.

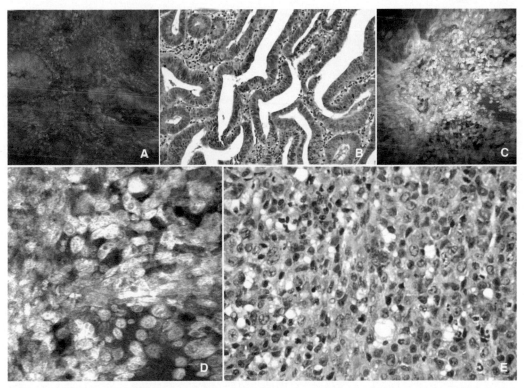

FIGURE 12-10 **A:** A confocal laser endomicroscopy (CLE) image of gastric mucosa with adenocarcinoma. There is obvious alteration of the normal foveolar pattern (compare with Fig. 12-8). However, some glandlike or tubular structures can be identified. The corresponding biopsy (**B**) showed a moderately differentiated adenocarcinoma, intestinal type. **C:** Another case of gastric adenocarcinoma as seen with CLE. In this case, there is total loss of the mucosal architecture, with no foveolar or glandlike structures seen. A higher magnification view (**D**) shows cells with variation in nuclear size and shape. There is good morphologic correlation with the mucosal biopsy (**E**), which showed a poorly differentiated adenocarcinoma, diffuse type.

NEAR-INFRARED RAMAN SPECTROSCOPY

A novel method that in due course may gain acceptance is Raman spectroscopy. Unlike the forms of image-enhanced endoscopy described above, which are in essence morphological methods of detecting subtle differences between normal mucosa and premalignant or early malignant conditions, Raman spectroscopy seeks to identify the molecular changes in tissue associated with cancer transformation by means of a vibrational analytic technique based on the inelastic scattering of laser excitation photons by the molecules of the sample.[29] The difference between the incident and scattered frequencies corresponds to the vibrational modes of molecules participating in the interaction. A two-dimensional diagram (known as a Raman spectrum) depicts the Raman molecular information visually by plotting the intensity of the scattered photons as a function of the frequency shift (Fig. 12-11).[29,30] A Raman spectrum of a given molecule consists of a series of peaks, each shifted by one of the characteristic vibrational frequencies of that molecule.[30] Each molecule has its own characteristic spectrum, and the intensity of a band is proportional to the concentration of the molecule from which the band arises.[30] Thus, the Raman spectrum

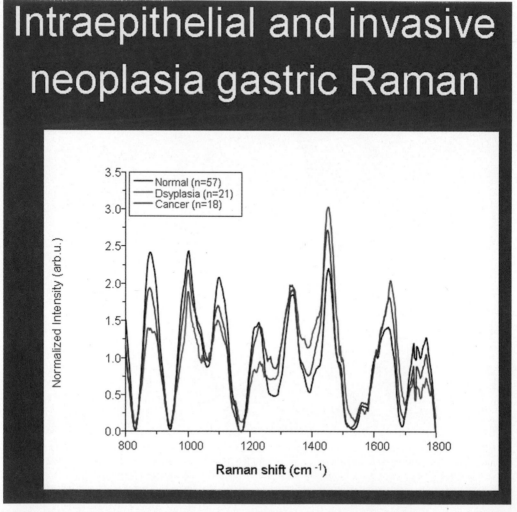

FIGURE 12-11 Comparison of mean Raman spectra acquired from normal ($n = 57$), dysplasia ($n = 21$), and cancer ($n = 18$) gastric tissues.

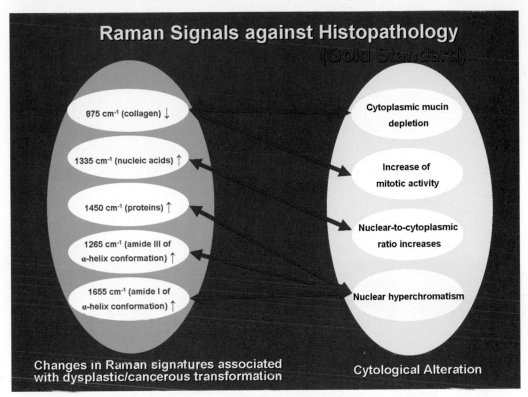

FIGURE 12-12   Correlation between the Raman signals and histopathologic results of gastric tissues.

can provide a "fingerprint" of a substance from which molecular structure and composition can be elucidated.[30] When compared with histopathology, which is the gold standard, there appear to be changes in Raman signatures associated with cytological alterations in dysplasia or cancerous transformations (Fig. 12-12).

With the use of near-infrared (NIR) lasers as excitation light sources, NIR Raman spectroscopy provides unique advantages for probing the molecular information in biological tissues. Water exhibits very low absorption at the working wavelength range, and tissues exhibit far less autofluorescence than with visible light excitation.[31] Less water absorption makes tissue components easy to detect and results in deeper light penetration into the tissue.[31,32] Less autofluorescence reduces the background interference in an already weak Raman signal.[32] As a result, NIR Raman spectroscopy has been widely studied for early detection of preneoplastic and invasive neoplastic tumors in a number of organ sites, including the stomach.[33–38]

Our group has investigated the potential of a rapid fiberoptic Raman system[39] coupled with powerful chemometric algorithms (e.g., principal component analysis, linear discriminant analysis, logistic regression, and classification and regression trees) for *ex vivo* gastric tissue diagnosis during an *en-face* orientation so as to mimic an in vivo clinical situation.[40–44] Raman spectral features related to collagen, histones, nucleic acids, and phospholipids have been found to change significantly with preneoplastic and neoplastic transformation.[41–43] By correlating the Raman biomolecular information, analytic algorithms with high predictive accuracies (~90%) were developed for diagnosis of gastric nonneoplastic lesions (e.g., *Helicobacter pylori* infection and intestinal metaplasia), preneoplasia (i.e., dysplasia) (Fig. 12-13), and neoplasia (e.g., intestinal-type and diffuse-type adenocarcinoma) (Fig. 12-14).[39–43] Our results have affirmed the feasibility of NIR Raman technique for detecting gastric nonneoplasia, preneoplastic tissue, and neoplasia.

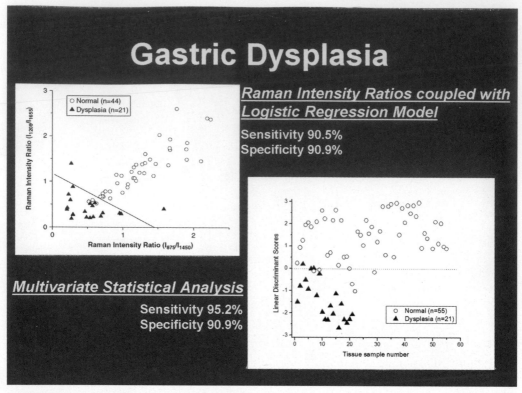

FIGURE 12-13 Raman difference spectrum between normal and dysplastic gastric tissues reveals biochemical/biomolecular changes associated with dysplastic transformation. The multivariate statistical analysis based on PCA-LDA model provides a diagnostic sensitivity of 95.2% and specificity of 90.9% with Raman technique for distinguishing dysplasia from normal gastric tissue.

With the successful *ex vivo* gastric Raman proof-of-concept demonstrations[40–44] and the recent development of a special miniaturized Raman probe (~2 mm) that could be effectively integrated into conventional endoscope (Fig. 12-15),[45] in vivo Raman investigation is currently ongoing for direct assessment of biochemical information of suspicious gastric lesions (e.g., dysplasia and carcinoma in situ) to improve tissue diagnosis during gastroscopic examinations.[46] NIR Raman endoscopic spectroscopy is expected to become a clinically promising tool for the rapid, noninvasive, in vivo diagnosis and detection of gastric precancer and early cancer at the molecular level.

ENDOSCOPIC ULTRASOUND

Endoscopic ultrasound (EUS) has been used to image gastric tumors for over two decades. During that time, EUS technology has improved, and experience with the technique has grown considerably. EUS imaging of the gastric wall allows differentiation of the different layers of the wall and thus is useful in diagnosing submucosal gastric tumors as well as in staging malignant gastric tumors.

The mucosa overlying gastric submucosal tumors, while raised, usually has a fairly normal endoscopic visual appearance. Biopsies from this overlying mucosa usually do not include significant submucosal tissue, and most often give no clue to the underlying lesion. EUS allows identification of submucosal tumors and can guide needle core biopsies or fine needle aspirations of these lesions.

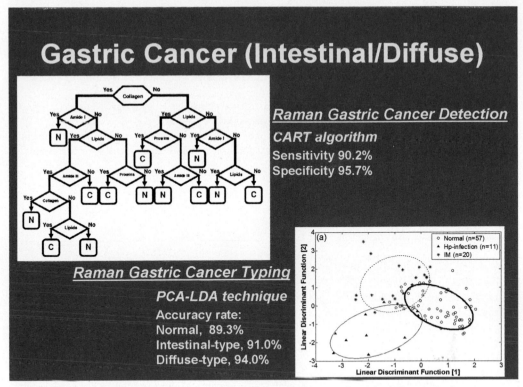

Gastric Cancer (Intestinal/Diffuse)

Raman Gastric Cancer Detection

CART algorithm
Sensitivity 90.2%
Specificity 95.7%

Raman Gastric Cancer Typing

PCA-LDA technique
Accuracy rate:
Normal, 89.3%
Intestinal-type, 91.0%
Diffuse-type, 94.0%

FIGURE 12-14 The classification and regression tree (CART) algorithms developed for differentiation between normal and cancer gastric tissues. Staging and typing of adenocarcinomatous gastric tissue using PCA-LDA and Raman spectroscopy techniques.

EUS staging of gastric cancers can assess the depth of tumor invasion, the layers of the gastric wall involved by tumor, and enlarged perigastric lymph nodes. However, meta-analyses of studies of EUS have shown that the technique has variable sensitivity and specificity for the detection of different levels of invasion of gastric cancer.[47,48] Likewise, EUS studies assessing lymph node status in gastric cancer have shown variable sensitivity and specificity.[49] Nonetheless, EUS remains useful and continues to be used for these purposes.

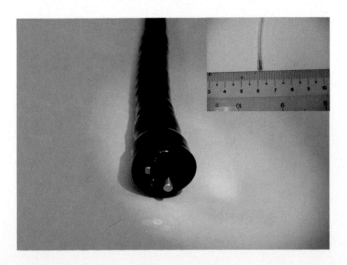

FIGURE 12-15 The 1.8 mm flexible fiberoptic Raman probe, which can fit into the instrument channel of medical endoscopes for in vivo tissue Raman measurements at endoscopy.

Acknowledgments

The authors would like to thank the following individuals for their gracious contribution of endoscopic photographs:

Professor Lawrence Ho Khek Yu, Department of Gastroenterology and Hepatology, National University Hospital, for the confocal laser endomicroscopy images (Figs. 12-7–12-10).

Associate Professor Jimmy So Bok Yan, Department of Surgery, National University Hospital, for the images of chromoendoscopy, autofluorescence imaging and narrow-band imaging and their corresponding white light endoscopic images (Figs. 12-1–12-5).

References

1. Tajiri H, Doi T, Endo H, et al. Routine endoscopy using a magnifying endoscope for gastric cancer diagnosis. *Endoscopy*. 2002;34:772–777.
2. Otsuka Y, Niwa Y, Ohmiya N, et al. Usefulness of magnifying endoscopy in the diagnosis of early gastric cancer. *Endoscopy*. 2004;36:165–169.
3. Yao K, Iwashita A, Tanabe H, et al. Novel zoom endoscopy technique for diagnosis of small flat gastric cancer: a prospective, blind study. *Clin Gastroenterol Hepatol*. 2007;5:869–878.
4. Dinis-Ribeiro M, da Costa-Periera A, Lopes C, et al. Magnification chromoendoscopy for the diagnosis of gastric intestinal metaplasia and dysplasia. *Gastrointest Endosc*. 2003;57:498–504.
5. Morales TG, Bhattacharyya A, Camargo E, et al. Methylene blue staining for intestinal metaplasia of the gastric cardia with follow-up for dysplasia. *Gastrointest Endosc*. 1998;48:26–31.
6. Sumiyama K, Kaise M, Nakayoshi T, et al. Combined use of a magnifying endoscope with a narrow band imaging system and a multibending endoscope for en bloc EMR of early stage gastric cancer. *Gastrointest Endosc*. 2004;60:79–84.
7. Kaltenbach T, Sano Y, Friedland S, et al. American Gastroenterological Association (AGA) Institute technology assessment on image-enhanced endoscopy. *Gastroenterology*. 2008;134:327–340.
8. Sakai Y, Eto R, Kasanuki J, et al. Chromoendoscopy with indigo carmine dye added to acetic acid in the diagnosis of gastric neoplasia: a prospective comparative study. *Gastrointest Endosc*. 2008;68:635–641.
9. Yamashita H, Kitayama, J, Ishigami H, et al. Endoscopic installation of indigo carmine dye with acetic acid enables the visualisation of distinct margin of superficial gastric lesion; usefulness in endoscopic treatment and diagnosis of gastric cancer. *Digest Liver Dis*. 2007;39:389–392.
10. Kawahara Y, Takenaka R, Okada H, et al. Novel chromoendoscopic method using an acetic acid-indigo carmine mixture for diagnostic accuracy in delineating the margin of early gastric cancers. *Dig Endosc*. 2009;21:14–19.
11. Ida K, Hashimoto Y, Kawai K. In vivo staining of gastric mucosa: its applications to endoscopic diagnosis of intestinal metaplasia. *Endoscopy*. 1975;7:18–24.
12. Fennerty MB, Sampliner RE, McGee DL, et al. Intestinal metaplasia of the stomach: identification by a selective mucosal staining technique. *Gastrointest Endosc*. 1992;38:696–698.
13. Areia M, Amaro P, Dinis-Ribeiro M, et al. External validation of a classification for methylene blue magnification chromoendoscopy in premalignant gastric lesions. *Gastrointest Endosc*. 2008;67:1011–1018.
14. Ohkawa A, Miwa H, Namihisa A, et al. Diagnostic performance of light-induced fluorescence endoscopy for gastric neoplasms. *Endoscopy*. 2004;36:515–521.
15. Uedo N, Iishi H, Tatsuta M, et al. A novel videoendoscopy system by using autofluorescence and reflectance imaging for diagnosis of esophagogastric cancers. *Gastrointest Endosc*. 2005;62:521–528.
16. Kato M, Kaise M, Yonezawa J, et al. Trimodal imaging endoscopy may improve diagnostic accuracy of early gastric neoplasia: a feasibility study. *Gastrointest Endosc*. 2009;70:899–906.
17. Uedo N, Ishihara R, Iishi H, et al. A new method of diagnosing gastric intestinal metaplasia: narrow band imaging with magnifying endoscopy. *Endoscopy*. 2006;38:819–824.
18. Nakayoshi T, Tajiri H, Matsuda K, et al. Magnifying endoscopy combined with narrow band imaging system for early gastric cancer: correlation of vascular pattern with histopathology (including video). *Endoscopy*. 2004;36:1080–1084.

19. Muto M, Horimatsu T, Ezoe Y, et al. Narrow-band imaging of the gastrointestinal tract. *J Gastroenterol.* 2009;44:13–25.

20. Larghi A, Lecca PG, Costamagna G. High-resolution narrow band imaging endoscopy. *Gut.* 2008;57: 976–986.

21. Hoffman A, Goetz M, Vieth M, et al. Confocal laser endomicroscopy: technical status and current indications. *Endoscopy.* 2006;38:1275–1283.

22. Nguyen NQ, Leong RWL. Current application of confocal endomicroscopy in gastrointestinal disorders. *J Gastroenterol Hepatol.* 2008;23:1483–1491.

23. Kiesslich R, Goetz M, Neurath MF. Virtual histology. *Best Pract Res Clin Gastroenterol.* 2008;22: 883–897.

24. Zhang J, Li Y, Zhao Y, et al. Classification of gastric pit patterns by confocal endomicroscopy. *Gastrointest Endosc.* 2008;67:843–853.

25. Yeoh KG, Salto-Tellez M, Khor CJL, et al. Confocal laser endoscopy is useful for in vivo rapid diagnosis of gastric neoplasia and pre-neoplasia. Digestive Disease Week 2005; Chicago, IL.

26. Guo YT, Li YQ, Yu T, et al. Diagnosis of gastric intestinal metaplasia with confocal laser endomicroscopy in vivo: a prospective study. *Endoscopy.* 2008;40:547–553.

27. Kakeji Y, Yamaguchi S, Yoshida D, et al. Development and assessment of morphologic criteria for diagnosing gastric cancer using confocal endomicroscopy: an ex vivo and in vivo study. *Endoscopy.* 2006;38:886–890.

28. Kitabatake S, Niwa Y, Miyahara R, et al. Confocal endomicroscopy for the diagnosis of gastric cancer in vivo. *Endoscopy.* 2006;38:1110–1114.

29. Hanlon EB, Manoharan R, Koo TW, et al. Prospects for in vivo Raman spectroscopy. *Phys Med Biol.* 2000;45:1–59.

30. Mahadevan-Jansen A, Richards-Kortum R. Raman spectroscopy for the detection of cancers and precancers. *J Biomed Opt.* 1996;1:31–70.

31. Manoharan R, Wang Y, Feld MS. Histochemical analysis of biological tissues using Raman spectroscopy. *Spectrochim Acta A.* 1996;52:215–249.

32. Huang Z, Lui II, McLean DI, et al. Raman spectroscopy in combination with background near-infrared autofluorescence enhances the in vivo assessment of malignant tissues. *Photochem Photobiol.* 2005;81:1219–1226.

33. Stone N, Kendall C, Sheperd N, et al. Near-infrared Raman spectroscopy for the classification of epithelial pre-cancers and cancers. *J Raman Spectrosc.* 2002;33:564–573.

34. Bakker Schut TC, Witjes MJ, Sterenborg HJ, et al. In vivo detection of dysplastic tissue by Raman spectroscopy. *Anal Chem.* 2000;72:6010–6018.

35. Molckovsky A, Song LM, Shim MG, et al. Diagnostic potential of near-infrared Raman spectroscopy in the colon: differentiating adenomatous from hyperplastic polyps. *Gastrointest Endosc.* 2003;57: 396–402.

36. Mahadevan-Jansen A, Mitchell MF, Ramanujam N, et al. Near-infrared Raman spectroscopy for in vitro detection of cervical precancers. *Photochem Photobiol.* 1998;68:123–132.

37. Lau DP, Huang Z, Lui H, et al. Raman spectroscopy for optical diagnosis in the larynx: preliminary findings. *Lasers Surg Med.* 2005;37:192–200.

38. Haka AS, Shafer-Peltier KE, Fitzmaurice M, et al. Diagnosing breast cancer by using Raman spectroscopy. *Proc Natl Acad Sci U S A.* 2005;102:12371–12376.

39. Huang Z, Zeng H, Hamzavi I, et al. Rapid near-infrared Raman spectroscopy system for real-time in vivo skin measurements. *Opt Lett.* 2001;26:1782–1784.

40. Teh SK, Zheng W, Ho KY, et al. Near-infrared Raman spectroscopy for gastric precancer diagnosis. *J Raman Spectrosc.* 2009;40:908–914.

41. Teh SK, Zheng W, Ho KY, et al. Diagnostic potential of near-infrared Raman spectroscopy in the stomach: differentiating dysplasia from normal tissue. *Br J Cancer.* 2008;98:457–465.

42. Teh SK, Zheng W, Ho KY, et al. Diagnosis of gastric cancer using near-infrared Raman spectroscopy and classification and regression tree techniques. *J Biomed Opt.* 2008;13:034013.

43. Teh SK, Zheng W, Ho KY, et al. Near-infrared raman spectroscopy for optical diagnosis in the stomach: identification of *Helicobacter-pylori* infection and intestinal metaplasia. *Int J Cancer.* 2009; DOI: 10.1002/ijc24935.

44. Teh SK, Zheng W, Ho KY, et al. Near-infrared Raman spectroscopy for early diagnosis and typing of adenocarcinoma in the stomach. *Br J Surgery.* 2009; DOI: 10.1002/bjs.6913.

45. Huang Z, Teh SK, Zheng W, et al. Integrated Raman spectroscopy and trimodal wide-field imaging techniques for real-time in vivo tissue Raman measurements at endoscopy. *Opt Lett.* 2009;34:758–760.

46. Huang Z, Mads SB, Teh SK, et al. In vivo early diagnosis and detection of gastric dysplasia using narrow-band image-guided Raman endoscopy. *J Biomed Opt.* 2010;15(3):037017.

47. Kwee RM, Kwee TC. The accuracy of endoscopic ultrasonography in differentiating mucosal from deeper gastric cancer. *Am J Gastroenterol.* 2008;103:1801–1809.

48. Puli SR, Batapati KRJ, Bechtold ML, et al. How good is endoscopic ultrasound for TNM staging of gastric cancers? A meta-analysis and systematic review. *World J Gastroenterol.* 2008;14:4011–4019.

49. Kwee RM, Kwee TC. Imaging in assessing lymph node status in gastric cancer. *Gastric Cancer.* 2009;12:6–22.

Molecular Pathology

Molecular Pathology of Gastric Neoplasms

13

▶ Shengle Zhang

INTRODUCTION

Amid the current rapid development in knowledge and technology of molecular oncology, gastric neoplasm, like other tumors, has been extensively investigated in molecular levels, that is, deoxyribonucleic acid (DNA), ribonucleic acid (RNA), and protein levels. As a result, this research has found that many genetic changes have been found to play key roles in carcinogenesis. Although the detailed mechanism remains unclear, "gain of function" alterations in protooncogene and "loss of function" in the tumor suppressor gene are considered to be two major causes of tumor development.

Genetic alterations in protooncogene are usually associated with amplification, mutation, and translocation, while genetic alterations in tumor suppressor genes are commonly related to deletion, mutation, and methylation. Not only are these genetic alterations associated with tumorigenesis but they are also very useful biomarkers in clinical application, such as tumor diagnosis, prognosis, and prediction of therapeutic response.[1,2] Personalized tumor treatment in the future would also depend on individual's genetic "signature."

More than 90% of total neoplasms in the stomach are carcinomas of epithelial origin. Primary gastric lymphoma is the second most common malignancy, and mesenchymal and neuroendocrine tumors are much less common.

Genetic alterations in carcinomas show different distributions or patterns from that of sarcomas or lymphomas.[3] A carcinoma could have multiple genetic changes. For example, gastric carcinomas might have E-cadherin gene mutations, epidermal growth factor receptor (EGFR) gene amplification/polysomy, and p53 gene deletion/methylation. Conversely, one genetic change could be seen in different carcinomas, such as p53 mutation in cancers of the breast, colon, lung, and pancreas. In addition, the frequencies of genetic alterations in carcinomas are low (usually <50%). Owing to the lack of organ specificity and lower frequency, genetic alterations in carcinoma are rarely used for diagnosis. However, genetic alterations could be used to indicate tumor prognosis and to predict a response to therapy. For instance, gastric carcinoma with a *CND1* gene mutation is associated with diffuse type of gastric cancer and a poor prognosis.

Unlike carcinomas, soft tissue sarcomas usually have more specific genetic alterations with higher frequency.[3] For example, >95% of synovial sarcomas have characteristic chromosome translocation of t(X;18)(p11;q11) and display unique gene fusions of *SYT-SSX1* or *SYT-SSX2*.[3] The gene fusions associated with translocations in soft tissue sarcomas are ideal biomarkers for the purpose of diagnosis, although sarcomas are not as common as carcinomas.[3]

Like sarcomas, lymphomas and leukemias usually have specific translocations as well.[4] For example, mantle cell lymphoma has t(11;14)(q13;q32) that displays *IGH-CCND1* gene fusion with >90% frequency. This translocation is an ideal biomarker not only for diagnosis but also for prognosis and predicting a response to therapy.

Recent studies showed that carcinoma, like sarcoma or lymphoma, would have gene fusion as well.[5] *TMPRSS2* gene fusion associated with translocations or deletions has been found in prostate cancers with high specificity and around 60% prevalence.[5] It is unclear, however, whether gastric cancer also carries specific gene fusion.

In this chapter, we discuss genetic alterations of inherited tumor syndrome, genetic alterations of sporadic neoplasms of the stomach, molecular techniques commonly used in clinical laboratories, and future perspectives.

GENETIC ALTERATIONS OF INHERITED TUMOR SYNDROME

The stomach is a commonly, but not exclusively, involved organ in a variety of inherited tumor syndromes. In this section, the following inherited tumor syndromes are reviewed: juvenile polyposis syndrome (JPS), Peutz-Jeghers syndrome (PJS), hereditary diffuse gastric cancer (HDGC), familial adenomatous polyposis (FAP), and hereditary nonpolyposis colorectal cancer syndrome (HNPCC) (Table 13-1).

Juvenile Polyposis Syndrome

JPS is an autosomal dominant disorder occurring in 1 out of every 100,000 to 160,000 individuals in whom polyps appear in the colon and stomach.[6] JPS occurring in infants involves the entire digestive tract and has the poorest prognosis.[7] In most other JPS patients, symptoms develop by age 20, although some patients with JPS are not diagnosed until their 30s. Common symptoms

Table 13-1	Summary of inherited tumor syndromes				
Syndrome	Prevalence	Inheritance	Gene Involved (Chromosomal Location)	Common Genetic Alterations	Detection Methods
Juvenile polyposis syndrome	1/100,000– 1/160,000	Autosomal dominant	*SMAD4* (18q21.1) *BMPR1A* (10q22.3) *PTEN* (10q23.3)	Deletion, insertion, missense, and nonsense mutations	DNA sequencing, MLPA
Peutz-Jeghers syndrome	1/29,000– 1/120,000	Autosomal dominant	*STK11/LKB1* (19p13.3)	Deletion, insertion, missense, and splicing mutations	DNA sequencing, MLPA
Hereditary diffuse gastric cancer	~10% of gastric cancer	Autosomal dominant	*CDH1* (16q22.1)	Frame-shift and missense mutations	DNA sequencing
Familial adenomatous polyposis	2–3/100,000	Autosomal dominant	*APC* (5q21)	Frame-shift, missense, and nonsense mutations, deletion and duplication	Protein truncation, linkage analysis, DNA sequencing
Lynch syndrome (HNPCC)	1%–3% of colon cancer	Autosomal dominant	*MLH1, MSH2, MSH6, PMS2, MSH3*	Deletion and duplication	Imminohisto chemistry, MSI, MLPA, DNA sequencing

DNA, deoxyribonucleic acid; HNPCC, hereditary nonpolyposis colorectal cancer; MLPA, multiplex ligation-dependent probe amplification; MSI, microsatellite instability.

include gastrointestinal (GI) bleeding, anemia, diarrhea, and abdominal pain. JPS is diagnosed clinically if any one of the following findings is present[7]:

- More than five juvenile polyps of the colorectum
- Multiple juvenile polyps of the upper and lower GI tract
- Any number of juvenile polyps and a family history of juvenile polyps

The polyps seen in JPS are regarded as hamartomatous polyps (juvenile polyps) that develop from an abnormal collection of tissue elements normally present at this site. Juvenile polyps show a normal-looking epithelium with inflammatory and dense stroma, and mucus-filled cystic glands in the lamina propria. Dysplasia can be identified in approximately 30% of patients with JPS,[8] and the lifetime malignancy rate ranges from 9% to 50%.[9] The incidence of gastric cancer is 21% in patients with the polyps in the stomach.[9] Early detection of genetic alterations associated with JPS allows for better treatment of polyps and surveillance of at-risk individuals.[9] Genetic alterations of *SMAD4* (18q21.1), *BMPR1a* (10q22.3), and *PTEN* (10q23.3) have been identified in 22%, 25%, and 5% of patients with JPS, respectively.[10]

Individuals with JPS and an *SMAD4* mutation are more likely to have a family history of upper GI polyps than are individuals with mutations in *BMPR1A* or those with no known mutations.[10] Individuals with either an *SMAD4* or a *BMPR1A* mutation are more likely to have more than ten lower GI polyps and a family history of GI cancer.[7] *SMAD4* and *BMPR1a* genetic alterations are currently evaluated in some tertiary medical centers or commercial laboratories to facilitate management of patients with JPS. Mutations in select exons of *SMAD4* have been reported in a combined syndrome of hereditary hemorrhagic telangiectasia (HHT) with JPS.[11] In families with the combined JPS/HHT syndrome and/or a known *SMAD4* mutation, predictive molecular genetic testing may be appropriate in patients before the age of 15 years to watch for potential complications of HHT that can begin in early childhood.[7]

Peutz-Jeghers Syndrome

PJS is an autosomal dominant syndrome associated with mucocutaneous hyperpigmentation and hamartomatous polyps. Peutz-Jeghers hamartomatous polyps are most prevalent in the small intestine. The density of polyps is greatest in the jejunum, followed by the ileum, stomach, and large bowel. The relative incidence of PJS is estimated at 1 of every 29,000 to 120,000 births. Patients with PJS are at increased risk of developing malignancies, beginning around the age of 10 years. It has been estimated that there are 84-, 213-, and 520-fold increased risks of patients developing colon, gastric, and small intestinal cancers, respectively, with a general cancer risk of 50% by the age of 65 years and a >90% lifetime risk.[12]

Seventy-five percent to ninety percent of patients with PJS carry germline mutation in *STK11* (*LKB1*), a tumor suppressor gene at 19p13.3 that encodes a serine/threonine kinase.[13] Tumorigenesis of PJS is often accompanied by additional somatic (biallelic) mutation, deletion, or inactivation in *STK11*.[12] Genetic testing is useful for confirming the diagnosis of PJS or to identify the presymptomatic first-degree relatives. If the familial mutation is identified, molecular genetic testing on the at-risk relatives can reduce morbidity and mortality by early diagnosis, appropriate surveillance, and treatment. Complete DNA sequencing of *STK11* is one of the most commonly used methods.[14]

For patients with PJS or individuals at risk of developing PJS, endoscopic surveillance for malignant transformation should be conducted every 1 to 2 years beginning in adolescence. Although surveillance is recommended, no published reports have proved its efficacy.[14]

Hereditary Diffuse Gastric Cancer

Clinical criteria for diagnosis of HDGC were established by the International Gastric Cancer Linkage Consortium (IGCLC) in 2004[15]:

- Two or more cases of gastric cancer in a family, with at least one diffuse gastric cancer diagnosed before age 50

- Three or more cases of gastric cancer in a family, diagnosed at any age, with at least one documented case of diffuse gastric cancer
- An individual diagnosed with diffuse gastric cancer before age 45
- An individual diagnosed with both diffuse gastric cancer and lobular breast cancer (no other criteria met)
- One family member diagnosed with diffuse gastric cancer and another with lobular breast cancer (no other criteria met)
- One family member diagnosed with diffuse gastric cancer and another with signet ring colon cancer (no other criteria met)

Around 10% to 15% of gastric cancers are familial. HDGC is an autosomal dominant disorder with high penetrance (about 80%), average onset in the fourth decade of life. Germline mutations, mainly frame-shift and missense mutations, in the CDH1 gene have been associated with HDGC.[16] There are two major histological variants of gastric cancer: diffuse-type gastric cancer (35%) and intestinal-type gastric cancer (50%). CDH1 mutations have been found only in diffuse-type gastric cancers. According to Cisco et al.,[17] four fifths of females and two thirds of males who are carriers of CDH1 gene mutations will develop HDGC by the age of 80 years.

The CDH1 gene, located at 16q22.1, encodes E-cadherin, a member of the cadherin super-family of calcium-dependent cell adhesion molecules.[18] Down-regulation of E-cadherin is observed in a number of epithelial-derived human cancers and promotes invasion through loss of epithelial cell–cell adhesion. Approximately 40% of HDGC kindred harbor germline mutations in CDH1. Down-regulation via promoter hypermethylation, along with mechanisms acting at transcriptional and posttranscriptional level, may act as the "second hit" in both inherited and sporadic diffuse cancers.[19] Patients with the CDH1 genetic alteration are also predisposed to develop lobular breast cancer and colon cancer. Women with the CDH1 mutation were found to have a 39% risk for lobular-type breast cancer.

With early detection (i.e., confined to mucosa and submucosa), >90% of patients with gastric cancer will be alive at 5 years compared with 10% to 20% of patients with advanced gastric cancer, even after potentially curative surgery has been carried out.[20] Patients with a clinical diagnosis of HDGC could be tested for the CND1 gene mutation. While the patients with the CND1 gene mutation should be managed with more frequent endoscopic surveillance and biopsies, their children and/or relatives could be tested for the carrier status of CND1 and therefore receive appropriate clinical management. Although it has been proposed that individuals who have a CDH1 cancer–predisposing mutation undergo routine surveillance for gastric cancer, the optimal management of individuals at risk for a cancer is controversial because of the unproven value of surveillance regimes.

Familial Adenomatous Polyposis

FAP is an autosomal dominant disorder with an estimated incidence of 2 to 3 out of every 100,000 individuals.[21] Florid polyposis throughout the colon will develop adenocarcinoma in 50% of patients with FAP by age 16 and in 95% by age 35. By age 50, almost all patients with untreated FAP in their colon will develop adenocarcinoma, accounting for approximately 1% of all colon cancers in the world.[21] The most familial adenomatous polyps are seen in the colon and the rectum, but they also can present in the upper gastrointestinal tract. Different from colon polyps, gastric polyps in FAP generally include two types: fundic gland polyps (occurring in 50% of cases) or adenomatous polyps (occurring in 10% of cases). In the stomach, the risk of transformation of FAP to cancer is low for both types of polyps.[21,22]

Goodman et al.[23] found that in a cohort of Japanese patients with FAP outside of the colon, 100% had adenomas and/or polyps in the duodenum and 50% had adenomas and/or polyps in the gastric antrum. However, in patients of North American origin with FAP, only 33% had duodenum adenomas and only 2% had gastric adenoma and/or polyps.[23] In the same study, a majority of stomach polyps in FAP were "fundic gland polyps."[23] It is generally believed that fundic gland polyps have little potential for malignant transformation, but the actual frequency of transformation in fundic gland polyps is probably high.[24] Lakshman et al.[24] found dysplastic changes in 16 (25%) of 64 fundic gland polyps in patients with FAP. In contrast, a different study reported neither dysplasia nor carcinoma in fundic gland polyps from non-FAP patients.[25] Therefore, the presence of fundic gland polyposis in FAP is not an entirely benign process.

FAP is associated with highly heterogeneous mutations in the *APC* gene (5q21), including frame-shift, missense, and nonsense mutations.[21] The normal *APC* gene product acts as a tumor suppressor protein that may participate in regulating the cell cycle and maintaining a normal level of apoptosis through interaction with a second protein, β-catenin. Several hundred different mutations have been described.[21] The most common consequence of these mutations is premature truncation of the *APC*-encoding protein. Marked polyposis with several thousand polyps is associated with mutation between codons 1250 and 1393. Of these mutations, the most common is a 5-base pair deletion at codon 1309. The attenuated form of FAP (<100 polyps) is associated with a mutation at the extreme 5 and 3 ends of the *APC* gene. A mutation at codon 1307 (the I1307K mutation) is present in about 6% of Ashkenazi Jews and produces a partial FAP phenotype. Mutations in codons 1554 and 1556 were reported as hot spots for gastric polyps.[26] For malignant transformation, additional somatic mutations or epigenetic alterations are usually required. Up to 30% of FAPs are associated with a de novo mutation in the *APC* gene without a family history of FAP.[22]

Genetic testing is the standard of care for management of FAP.[14] The test can be used to confirm the clinical diagnosis of FAP, establish the FAP genotype in the family, and identify at-risk asymptomatic or presymptomatic mutation carriers in family members. Genetic testing facilitates the management of FAP and would be more cost-effective than would be repeated endoscopic screening for at-risk family members.[14]

APC gene mutations can be evaluated by protein truncation assay, linkage analysis, and/or direct DNA sequencing.[14] Protein truncation assay can detect approximately 80% of the structural defects of *APC*-encoding protein caused by highly heterogeneous gene mutations. However, this assay does not reveal the specific mutations or genetic linkage required to identify carrier status in family members.[14]

Linkage analysis requires the participation of affected and unaffected family members but provides an alternative for families with FAP who do not have identifiable *APC* gene alteration by protein truncation test or direct DNA sequencing. The linkage of a specific haplotype with FAP in a family provides >95% accuracy in identifying carriers.[14]

Highly heterogeneous gene mutations necessitate multiple polymerase chain reactions (PCRs) with primers covering big areas for direct DNA sequencing.[14] The sensitivity for DNA sequencing is reported to be 90% to 99%. Many individuals with polyposis who test negative for a mutation in the *APC* gene may have an autosomal recessive disorder caused by a germline mutation in *MYH*.[27] Therefore, *MYH* alteration is often evaluated in conjunction with *APC*.

For a family with classic FAP, genetic testing usually is suggested for children 10 years or older, while endoscopic surveillance is recommended to begin at 10 to 12 years.[28]

Lynch Syndrome (HNPCC)

HNPCC, also known as Lynch syndrome, is an autosomal dominant syndrome with 1% to 2% incidence in patients with colon cancer. HNPCC predisposes a person to malignancy, including a lifetime risk of up to 80% for colorectal cancer (CRC), 20% to 60% for endometrial cancer, and 11% to 19% for gastric cancer.[29] HNPCC's predisposition to malignancy is associated with mutations in any of the mismatch repair (MMR) genes, which would accelerate DNA microsatellite instability (MSI). *MMR* genetic alterations can be found in 90% of tumors from HNPCC patients with germline mutations and in 10% to 15% of sporadic cancers.[30] At least five *MMR* genes cause HNPCC, with approximately 90% of mutations in the *MLH1* and *MSH2* genes and 7% to 10% in the *MSH6* gene.[31] Mutations are seen less frequently in the *PMS2* gene (<5%) and are rarely reported in the *PMS1* gene. Mutations in *MSH6* and *PMS2* genes tend to attenuate HNPCC, which has an older age of cancer onset.[30]

Gastric cancers associated with HNPCC are predominantly intestinal type and less involved with the *Helicobacter pylori* infection.[20] Occurrence of gastric cancer in patients younger than 60 years should indicate the possibility of HNPCC.[32] Patients with HNPCC CRC have a better prognosis than do those with sporadic colorectal carcinoma.[33]

Identifying *MMR* genetically associated alterations has a considerable clinical impact on the diagnosis, screening, and prevention of HNPCC.[29,34] Amsterdam Clinical Criteria II is often used to decide whether molecular testing should be pursued:

- Three or more affected family members with an HNPCC-related cancer and at least one family member must be a first-degree relative of the other two
- Two successive affected generations
- One or more CRCs must be diagnosed before the age of 50 years

However, up to 39% of families with mutations in the HNPCC genes do not meet Amsterdam Criteria.[34]

Preliminary molecular testing on HNPCC can be performed to evaluate MSI by PCR and/or abnormal MMR protein by immunohistochemistry (IHC). The presence of MSI in a tumor specimen is not indicative of a particular gene defect, and neither MSI nor IHC can distinguish between sporadic and HNPCC-related cancers. However, IHC results indicating the absence of a specific MMR protein can be used to determine which targeted mutation analysis should be performed.[35]

A comprehensive analysis of the entire *MLH1, MSH2,* and *MSH6* genes is recommended for diagnostic testing of HNPCC.[34] Other clinical applications include screening and preimplantation diagnosis. Prenatal testing and testing individuals younger than 18 years are generally not recommended. Identifying the carriers means increased colonoscopic surveillance for the detection of CRC at earlier stages, which can prevent >60% of CRC and reduce mortality by 60%.[36] Routine surveillance for the carriers of the *MMR* mutation includes colonoscopy every 1 to 2 years starting at age 20 to 25 or 10 years before the earliest age of diagnosis in the family, whichever is earlier.[36]

Analysis of the *MMR* genetic alteration can be performed using comprehensive direct DNA sequencing for those patients with unknown mutations or by using a specific test on the *MLS1, MSH2,* or *MSH6* genes for those with known familial genetic mutation. However, the clinical utility and methodology of analysis on MSI, MMR protein expression, and mutations are not as well established in gastric carcinoma associated with HNPCC as they are in colorectal adenocarcinoma. A standardized method for MSI detection in gastric cancer has been proposed, but whether it will become the treatment standard remains unknown.[37] In addition, the relative rarity of gastric cancer in HNPCC families makes the cost-effectiveness of endoscopic screening questionable.[32]

Other Rare Inherited Tumor Syndromes in Stomach

Although not frequent, gastric carcinoma could be part of other inherited tumor syndromes such as Li-Fraumeni cancer syndrome, Cowden syndrome, familial breast cancer, and MEN-1, which are associated with genetic alteration in p53 gene, *PTEN* gene, *BRCA1/2* gene, and *MEN-1* gene, respectively.[38,39]

GENETIC ALTERATIONS OF SPORADIC NEOPLASMS IN STOMACH

Gastrointestinal Stromal Tumor

Gastrointestinal stromal tumor (GIST) is the most common mesenchymal tumor in the gastrointestinal tract and is believed to originate from the interstitial cells of Cajal or their precursors. GISTs are most commonly seen in the stomach (60%–70%) but also occur in the small intestine (20%–30%), colorectum, and esophagus (colorectum and esophagus together <10%).[39] Expression of CD117 (c-kit protein) by immunoreactivity has been considered as a characteristic

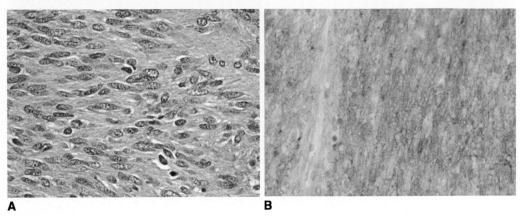

A   **B**

FIGURE 13-1 **A:** Gastrointestinal stromal tumor (case 1) with H&E stain, showing spindle cell in histology. **B:** Gastrointestinal stromal tumor (case 1) with CD117 immunostain, showing cytoplasmic positivity.

molecular marker for diagnosis of GISTs and can be identified in approximately 95% of GIST cases. The GISTs with CD117 expression are usually spindle cell or epithelioid in histology. Expression of CD117 has also been used as a criterion of eligibility for GIST treatment with tyrosine kinase inhibitor (TKI) such as imatinib.[40] GISTs also express CD34 and nestin proteins by IHC with less specificity. GISTs with negative or weak CD117 expression often show *PDGFRA* genetic alteration and are usually epithelioid in morphology (Figs. 13-1 and 13-2).

Although a variety of genetic alterations have been found in GISTs, *KIT* and *PDGFRA* gene mutations are the most important alterations with the most crucial clinical implications.[41] Both *KIT* and *PDGFRA* genes are located at 4q12 and encode highly homologous receptor tyrosine kinase proteins. Mutations of *KIT* and *PDGFRA*, which are usually mutually exclusive, can cause constitutive activation of this receptor tyrosine kinase, resulting in increased cell proliferation and survival. *KIT* mutation can be identified in approximately 80% of GISTs: 66% at exon 11, 13% at exon 9, 1.2% at exon 13, and 0.6% at exon 17. *PDGFRA* mutation can be identified in approximately 8% of GISTs: 5.6% at exon 18, 1.5% at exon 12, and 0.3% at exon 14.[50] The genetic alterations of *KIT* and *PDGFRA* include in-frame deletions, point mutations, duplications, and insertions. The presence of any *KIT* and/or *PDGFRA* mutations is significantly associated with high risk/malignant GISTs.[41]

Different mutation types in GIST may be associated with different clinicopathologic features and responses to TKI therapy. GISTs with mutations in *PDGFRA* are mostly commonly seen in

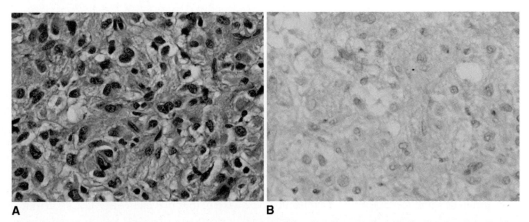

A   **B**

FIGURE 13-2 **A:** Gastrointestinal stromal tumor (case 2) with H&E stain, showing epithelioid cell in histology. **B:** Gastrointestinal stromal tumor (case 2) with CD117 immunostain, showing very weak positivity. However, *PDGFRA* gene mutation at exon 18 (D824) present.

the stomach with epithelioid histological appearance.[41] In general, the *KIT* mutation at exon 11 showed longer event-free survival and more sensitivity to TKI therapy than that shown at exon 9 or wild type. Conversely, mutations at *KIT* exon 17 and *PDGFRA* exon 18 showed resistance to TKI therapy.[41,42]

Molecular analysis of *KIT* and *PDGFRA* genes and their expression has been used for diagnosis and management of GIST. Although CD117 expression by immunostain has diagnostic value for GIST, approximately 5% of GISTs are negative and make diagnosing GIST a challenge in these cases. Studies showed that majority of the CD117-negative GISTs were positive for *PDGFRA* expression,[43] which would be useful for diagnosis of CD117-negative GIST. Detections of *KIT* and *PDGFRA* gene mutations are usually not used for diagnosis but are used to postulate the patient's prognosis and therapeutic response to TKIs. Direct DNA sequencing is a commonly employed method for *KIT* and *PDGFRA* mutations.[41,42]

Lymphomas of Mucosa-Associated Lymphoid Tissue

Primary gastric lymphomas are defined as lymphomas originating from the stomach and contiguous lymph nodes. The majority of gastric lymphomas are high-grade B-cell lymphomas, some of which have progressed from low-grade lymphomas of MALT. Although a variety of lymphomas, such as diffuse large B-cell lymphoma, Burkitt lymphoma, and T-cell lymphoma, can occur in the stomach as a primary or secondary site, B-cell MALT lymphoma is almost exclusively a low-grade lymphoma in the stomach and has been well studied at the molecular level.[39]

Chromosomal translocation t(11;18)(q21;q21), t(1;14)(p22,q32), t(14;18)(q32;q21), and t(3;14)(p14.1;q32), rendering gene fusion of *API2-MALT1*, *BCL10-IGH*, *IGH-MALT1*, and *IGH-FOXP1*, respectively, have been identified in MALT lymphoma. Among them, t(11;18)(q21;q21) and t(1;14)(p22,q32) are specific for MALT lymphoma and can be found in 22% and 4% of the MALT cases, respectively. Gene fusions of *API2-MALT1*, *BCL10-IGH*, and *IHG-MALT1* result in the constitutive activation of NF-κB, which may represent a common pathway for MALT lymphomagenesis.[44,45]

H. pylori infection is seen in 70% to 90% of low-grade MALT lymphoma and 25% to 35% of high-grade lymphoma.[44,45] In a clinical setting, eradication of *H. pylori* can lead to complete regression of 60% to 80% of gastric MALT lymphomas. However, MALT lymphomas with *API2-MALT1* or *BCL10-IGH* fusion are rarely associated with *H. pylori* infection and therefore do not respond well to *H. pylori* eradication therapy. In addition, MALT lymphomas with *API2-MALT1* usually display a low-grade histology with a stable clinical course and rarely progress to high-grade lymphomas.[44,45]

T-cell and B-cell gene rearrangement by PCR can be used to detect monoclonality of lymphoma, although subtypes of lymphoma cannot be determined. Owing to the low frequency of gene rearrangements in MALT lymphoma, this test is not ideal for the purpose of diagnosis. However, *API2-MALT1* and *BCL10-IGH* gene fusions are associated with resistance to *H. pylori* eradication therapy and could be used to manage MALT lymphomas. The gene fusions can be detected by reverse transcriptase polymerase chain reaction (RT-PCR), fluorescence in situ hybridization (FISH), or Southern blot. Both fresh and paraffin tissues can be used for RT-PCR and FISH, while fresh tissue is required for Southern blot. The Southern blot method requires much DNA and is time-consuming and would therefore not be practical as a clinical assay.

Sporadic Gastric Carcinoma

A variety of genetic alterations have been identified in sporadic gastric carcinoma, such as in genes of *TP53*, *E-cadherin (CDH1)*, *c-erbB-2*, *DCC* and *c-met*, MSI, and loss or gain of chromosomal regions (3p, 4, 5q, 6q, 9p, 17p).[38,39] Intestinal type and diffuse type of gastric carcinoma show different genetic alterations. The intestinal type has a higher prevalence of MSI, *TP53* mutation, and *APC* deletion, while the diffuse type has higher frequency of *CDH1* mutation and higher expression of *c-met*.[38,39,46] Some of these genetic alterations may be associated with environmental factors such as *H. pylori* infection and high nitrite ingestion.[39,47]

Table 13-2	Summary of common gastric sporadic neoplasms and their genetic alterations			
Tumor	Tumor Prevalence	Gene Involved	Common Genetic Alterations	Detection Methods
Gastric carcinoma	~60/100,000 in general population	*P53, CDH1, c-erbB-2, c-met, MLH1, MSH2, MSH6, PMS2, MSH3,* loss or gain of 3p, 4, 5q, 6q, 9p, 17p	Point mutations, deletions, duplications, insertions, and gains	PCR, DNA sequencing, and FISH
Gastrointestinal stromal tumor (GIST)	~2.2% of malignant gastric tumors	*KIT* (4q12) *PDGFRA* (4q12)	In-frame deletions, point mutations, duplications, and insertions	Immunohis-tochemistry for c-Kit and PDGFAR protein expression. DNA sequencing for *KIT* and *PDGFRA* gene alterations
Lymphomas of MALT	~8% of malignant gastric tumors	Gene fusions of *API2-MALT1, IGH-BCL10, IGH-MALT1,* and *IGH-FOXP1*	t(11;18)(q21;q21), t(1;14)(p22,q32), t(14;18)(q32;q21), and t(3;14) (p14.1;q32)	RT-PCR, DNA sequencing, and FISH

Although the genetic alterations mentioned previously are associated with the carcinogenesis of gastric cancer, almost all of them can also be identified in cancers of other organs, such as *TP53, c-erbB-2,* and *CDH1* in breast cancer. In addition, the prevalence of these genetic alterations is low, usually <50%. Therefore, these genetic alterations are not ideal molecular markers to set up specific and sensitive assays for the purpose of diagnosis. Clinical utility of these gene alterations for tumor prognosis and prediction to therapeutic response requires additional study. Common gastric sporadic neoplasms and their genetic alterations are summarized in Table 13-2.

MOLECULAR TECHNIQUES COMMONLY USED IN CLINICAL LABORATORIES

Common genetic alterations in neoplasms include deletion, mutation, translocation, and ampli-fication. PCR can be used to detect gene rearrangement, mutation, deletion, and translocation, while FISH can be used for deletion, translocation, and amplification. Other advanced techniques such as DNA/RNA microarray, comparative genomic hybridization (CGH), and proteomics have great potential for clinical application but are not yet being used routinely.[48,49]

Polymerase Chain Reaction

Regular PCR can be used to detect B- or T-cell gene rearrangement, point mutation, and deletion. RT-PCR can be used to detect gene fusions caused by chromosome translocation. Real-time PCR is a close system and can play a role like the other PCRs but with more efficiency and less chance of contamination. Multiplex ligation-dependent probe amplification (MLPA) is a variation of PCR that permits multiple targets to be amplified with only a single primer pair. Each probe consists of two oligonucleotides, which recognize adjacent target sites on the DNA. One probe oligonucleotide contains the sequence recognized by the forward primer, and the other probe contains the sequence recognized by the reverse primer. Only when both probe oligonucleotides are hybridized to their respective targets can they be ligated into a complete probe. The advantage of splitting the probe into two parts is that only the ligated oligonucleotides, but not the unbound probe oligonucleotides, are amplified. PCR products can be used for direct DNA sequencing to detect point mutations, small deletions, and insertions.[48,49]

FISH

FISH is a morphology-based assay that is simple and reliable and can be used to detect deletion, translocation, and amplification.[48,49] FISH needs only a small amount of tissue (<200 cells) with no carryover or crossover contamination, like that seen in the PCR procedure. Gene break-apart FISH probes have been successfully used to detect gene break-apart associated with chromosomal translocation. However, FISH has a longer turnaround time owing to overnight incubation and cannot be used to detect point mutation.[38,39]

FUTURE PERSPECTIVES

With advanced molecular techniques (including DNA/RNA microarrays, CGH, proteomics, and DNA sequencing), more new genetic alterations in neoplasms have been discovered at a fast pace. Some of these genetic alterations have been used in tumor diagnosis, prognosis, and prediction of therapeutic response. Although tumor-specific gene fusions caused by translocation are usually seen in sarcomas and lymphomas, recent studies using advanced molecular techniques have revealed that prostate cancer contains *TMPRSS2* gene fusions with *ETS* transcription factor family in approximately 60% of prostate cancer but none in the corresponding normal tissue.[5]

For the first time, our medical scientists have demonstrated that gene fusion also exists in carcinoma of epithelial origin.[5] We speculate that gene fusions can occur in other types of carcinomas, including gastric cancer. In addition, the costs of the molecular studies (including DNA/RNA microarrays, PCR, and FISH) have significantly decreased in recent years. We expect rapid development in molecular diagnostics of neoplasms in coming years, and these advancements will help physicians to more extensively and more effectively engage in management of gastric cancer, specifically through diagnosis, prognosis, and predication of therapy response.[50]

References

1. Pierotti MA, Sozzi G, Croce CM. Oncogenes. In: Kufe DW, Pollock RE, Weichselbaum RR, et al., eds. *Cancer medicine.* 6th ed. Hamilton, ON: BC Decker; 2003:73–85.
2. Park BH, Vogelstein B. Tumor-suppressor genes. In: Kufe DW, Pollack RE, Weichselbaum RR, et al., eds. *Cancer medicine.* 6th ed. Hamilton, ON: BC Decker; 2003:87–106.
3. Kaul KL. Solid tumors. In: Leonard DGB, ed. *Molecular pathology in clinical practice.* Springer, New York; 2006:269–313.
4. Bagg A. Neoplastic hematopathology In: Leonard DGB, ed. *Molecular pathology in clinical practice.* Springer, New York; 2006:321–383.
5. Tomlins SA, Rhodes DR, Perner S, et al. Recurrent fusion of TMPRSS2 and ETS transcription factor genes in prostate cancer. *Science.* 2005;310:644–648.
6. Chow E, Macrae F. Review of juvenile polyposis syndrome. *J Gastroenterol Hepatol.* 2005;20:1634–1640.
7. Haidle JL, Howe JR. *Juvenile polyposis syndrome.* Genereviews, September, 2008. Available at: http://www.ncbi.nlm.nih.gov/bookshelf/br.fcgi?book=gene&part=jps
8. Wu TT, Rezai B, Rashid A, et al. Genetic alterations and epithelial dysplasia in juvenile polyposis syndrome and sporadic juvenile polyps. *Am J Pathol.* 1997;150:937–947.

9. Merg A, Howe JR. Genetic conditions associated with intestinal juvenile polyps. *Am J Med Genet C Semin Med Genet.* 2004;129:44–55.

10. Fearon ER, Bommer GT. Molecular biology of colorectal cancer. In: DeVita VT, Lawrence TS, Rosenberg SA, eds. *Cancer: principles and practice of oncology.* 8th ed. Philadelphia, PA: Lippncott Williams & Wilkins; 2008:1218–1223.

11. Gallione CJ, Richards JA, Letteboer TG, et al. SMAD4 mutations found in unselected HHT patients. *J Med Genet.* 2006;43:793–797.

12. Mais DD, Nordberg ML. Gastrointestinal tumor syndromes. In: Mais DD, Nordberg ML, eds. *Quick compendium of molecular pathology.* Chicago, IL: ASCP Press; 2009:214.

13. Jenne DE, Reimann H, Nezu J, et al. Peutz-Jeghers syndrome is caused by mutations in a novel serine threonine kinase. *Nat Genet.* 1998;18:38–43.

14. Neibergs HL, Massey AT. Familial adenomatous polyposis and Turcot and Peutz-Jeghersmes. In: Leonard DGB, ed. *Molecular pathology in clinical practice.* Springer, New York; 2006:215–222.

15. Brooks-Wilson AR, Kaurah P, Suriano G, et al. Germline E-cadherin mutations in hereditary diffuse gastric cancer: assessment of 42 new families and review of genetic screening criteria. *J Med Genet.* 2004;41:508–517.

16. Guilford P, Hopkins J, Harraway J, et al. E-cadherin germline mutations in familial gastric cancer. *Nature.* 1998;392:402–405.

17. Cisco RM, Ford JM, Norton JA. Hereditary diffuse gastric cancer: implications of genetic testing for screening and prophylactic surgery. *Cancer.* 2008;113(7 suppl):1850–1856.

18. Robertson EV, Jankowski JA. Genetics of gastroesophageal cancer: paradigms, paradoxes, and prognostic utility. *Am J Gastroenterol.* 2008;103:443–449.

19. Grady WM, Willis J, Guilford PJ, et al. Methylation of the CDH1 promoter as the second genetic hit in hereditary diffuse gastric cancer. *Nat Genet.* 2000;26:16–17.

20. Kelsen DP, Van De Velde CJH, Minsky BD. Gastric cancer management. In: Kelsen DP, Daly JM, Kern SE, eds. *Principles and practice of gastrointestinal oncology.* 2nd ed. Philadelphia, PA: Lippincott Williams & Wilkins; 2008:287; chap 23.

21. Moisio A-L, Jarvinen H, Peltomaki, et al. Genetic and clinical characterization of familial adenomatous polyposis: a population based study. *Gut.* 2002;50:845–850.

22. Mais DD, Nordberg ML. Gastrointestinal tumor syndromes. In: Mais DD, Nordberg ML, ed. *Quick compendium of molecular pathology.* Chicago, IL: ASCP Press; 2009:210–211.

23. Goodman AJ, Dundas SAC, Scholefield JH, et al. Gastric carcinoma and familial adenomatous polyposis (FAP). *Int J Colorect Dis.* 1988; 3:201–203.

24. Lakshman V, Shah AN, Ryan CK, et al. The presence of dysplasia and carcinoma in gastric fundic gland polyps in patients with familial adenomatous polyposis. *Gastroenterology.* 1997;112:A599.

25. Odze RD. Gastric fundic gland polyps: are they preneoplastic lesion? *Gastroenterology.* 1998;114: 422–423.

26. Groves C, Lamlum H, Crabtree M, et al. Mutation cluster region, association between germline and somatic mutations and genotype-phenotype correlation in upper gastrointestinal familial adenomatous polyposis. *Am J of Pathol.* 2002;160:2055–2061.

27. Sieber OM, Lipton L, Crabtree M, et al. Multiple colorectal adenomas, classic adenomatous polyposis, and germ-line mutations in MYH. *N Eng J Med.* 1995;332:839–834.

28. American Gastroenterological Association. AGA technical review on hereditary colorectal cancer and genetic testing. *Gastroenterology.* 2001;121:198–213.

29. Lynch HT, Smyrk TC, Watson P, et al. Genetics, nature history, tumor spectrum, and pathology of hereditary nonpolyposis colorectal cancer: an updated review. *Gastroenterology.* 1993;104:1535–1549.

30. Boland CR, Koi M, Chang DK, et al. The biochemical basis of microsatellite instability and abnormal in immunohistochemistry and clinical behavior in Lynch syndrome: from bench to bedside. *Fam Cancer.* 2008;7:41–52.

31. Peltomaki P. Role of DNA mismatch repair defects in the pathogenesis of human cancer. *J Clin Oncol.* 2003;21:1174–1179.

32. Aarnio M, Salovaara R, Lauri A, et al. Features of gastric cancer in hereditary non-polyposis colorectal cancer syndrome. *Int J Cancer.* 1997;74:551–555.

33. Sankila R, Aaltonen LA, Jarvinen HJ, et al. Better survival rates in patients with MLH1-associated hereditary colorectal cancer. *Gastroenterology.* 1996;110:943–947.

34. Syngal S, Fox EA, Eng C, et al. Sensitivity and specificity of clinical criteria for hereditary non-polyposis colorectal cancer associated mutations in MSH2 and MLH1. *J Med Genet.* 2000;37:641–645.

35. Wahlberg SS, Schmeits J, Thomas G, et al. Evaluation of microsatellite instability and immunohistochemistry for the prediction of germ-line MSH2 and MLH1 mutations in hereditary nonpolyposis colon cancer families. *Cancer Res.* 2002;62:3485–3492.

36. de Jong AE, Nagengast FM, Kleibeuker JH, et al. What is the appropriate screening protocol in Lynch syndrome? *Fam Cancer.* 2006;5:373–378.

37. Musulen E, Moreno V, Reyes G, et al. Standardized approach for microsatellite instability detection in gastric carcinoma. *Hum Pathol.* 2004;35:335–342.

38. Pfeifer JD. Gastrointestinal tract. In: Pfeifer JD, ed. *Molecular genetic testing in surgical pathology.* Philadelphia, PA: Lippincott Williams & Wilkins; 2006:303–306.

39. Fenoglio-Preiser C, Carneiro F, Correa P, et al. Gastric carcinoma. In: Hamilton SR, Aaltonen LA, eds. *Pathology and genetics tumours of the digestive system.* Lyon: IARC Press; 2000:39–67.

40. Fletcher CD, Berman JJ, Corless C, et al. Diagnosis of gastrointestinal stromal tumors: a consensus approach. *Hum Pathol.* 2002;33:459–465.

41. Miettinen M, Lasota J. Gastrointestinal stromal tumors. Review on morphology, molecular pathology, prognosis, and differential diagnosis. *Arch Pathol Lab Med.* 2006;130:1466–1478.

42. Corless CL, Fletcher JA, Heinrich MC. Biology of gastrointestinal stromal tumors. *J Clin Oncol.* 2004;22:3813–3825.

43. Peterson MR, Piao Z, Weidner N. Strong PDGFRA positivity is seen in GISTs but not in other intra-abdominal mesenchymal tumors: immunohistochemical and mutational analyses. *Appl Immunohistochem Mol Morphol.* 2006;14:390–396.

44. Inagaki H. Mucosa-associated lymphoid tissue lymphoma: molecular pathogenesis and clinicopathologic significance. *Pathol Int.* 2007;57:474–484.

45. Ming-Qing DU. MALT lymphoma: recent advances in aetiology and molecular genetics. *J Clin Exp Hematopathol.* 2007;47:31–42.

46. Ming S-C. Cellular and molecular pathology of gastric carcinoma and precursor lesions: a critical review. *Gastric Cancer.* 1998;1:31–50.

47. Stoicov C, Saffari R, Cai X, et al. Molecular biology of gastric cancer: Helicobacter infection and gastric adenocarcinoma: bacterial and host factors responsible for altered growth signaling. *Gene.* 2004; 341:1–17.

48. Smith-Zagone M, Pulliam JF, Farkas DH. Molecular pathology methods. In: Leonard DGB, ed. *Molecular pathology in clinical practice.* Springer, New York; 2006:553–575.

49. Frayling IM, Payne DA, Highsmith WE, et al. Molecular diagnostic technologies. In: Coleman WB, Gregory J, ed. *Molecular diagnostics for clinical laboratorian.* 2nd ed. New Jersey: Humana Press; 2005; 65–149.

50. Mansour JC, Schwarz RE. Molecular mechanisms for individualized cancer care (review). *J Am Coll Surg.* 2008;207:250–258.

Epigenetic Abnormalities of Gastric Cancer

14

► Annie On On Chan
► Asif Rashid

INTRODUCTION

Epigenetics refers to changes in the phenotype (appearance) or expression of genes that are caused by mechanisms other than changes in the underlying DNA sequence. Neoplastic cells have three paradoxical changes in DNA methylation[1]: increased expression or activity of DNA methyltransferases,[2] global hypomethylation,[3] and de novo CpG-island methylation.[1,2] Global reductions in the levels of 5-methylcytosine in a gene (hypomethylation) have been associated with tumorigenesis. Methylation of cytosine at CpG sequences is the only known DNA modification in human cells that can silence tumor suppressor genes in cancer. CpG methylation is an alternative to gene mutations and allelic losses as a mechanism for gene silencing, as demonstrated for a variety of genes, including the *von Hippel-Lindau, human mut L homologue 1 (hMLH1)* and *p16* tumor suppressor genes.[2] The primary evolutionary significance of DNA methylation has not been fully elucidated, but the leading hypothesis is that it evolved to silence and suppress the harmful effects of viruses and repeated DNA sequences.[3] Methylation of cytosines within CpG islands is associated with loss of protein expression by repression of transcription and is observed in normal physiological conditions such as aging, X chromosome inactivation, and imprinting.[1,2] CpG islands are 0.5- to 2-kilobase regions that are rich in the cytosine guanine dinucleotides and present in the 5′ regions of about half of all human genes.[4] Epigenetic silencing of tumor suppressor genes by CpG-island methylation is recognized as one of the most important mechanisms in carcinogenesis and is thought to initiate or act at an early stage of carcinogenesis. Gene silencing by CpG-island methylation is mediated in part by alterations in histone acetylation or methylation. The inactivation of chromatin by histone deacetylation suppresses transcription of tumor suppressor genes and likely also plays an early role in carcinogenesis.

Although decreasing in incidence, gastric cancer remains a major medical problem and is the second most common cause of cancer-related deaths worldwide. The incidence of gastric cancer is determined largely by environmental rather than genetic factors. The identification and subsequent classification of *Helicobacter pylori* infection as a type I carcinogen by the World Health Organization (WHO) were a major milestone in our understanding of the etiology of gastric cancer. Gastric cancer progresses through a series of morphological steps, from gastritis to early precancerous lesions to intestinal metaplasia and dysplasia to adenocarcinoma. The earliest alterations in the gastric mucosa involve epigenetic changes such as hypermethylation, which results in gene inactivation. This chapter focuses on the epigenetic changes along with environmental factors that contribute to gastric carcinogenesis.

CpG-ISLAND METHYLATION OF TUMOR SUPPRESSOR GENES IN GASTRIC CANCER AND NONNEOPLASTIC MUCOSAE

A large number of genes, including tumor suppressor genes, have been reported to be methylated in nonneoplastic mucosae, precursor lesions, and gastric cancers.[5–8] Some of these genes include *adenomatous polyposis coli, Cox-2, death-associated protein kinase, glutathione S-transferase P1, E-cadherin, hMLH1, O⁶-methylguanine methyltransferase, p14, p16, RAS association family 1A, thrombospondin 1*, and *tissue inhibitors of metalloproteinase 3*. Methylation of these genes has been shown to accumulate in the multistep gastric carcinogenesis process[5] and is associated with the increased expression of DNA methyltransferase 1 in gastric cancers.[8]

CpG-island methylation is dependent on the gene involved, the age of the patient, the underlying inflammatory conditions, and the site and histology of the nonneoplastic or neoplastic lesions. Similar patterns of age-related and cancer-specific methylation were observed in other epithelial malignancies besides gastric cancer.[5] Some genes, such as *death-associated protein kinase*, are methylated with similar frequencies in nonneoplastic mucosae, precursor lesions, and invasive carcinomas.[5] In contrast, other genes, such as the *E-cadherin, p16*, and *hMLH1* tumor suppressor genes, show a stepwise increase in the frequency of methylation as the disease progresses from normal mucosa to invasive carcinoma.[5,7] Methylation of some genes in nonneoplastic mucosae increases with the age of the patient and is more frequent in patients with gastric cancer than in those without gastric cancer.[5] This age-associated increase in methylation in gastric nonneoplastic mucosae is observed for some genes, such as *E-cadherin* and *p16*, whereas others, such as *hMLH1*, show no increase in methylation.[7]

E-CADHERIN METHYLATION IN THE STOMACH

Of the genes that play a major role in gastric carcinogenesis, *E-cadherin*, a transmembrane glycoprotein that mediates cell adhesion, is one of the most well-studied.[9] *E-cadherin* methylation has been reported in more than half of gastric cancers and is more common in diffuse-type carcinomas. Among patients with gastric cancers, those with intestinal metaplasia and invasive carcinomas have reduced expression of E-cadherin owing to *E-cadherin* methylation, suggesting that the loss of E-cadherin and its cell adhesion function plays a part in early gastric carcinogenesis.[10] *E-cadherin* methylation has also been found in the nonneoplastic gastric mucosae of gastric cancer patients.[7,10]

Interestingly, *E-cadherin* methylation has also been found in nonneoplastic mucosae (without intestinal metaplasia) from one third of dyspepsia patients without gastric cancer and is associated with *H. pylori* infection.[11] *E-cadherin* methylation has been found in the mucosae of approximately half of all patients with *H. pylori* infection (without intestinal metaplasia), and this methylation is reversible in at least two thirds of the patients when the infection is eradicated.[11] In contrast, the methylation of other genes is not reversed by the eradication of *H. pylori* infection. Thus, it appears that *H. pylori* infection can induce reversible epigenetic alterations of the *E-cadherin* gene.

METHYLATION BY CHRONIC INFLAMMATORY CONDITIONS AND GASTRIC CARCINOGENESIS

CpG-island methylation is increased in patients with chronic inflammatory conditions and may contribute to the pathogenesis of tumors that develop in patients with these conditions. In the stomach, *H. pylori* and Epstein-Barr virus infections are associated with increased methylation in nonneoplastic mucosae, and studies have shown that increased CpG-island methylation in the affected nonneoplastic mucosae is a precursor to gastric cancer.[12,13] Thus, methylation may be one of the primary molecular mediators of gastric cancer and gastric cancer precursors arising in patients with inflammatory conditions, and this methylation is gene and precursor lesion dependent.

H. pylori infection also induces aberrant methylation in other genes and loci besides *E-cadherin* in nonneoplastic mucosae and precursor lesions.[11,14] Methylation of eight CpG loci was higher in nonneoplastic mucosa of healthy volunteers with *H. pylori* infection or in nonneoplastic mucosa from gastric cancer patients without *H. pylori* infection than in healthy volunteers without infection.[14] In contrast, there was a large variation in the methylation patterns between nonneoplastic mucosae from gastric cancer patients with *H. pylori* infection and healthy volunteers with the infection, but only one of the eight loci showed a significant difference in methylation patterns. In a population-based study, *p16* methylation was higher in patients with *H. pylori* infection who had superficial gastritis, chronic atrophic gastritis, intestinal metaplasia, dysplasia, and dysplasia characterized as indeterminate than in patients with similar lesions but without infection.[15] Similarly, *H. pylori* infection was an independent risk factor for *RUNX3* methylation in the nonneoplastic mucosae from patients with gastric cancer.[16] In another study, *H. pylori* infection was associated with promoter methylation of the *E-cadherin, adenomatous polyposis coli, Cox-2, p16,* and *hMLH1* genes.[17] While *E-cadherin* methylation was an early event in *H. pylori*–induced gastritis, *hMLH1* methylation occurred later, along with the development of intestinal metaplasia. More importantly, eradication of *H. pylori* significantly reduced gene methylation, which delayed or reversed *H. pylori*–induced gastric carcinogenesis.[17]

The mechanisms underlying the methylation of *E-cadherin* and other genes in patients with *H. pylori* infection are not completely understood, but the methylation appears to be mediated by inflammatory cytokines. Methylation of four genes, including *E-cadherin*, was more frequent in gastric cancer patients who had *H. pylori* infection and interleukin-1β polymorphisms, which are associated with increased production of the cytokine.[18] This finding was further corroborated by a study that showed that, when gastric cancer cells were incubated with interleukin-1β or cocultured with *H. pylori*, methylation of *E-cadherin* was induced, and this phenomenon was reversed by an interleukin-1β inhibitor.[19] Similarly, in another in vitro study, macrophages were stimulated by *H. pylori* or lipopolysaccharide to produce nitric oxide, which induced the methylation of *RUNX3* in a gastric cell line, and this methylation was inhibited by a nitric oxide inhibitor.[20]

Approximately 10% of gastric carcinomas worldwide are associated with Epstein-Barr virus infection and are more frequent in younger patients (**<60 years old**), men, Caucasians, and Hispanics. The Epstein-Barr virus–associated gastric carcinomas more frequently develop in the cardia or body of the stomach and have a "lymphoepithelial" carcinoma histology characterized by intratumoral and peritumoral lymphocytosis. In addition, the majority of Epstein-Barr virus–associated gastric cancers have high levels of CpG-island methylation.[21,22]

THE CpG-ISLAND METHYLATOR PHENOTYPE IN GASTRIC CARCINOMAS

Similar to colorectal cancers, approximately 30% to 50% of gastric cancers have a CpG-island methylator phenotype (CIMP-high) characterized by concordant methylation of multiple genes or loci, including the *p16* and *hMLH1* genes and multiple tumor-specific CpG islands (methylated in tumor 1 [MINT1], MINT2, MINT12, MINT25, and MINT31), which have been identified as de novo methylation sites in colorectal carcinomas.[23–25] The CIMP-high phenotype has also been reported in precursor lesions of gastric carcinomas. It is present in 15% of intestinal metaplasias and approximately 50% of dysplasias or adenomas in patients with or without gastric cancers.[24] This suggests that CIMP-high is an early event in gastric carcinogenesis.

The CIMP-high gastric carcinomas have been associated with higher stage tumors in one study[26] and with proximal tumor location, diffuse tumor type, and less advanced disease stage in another study.[27]

The microsatellite instability–high phenotype, which is characterized by allelic shifts in 30% to 40% of microsatellite markers, is present in approximately 30% of gastric carcinomas and is caused by the methylation-induced silencing of *hMLH1*,[28] especially in CIMP-high carcinomas, which have methylation of the *hMLH1* gene promoter.[23] These tumors have alterations in simple repetitive sequences that are contained within a number of target genes associated with cell proliferation, apoptosis, or DNA mismatch repair, including *transforming growth factor β type II receptor, Bcl-2–associated X (Bax), hMSH3,* and *E2F-4.*[29] Methylation of the *hMLH1* promoter has also been described in the nonneoplastic gastric epithelium adjacent to gastric cancers with the microsatellite instability–high phenotype.[30] This methylation field defect may increase the risk of synchronous or metachronous neoplasia, as the microsatellite instability–high phenotype has also been observed in patients with multiple gastric cancers.[31]

METHYLATION AND PROGNOSIS IN GASTRIC CANCER

Similar to other tumors, CpG-island methylation and CIMP have been associated with prognosis in gastric cancers. Patients whose resected gastric cancers have methylation of the MINT31 locus have better prognoses than those whose tumors are unmethylated at MINT31.[25] Similarly, patients whose resected gastric cancers are CIMP-high have better prognoses than those whose tumors are CIMP-low or negative. However, neither MINT31 methylation nor CIMP-high phenotype is an independent predictor of survival.[25] In contrast, another study showed that methylation of *protocadherin 10* in the nonneoplastic mucosae of patients with gastric cancer was an independent predictor of poor prognosis.[32]

HISTONE ACETYLATION

DNA methylation affects gene expression by altering chromatin states, and recently, the molecular mechanisms have been clarified. A seminal observation was that dense DNA methylation results in local histone deacetylation through the recruitment of a protein complex that includes histone deacetylases and other chromatin modifiers.[33–35] This protein complex is recruited and targeted to hypermethylated promoters by methyl-binding proteins.[4] It has now become clear that the switch from the unmethylated to methylated states sets up a cascade of events that result in sequential modifications of histones (deacetylation, methylation, binding of chromatin regulatory proteins such as HP1, etc.), culminating in the silencing of genes.[4]

Inactivation of chromatin by the deacetylation and methylation of several lysines in histone H3 and H4 is involved in the transcriptional repression of several tumor suppressor genes, including *p21WAF1/CIP1*. Hypoacetylation of histones H3 and H4 in the *p21WAF1/CIP1* promoter region is observed in >50% of gastric cancer tissue samples by chromatin immunoprecipitation.[36] Using an antiacetylated histone antibody, the global acetylation status of histones can be analyzed by immunohistochemical analysis of gastric cancer tissue specimens.[37] The level of acetylated histone H4 expression is reduced in 70% of gastric cancers in comparison with nonneoplastic mucosae, indicating that there is global hypoacetylation in gastric cancer. Reduced expression of acetylated histone H4 correlates well with advanced tumor stage, deep tumor invasion, and lymph node metastasis.[37] In fact, trichostatin A, a histone deacetylase inhibitor, induced growth arrest and apoptosis and suppressed the invasion of gastric cancer cell lines.[37,38] In another study, trimethylation of lysine 9 of histone H3 (H3K9) positively correlated with tumor stage and cancer recurrence, and a higher level of H3K9 trimethylation was an independent predictor of survival.[39]

CLINICAL APPLICATIONS

Epigenetic alterations in gastric cancer tissue and precursor lesions to gastric cancer have raised expectations that methylation assessment–based methodologies can be used for prevention, risk assessment, early detection, determination of prognosis, identification of therapeutic targets, and assessment of response to therapy. For early detection, DNA methylation has been proposed as a particularly good early biomarker of disease activity. For stomach cancer, this could take the form of detecting methylation in nonneoplastic mucosae,[14,40,41] gastric washes,[42] or sera[43,44] to assess risk or for early detection of gastric cancer. While proof of concept for these approaches has been established, the sensitivity and, importantly, specificity of these findings remain to be established.

The most provocative clinical implication of this work relates to targeting epigenetic changes as a treatment for gastric malignancies. Inhibitors of DNA methyltransferases reactivate gene expression in vitro in various gastrointestinal (GI) malignancies, and histone deacetylase inhibitors potentiate this effect. 5-Aza-2′-deoxycytidine is a potent inhibitor of DNA methylation in vitro and has shown promise in hematological malignancies in vivo.[45]

CONCLUSION

Research into the epigenetic changes in gastric malignancies has opened fascinating new windows related to the etiology of and the molecular pathways that lead to neoplastic transformation. The concept that epigenetic changes could be a parallel and potentially equal pathway to genetic changes in driving clonal selection has profound epidemiologic and clinical implications, and therapy targeted at epigenetic changes holds much promise for the future treatment of gastric cancer.

References

1. Jones PA, Laird PW. Cancer epigenetics comes of age. *Nat Genet.* 1999;21:163–167.
2. Baylin SB, Herman JG, Graff JR, et al. Alterations in DNA methylation: a fundamental aspect of neoplasia. *Adv Cancer Res.* 1998;72:141–196.
3. Yoder JA, Walsh CP, Bestor TH. Cytosine methylation and the ecology of intragenomic parasites. *Trends Genet.* 1997;13:335–340.
4. Bird A. DNA methylation patterns and epigenetic memory. *Genes Dev.* 2002;16:6–21.
5. Kang GH, Shim YH, Jung HY, et al. CpG island methylation in premalignant stages of gastric carcinoma. *Cancer Res.* 2001;67:2847–2851.
6. To KF, Leung WK, Lee TL, et al. Promoter hypermethylation of tumor-related genes in gastric intestinal metaplasia of patients with and without gastric cancer. *Int J Cancer.* 2002;102:623–628.
7. Waki T, Tamura G, Tsuchiya T, et al. Promoter methylation status of E-cadherin, hMLH1, and p16 genes in non-neoplastic gastric epithelia. *Am J Pathol.* 2002;161:399–403.
8. Etoh T, Kanai Y, Ushijima S, et al. Increased DNA methyltransferase 1 (DNMT1) protein expression correlates significantly with poorer tumor differentiation and frequent DNA hypermethylation of multiple CpG islands in gastric cancers. *Am J Pathol.* 2004;164:689–699.
9. Tamura G, Yin J, Wang S, et al. E-cadherin gene promoter hypermethylation in primary human gastric carcinomas. *J Nat Cancer Inst.* 2000;92:569–573.
10. Chan AO, Lam SK, Wong BCY, et al. Promoter methylation of E-cadherin gene in gastric mucosa associated with *Helicobacter pylori* infection and in gastric cancer. *Gut.* 2003;52:502–506.
11. Chan AO, Peng JZ, Lam SK, et al. Eradication of *Helicobacter pylori* infection reverses E-cadherin promoter hypermethylation. *Gut.* 2006;55:463–468.
12. Kang GH, Lee HJ, Hwang KS, et al. Aberrant CpG island hypermethylation of chronic gastritis, in relation to aging, gender, intestinal metaplasia, and chronic inflammation. *Am J Pathol.* 2003;163:1551–1556.

13. Etoh T, Kanai Y, Ushijima S, et al. Increased DNA methyltransferase 1 (DNMT1) protein expression correlates significantly with poorer tumor differentiation and frequent DNA hypermethylation of multiple CpG islands in gastric cancers. *Am J Pathol.* 2004;164:689–699.

14. Maekita T, Nakazawa K, Mihara M, et al. High levels of aberrant DNA methylation in *Helicobacter pylori*-infected gastric mucosae and its possible association with gastric cancer risk. *Clin Cancer Res.* 2006; 12:989–995.

15. Dong CX, Deng DJ, Pan KF, et al. Promoter methylation of p16 associated with *Helicobacter pylori* infection in precancerous gastric lesions: a population-based study. *Int J Cancer.* 2009;124:434–439.

16. Kitajima Y, Ohtaka K, Mitsuno M, et al. *Helicobacter pylori* infection is an independent risk factor for Runx3 methylation in gastric cancer. *Oncol Rep.* 2008;19:197–202.

17. Perri F, Cotugno R, Piepoli A, et al. Aberrant DNA methylation in non-neoplastic gastric mucosa of *H. pylori* infected patients and effect of eradication. *Am J Gastroenterol.* 2007;102:1361–1371.

18. Chan AO, Chu KM, Huang C, et al. Association between *Helicobacter pylori* infection and interleukin 1beta polymorphism predispose to CpG island methylation in gastric cancer. *Gut.* 2007;56:595–597.

19. Qian X, Huang C, Cho CH, et al. E-cadherin promoter hypermethylation induced by interleukin-1beta treatment or *H. pylori* infection in human gastric cancer cell lines. *Cancer Lett.* 2008;263:107–113.

20. Katayama Y, Takahashi M, Kuwayama H. *Helicobacter pylori* causes runx3 gene methylation and its loss of expression in gastric epithelial cells, which is mediated by nitric oxide produced by macrophages. *Biochem Biophys Res Commun.* 2009;388:496–500.

21. Chang MS, Uozaki H, Chong JM, et al. CpG island methylation status in gastric carcinoma with and without infection of Epstein-Barr virus. *Clin Cancer Res.* 2006;12:2995–3002.

22. Lee J-H, Kim S-H, Han S-H, et al. Clinicopathologic and molecular characteristics of Epstein-Barr virus-associated gastric cancer: a meta-analysis. *J Gastroenterol Hepatol.* 2009;24:354–365.

23. Toyota M, Ahuja N, Suzuki H, et al. Aberrant methylation in gastric cancer associated with the CpG island methylator phenotype. *Cancer Res.* 1999;59:5438–5442.

24. Lee J-K, Park S-J, Abraham SC, et al. Frequent CpG island methylation in precursor lesions and early gastric adenocarcinomas. *Oncogene.* 2004;23:4646–4654.

25. An C, Choi IS, Yao JC, et al. Prognostic significance of CpG island methylator phenotype and microsatellite instability in gastric carcinoma. *Clin Cancer Res.* 2005;11:656–663.

26. Oue N, Mitani Y, Motoshita J, et al. Accumulation of DNA methylation is associated with tumor stage in gastric cancer. *Cancer.* 2006;106:1250–1259.

27. Kusano M, Toyota M, Suzuki H, et al. Genetic, epigenetic, and clinicopathologic features of gastric carcinomas with the CpG island methylator phenotype and an association with Epstein-Barr virus. *Cancer.* 2006;106:1467–1479.

28. Fleisher AS, Esteller M, Wang S, et al. Hypermethylation of the hMLH1 gene promoter in human gastric cancers with microsatellite instability. *Cancer Res.* 1999;59:1090–1095.

29. Kim JJ, Baek MJ, Kim L, et al. Accumulated frameshift mutations at coding nucleotide repeats during the progression of gastric carcinoma with microsatellite instability. *Lab Investig.* 1999;79:1113–1120.

30. Endoh Y, Tamura G, Ajioka Y, et al. Frequent hypermethylation of the hMLH1 gene promoter in differentiated-type tumors of the stomach with the gastric foveolar phenotype. *Am J Pathol.* 2000; 157:717–722.

31. Guo RJ, Arai H, Kitayama Y, et al. Microsatellite instability of papillary subtype of human gastric adenocarcinoma and hMLH1 promoter hypermethylation in the surrounding mucosa. *Pathol Int.* 2001; 51:240–247.

32. Yu J, Cheng YY, Tao Q, et al. Methylation of protocadherin 10, a novel tumor suppressor, is associated with poor prognosis in patients with gastric cancer. *Gastroenterology.* 2009;136:640–651.

33. Kass SU, Landsberger N, Wolffe AP. DNA methylation directs a time-dependent repression of transcription initiation. *Curr Biol.* 1997;7:157–165.

34. Nan X, Ng HH, Johnson CA, et al. Transcriptional repression by the methyl-CpG-binding protein MeCP2 involves a histone deacetylase complex. *Nature.* 1998;393:386–389.

35. Jones PL, Veenstra GJ, Wade PA, et al. Methylated DNA and MeCP2 recruit histone deacetylase to repress transcription. *Nat Genet.* 1998;19:187–191.

36. Mitani Y, Oue N, Hamai Y, et al. Histone H3 acetylation is associated with reduced p21WAF1/CIP1 expression in gastric carcinoma. *J Pathol.* 2005;205:65–73.

37. Yasui W, Oue N, Ono S, et al. Histone acetylation and gastrointestinal carcinogenesis. *Ann N Y Acad Sci.* 2003;983:220–231.

38. Suzuki T, Kuniyasu H, Hayashi K, et al. Effect of trichostatin A on cell growth and expression of cell cycle- and apoptosis-related molecules in human gastric and oral carcinoma cell lines. *Int J Cancer*. 2000; 88:992–997.
39. Park YS, Jin MY, Kim YJ, et al. The global histone modification pattern correlates with cancer recurrence and overall survival in gastric adenocarcinoma. *Ann Surg Oncol*. 2008;15:1968–1976.
40. Tahara T, Arisawa T, Shibata T, et al. Risk prediction of gastric cancer by analysis of aberrant DNA methylation in non-neoplastic gastric epithelium. *Digestion*. 2007;75:54–61.
41. Castellvi-Bei S, Castells A. Aberrant DNA methylation in non-tumor gastric mucosa: a potential marker of early detection of gastric mucosa? *Gastroenterology*. 2006;135:1647–1649.
42. Watanabe Y, Kim HS, Castoro RJ, et al. Sensitive and specific detection of early gastric cancer with DNA methylation analysis of gastric washes. *Gastroenterology*. 2009;136:2149–2158.
43. Wang YC, Yu ZH, Liu C, et al. Detection of RASSF1A promoter hypermethylation in serum from gastric and colorectal adenocarcinoma patients. *World J Gastroenterol*. 2008;14:3074–3080.
44. Abbaszadegari MR, Moaven O, Sima HR, et al. p16 promoter hypermethylation: a useful serum marker for early detection of gastric cancer. *World J Gastroenterol*. 2008;14:2055–2060.
45. Issa JP. Decitabine. *Curr Opin Oncol*. 2003;15:446–451.

15

Molecular Biomarkers of Gastric Adenocarcinoma

▶ John J. Liang

▶ Dongfeng Tan

INTRODUCTION

Gastric cancer is a global health problem with a high rate of incidence and mortality. It is the second most common cause of death from cancer, with an estimated 700,000 deaths each year worldwide.[1] Its incidence varies widely from country to country (see Chapter 2). The Laurén classification is the most widely used histologic classification of gastric cancer. In 1965, Laurén[2] classified gastric carcinoma into the intestinal and diffuse subtypes. The intestinal type is strongly associated with *Helicobacter pylori* infection and commonly arises within a background of chronic gastritis, glandular atrophy, and intestinal metaplasia (see Chapter 3). In contrast, diffuse-type adenocarcinomas often present with diffuse thickening of the stomach wall rather than a mass.

Although gastric carcinoma has shown a decline in frequency in the United States and Western Europe,[1] it is still very common in developing countries. The prognosis for gastric carcinoma traditionally has been poor, mainly due to an advanced stage at diagnosis, with a 5-year survival rate of <5%. In contrast, very early gastric cancer is a curable disease, and the 5-year survival rate of surgically treated early gastric cancer approaches 90% to 95%. Therefore, it is crucial to identify clinically useful molecular markers that can detect gastric cancer at an early stage. Recent studies have demonstrated that many factors are involved in the progression of gastric neoplasia, including genetic and environmental factors (*H. pylori* infection, diet, and smoking) and predisposing lesions, among others. Adenocarcinoma of the cardia and Barrett-associated adenocarcinomas of the esophagus share similar backgrounds, temporal trends, molecular profiles, and behavioral patterns, which have recently been reviewed.[4] In this chapter, we focus on molecular genetics and potential diagnostic molecular biomarkers in noncardia/distal gastric carcinoma.

MOLECULAR MODELS OF GASTRIC ADENOCARCINOMA

The intestinal type of gastric carcinoma that predominates in geographical regions with high incidence is more frequently observed in older patients (>65 years old) and develops from precursor lesions associated with intestinal metaplasia and dysplasia. In contrast, the incidence of the diffuse type is relatively constant, and the tumors have no identifiable precursor lesions. Diffuse cancer occurs more commonly in young patients, is multifocal, and is rarely associated with intestinal metaplasia. Recent studies have demonstrated that many genetic alterations are involved in the development and progression of gastric cancer.[3] It appears that there are different genetic pathways leading to intestinal- and diffuse-type gastric adenocarcinoma (GAC). In 1992, Correa[5] postulated a multistep and multifactorial model of intestinal-type GAC, involving development of chronic gastritis, atrophy, intestinal metaplasia, and dysplasia and eventually GAC. A number of molecular abnormalities have been identified, including microsatellite instability (MSI), inactivation of tumor suppressor genes, activation of oncogenes, and reactivation of telomerase.[3] On the basis of the findings from prophylactic gastrectomy specimens, Carneiro et al.[6] proposed a model for the development of diffuse-type GAC in E-cadherin (CDH1) mutation carriers, involving development of nonatrophic gastritis, in situ signet ring cell carcinoma, pagetoid spread of signet ring cells, and invasive GAC. It is believed that the histology of gastric mucosa is normal in CDH1 mutation carriers until the second CDH1 allele is inactivated by multiple factors.

PROMISING MARKERS IN EVALUATION OF PREMALIGNANT LESIONS

Intestinal-type GAC typically arises in the setting of chronic gastritis. The progression from atrophic gastritis, intestinal metaplasia, and dysplasia to GAC is dependent on continued chronic inflammation.[7] Several genetic changes with p16 methylation in intestinal metaplasia have been shown in association with *H. pylori* infection in gastric precancerous lesions.[8] Murata-Kamiya et al. found that E-cadherin expression in *H. pylori*–infected gastric mucosa was decreased compared with that in the control group. The cytoplasmic and nuclear accumulation of β-catenin induced by interaction of CagA with CDH1 has been implicated in the development of intestinal metaplasia.[9] Zavros et al.[10] demonstrated that down-regulation of Sonic hedgehog (Shh) by *H. pylori* leads to the disruption of glandular structure and the gain of a more intestinal phenotype through up-regulation of intestine-related genes, such as CDX2, MUC2, and villin. Gastric intestinal metaplasia can be induced through ectopically expressed Cdx2 in mouse models.[11] Studies by Wang and coworkers showed that overexpression of Shh was significantly correlated with premalignant lesions and carcinoma.[12] Shh expression was associated with clinical stage, direct tumor invasion, and differentiation of tumor cells.[12] These studies suggest that Shh expression is involved in gastric carcinogenesis. The genetic and epigenetic changes in intestinal metaplasia and premalignant lesions could be used as surrogate markers for the evaluation of GAC risk and clinical malignant potential.

MSI, HYPERMETHYLATION, AND TARGET GENES

MSI is a marker of the presence of replication errors in simple repetitive microsatellite sequences due to DNA mismatch repair (MMR) deficiency. MMR proteins include the MutS proteins hMSH2, hMSH3, and hMSH6 and the MutL proteins hMLH1, hPMS1, hPMS2, and hMLH3.[13] Tumors are classified as MSI-high (MSI-H) when at least 30% of the microsatellite markers examined show MSI, whereas tumors with <30% of the markers showing instability are described as MSI-low (MSI-L). Those with no instability at any loci examined are considered stable (MSS). Several studies have reported that MSI is present in both familial and sporadic GAC and that about 20% to 30% of GACs have MSI.[14] MSI occurs at the stage of chronic gastritis, several years before a diagnosis of GAC.[15] Therefore, MSI analysis is promising as a valuable marker of the risk of progression to cancer.

MSI analysis of colonic carcinomas showed that MSI-H tumors were associated significantly with inactivation of hMLH1.[16] Genome-wide hypomethylation and selective hypermethylation of DNA sequences have been recognized as hallmarks of human cancers.[17] Recent studies have demonstrated that hypermethylation of gene promoters occurs along the pathway from chronic gastritis, intestinal metaplasia, and adenoma to GAC.[18] Loss of expression of hMLH1 associated with promoter hypermethylation is the underlying mechanism causing MSI in gastric adenomas and early gastric cancer, similar to findings for advanced gastric cancers. Baek and co-workers found, by using immunohistochemistry, that about 87% to 88% of MSI-positive gastric adenoma and GAC show absent or decreased hMLH1 expression and that all of these tumors have methylation of the hMLH1 gene promoter.[19a] Carvalho et al.[19b] reported that hypermethylation was detected in about 30% of COX2 and hMLH1 and in about 50% to 60% of CDH1 and MGMT gene promoters in sporadic GAC. These results indicate that inactivation of different gene promoters by hypermethylation plays an important role in carcinogenesis of GAC. MSI-H GAC is associated with antral location, intestinal-type differentiation, relatively old patients, and a better prognosis.[20] In a large series of GAC studies, MSI was detected in 16% of cases and was significantly associated with long survival. Therefore, MSI analysis has clinical prognostic utility (see Chapter 17).

There are hundreds of thousands of mutations in MSI carcinomas due to genetic instability. Approximately 70% of TGFβRII genes, 25% of IGFIIR genes, and 30% of BAX genes were found to be mutated in GAC.[21] Transforming growth factor-β (TGF-β) family members are involved in the regulation of cell proliferation, differentiation, motility, and apoptosis. TGF-β action starts after its secretion in the extracellular matrix as a latent protein complex. TGF-β signaling is initiated by the binding of TGF-β ligands to type II TGF-β receptors (TGFβRII). Once bound to TGF-β, TGFβRII recruits and phosphorylates the type I TGF-β receptor TGFβRI, which stimulates TGFβRI protein kinase activity.

The high frequency of TGFβRII gene mutations suggests that the alteration of TGFβRII gene mutations occurs earlier than for IGFIIR, BAX, and TCF-4 genes in gastric carcinogenesis and that it is associated with intestinal-type GAC.[22] There are two types of TGF-β serine/threonine kinase receptors: type I and type II, both necessary for downstream signal transduction. Mutations of the type II receptors can interrupt the signal transduction passway, resulting in growth stimulation rather than growth restriction. In one study, frame-shift mutations of TGFβRII were detected in 38% of MSI-H adenomas, but no frame-shift mutations of hMSH6 and IGFIIR were observed.[23] Kim et al.[24] reported that MSI-positive adenomas coexisting with cancer showed a higher mutation rate of the TGFβRII gene than those not coexisting with cancer (88% compared with 40%), suggesting that gastric adenoma with TGFβRII gene mutation may be more likely to transform into carcinoma.

IGFIIR is a multifunctional protein with important functions in lysosomal enzyme trafficking, endocytosis, and activation of TGF-β.[25] Mutations of IGFIIR poly(G) 8 were detected in about 30% of MSI gastric tumors and were significantly associated with low frequency of lymph node metastasis and serosal invasion.[26] These findings raise the possibility that the IGFIIR mutation is a prognostic marker for GAC.

INACTIVATION OF TUMOR SUPPRESSOR GENES

APC and p53

Up to 60% of intestinal-type gastric tumors and approximately 25% of gastric adenomas harbor mutation and/or loss of heterozygosity (LOH) of *APC,* but such are rare in diffuse-type GAC.[27] Consistently, β-catenin mutations have also been detected in intestinal-type gastric tumors but are absent from diffuse-type tumors.[28] Furthermore, Abraham et al.[29] reported that 91% of intestinal-type adenomas harbored at least one detectable genetic alteration, including APC alterations, MSI-H, or K-ras mutations. In that study, APC mutations, including stop codon and frame-shift mutations, were reported in 46% and 5q allelic loss in 33% of informative cases of gastric adenoma. APC gene mutations were detected in 67% of the gastric adenomas/dysplasia with low levels of MSI but in none of the adenomas/dysplasia with the MSI-H phenotype.[29] These data suggest that MSI-H and MSI-L tumors may have different molecular pathways.

The tumor protein 53 gene (*p53*) is one of the most frequently mutated tumor suppressor genes in human carcinogenesis and plays a pivotal role in the cellular response to stress by inducing cell growth arrest or apoptosis. It is conceivable that functional variants in *TP53,* which differ in their biological functions, may influence the initiation and progression of normal tissues to malignancies. p53 gene alterations were detected in 38% of intestinal metaplasia, 58% of dysplasia, and 67% of GAC.[30] A study by Lee et al.[31] found that APC mutations occurred in 74% of flat dysplasia, 77% of adenomas, and 45% of GAC. Among those cases, 71% of mutations occurred at exons 5 to 8, leading to G:C to A:T transitions.[52] These data suggest that mutation of the p53 gene is an early event in gastric carcinogenesis.

ACTIVATION OF ONCOGENES

KRAS and BRAF Mutations

K-ras and related B-raf are members in the MAPK-ERK pathway, which mediates cellular responses to varied signals regulating cell growth, differentiation, and programmed cell death. Mutation of K-ras gene results in activation of the gene, leading to uncontrolled cell growth. K-ras mutations have been frequently observed in several human malignancies, including lung cancer, colon cancer, and prostate cancer, while K-ras mutation has been infrequently reported in gastric cancer. Hunt et al. reported that K-ras mutations were detected in 14% of biopsies from patients with atrophic gastritis; however, there was no predictive value for progression of preneoplastic changes or malignancy.[32] In addition, K-ras mutations were reported in <10% of adenomas, flat dysplasia, and carcinomas.[31]

B-raf, like K-ras, is a component of the RAF family of serine/threonine kinases, and consequently, activated B-raf promotes cell proliferation. BRAF mutations are inversely associated with KRAS mutation.[33] In contrast to KRAS, BRAF mutations do not occur in MSI-H GAC and are also very rare in MSS GAC.[34] One study found that only one (0.8%) of 124 MSS GAC had BRAF V600E mutations.[34] These findings indicate that KRAS but not BRAF mutations are involved in the carcinogenesis of GAC.

PIK3CA

The phosphatidylinositol 3-kinase (PI3K)/Akt signaling pathway plays an important role in the regulation of cell growth, proliferation, and survival and is involved in human tumorigenesis. PI3Ks are composed of heterodimers of a p85 regulatory subunit and one of the several p110 catalytic subunits. Among several isoforms of the catalytic subunits, only the a type has been shown to harbor oncogenic mutations or amplifications in its gene (PIK3CA) in human cancers. PIK3CA mutations were present in 4% to 25% of GAC, in 19.2% of MSI, and rarely in MSS.[35] In addition, PIK3CA alterations were found in both early and advanced specimens, suggesting an important role in the development and progression of GAC. Genomic amplification of PIKsCA was reported to occur in 36.4% of GAC and was strongly associated with increased expression of PIK3CA transcript and elevation of phophor-AKT.[36] PIK3CA is a promising molecular marker for early detection or for monitoring tumor progression and is a potential therapeutic target for specific inhibitors of the p110a subunit.

TELOMERASE REACTIVATION

Telomerase is a unique ribonucleoprotein enzyme that maintains telomere length through the addition of TTAGGG repeats.[37] The major components of telomerase are human telomerase RNA (hTR or TERC) and telomerase-associated protein 1 and its catalytic subunit (hTERT). Using TERC as a template, hTERT can add a six-nucleotide repeating sequence, TTAGGG, to the 3′ end of chromosomes, which elongates telomeres. Studies have found that telomerase is expressed in 85% to 90% of malignant tumors but is usually absent in normal somatic cells.[38] In addition, the nucleolar expression of hTERT has been shown to be associated with prognosis in patients with colon, lung, stomach, and urothelial cancers. hTERT-induced Mac-2 binding protein (Mac-2BP) was significantly elevated in the serum of gastric cancer patients and was also significantly associated with distant metastasis ($p = 0.05$) and higher tumor stage ($p = 0.04$), indicating that hTERT-induced Mac-2BP may be a useful marker for detecting the malignant progression of metastatic stomach cancers.[39]

E-CADHERIN, SECOND-HIT INACTIVATION, AND EGFR ACTIVATION

The CDH1 gene maps to chromosome 16q22.1 and encodes a calcium-dependent transmembrane cellular adhesion protein, which interacts with cytoskeleton actin filaments through catenins in regulating intracellular signaling and which promotes tumor growth through the Wnt signaling pathway. E-cadherin consists of five cadherin repeats (EC1–EC5) in the extracellular domain, one transmembrane domain, and an intracellular domain that binds p120-catenin and β-catenin. The intracellular domain contains a highly phosphorylated region vital to β-catenin binding and therefore to E-cadherin function. Loss of E-cadherin function or expression has been implicated in cancer progression and metastasis. It is estimated that about 30% to 40% of the families with hereditary diffuse gastric cancer (HDGC) have E-cadherin germline mutations with high susceptibility to early development of diffuse-type GAC.[40] In addition, somatic mutations of E-cadherin have also been detected in 40% to 83% of sporadic diffuse-type GAC. These results suggest that CDH1 may act as a tumor suppressor in diffuse gastric cancer and that its loss of function may predispose to gastric cancer.

Heterozygous carriers of CDH1 germline mutations are commonly asymptomatic at least until the second decade of life, when the remaining wild-type alleles of the E-cadherin gene are inactivated.[41] Studies of families with HDGC have shown that E-cadherin mutations are present in the whole sequence of the gene, with an absence of preferential hot spots; about 80% of these mutations are nonsense, slice-site, and frameshift, with 20% being missense mutations.[42,43]

Machado et al.[44] detected E-cadherin mutations in nine (56%) of 16 sporadic diffuse-type GACs but in none of seven intestinal-type GACs. E-cadherin promoter hypermethylation was present in 67% of cases with E-cadherin mutations.[44] In contrast, LOH is rarely present in sporadic diffuse-type GAC.[44] These data suggest that E-cadherin promoter hypermethylation is likely the second-hit inactivation mechanism in the sporadic diffuse-type GAC with E-cadherin gene mutations. Studies of HDGC cases showed that E-cadherin promoter hypermethylation occurs in about 40% of HDGC patients, with a relatively higher frequency of LOH than in sporadic diffuse-type GAC. Additional studies are needed to further characterize second-hit mechanisms of E-cadherin inactivation and the potential of demethylating drugs in targeted gene therapy in diffuse-type GAC.

As a membrane receptor, E-cadherin interacts with a number of the receptor tyrosine kinases (RTKs). The interaction of E-cadherin with epidermal growth factor receptor (EGFR) seems to require an intact extracellular E-cadherin domain based on constructs with various domain deletions.[45] This observation is further supported by the identification of E-cadherin gene mutations in patients with HDGC.[46] Mateus et al.[46] reported that the stability of EGFR/E-cadherin heterodimer was interrupted by the presence of single-point mutations in the extracellular domain (T340A and A634V) but not by the presence of intracellular E-cadherin alterations. The instability of EGFR/E-cadherin heterodimer resulted in EGFR activation, leading to cell proliferation and migration.[47]

RTKs, EGFR, AND ERBB2

EGFR and ERBB are glycoproteins with extracellular, transmembrane, and intracellular domains. The ligands bind the extracellular domain, and the intracellular domain carries tyrosine kinase activity. Overexpression or aberrant activation of EGFR has been reported in various cancers, including lung, breast, bladder, and prostatic cancers.[48,49] EGFR mutations were recently reported in about 3% of GACs and were associated with increased EGFR copy number, tumor size, and invasive behavior. These findings point to promising targets for therapeutic intervention.

Overexpression of ERBB2 has been reported in numerous cancers, including breast, lung, ovarian, and gastric cancers.[50,51] The overexpression of ERBB2 in GAC, as determined by using immunohistochemistry and fluorescence in situ hybridization techniques, was reported to range between 8% and 23% and was associated with invasive behavior.[52,53] The clinical utilities of overexpression of ERBB2 in GAC are promising.[54]

GENETIC SUSCEPTIBILITY TO GASTRIC CANCER

It is evident that gastric cancer is a disease of gene–environment interactions, as suggested by the varying geographic patterns of its incidence. For example, even in areas with high rates of *H. pylori* infection, only a small proportion of infected individuals develop gastric cancer, suggesting genetic susceptibility plays a role in the gastric cancer development. Genetic susceptibility to gastric cancer can be investigated by common genetic variants, such as single nucleotide polymorphisms (SNPs), in various genes that regulate multiple biological pathways. It has been found that the susceptibility to gastric carcinogenesis has a substantial influence on the population attributable risk by modulating the effects of environmental risk factors.

GSTM1 is a member of the GST family that facilitates the binding of glutathione (GSH), a nucleophilic tripeptide, to carcinogens, leading to detoxification of several known chemical compounds. The loss/absence of *GSTM1* expression, due to an inherited homozygous deletion of the *GSTM1* gene in the general population, may confer an increased cancer risk because of the deletion carriers' inability to detoxify several xenobiotics, causing a decreased defense against cellular damage.[55] Because in vitro studies have shown that *H. pylori* causes oxidative damage in gastric epithelial cells, the *GSTM1*-null genotype probably facilitates *H. pylori*–caused oxidative damage and therefore may be considered a risk factor for gastric cancer. A meta-analysis study using a pool of 25 GSTM1 studies found that the *GSTM1*-null genotype elevated the gastric cancer risk by 1.33-fold.[56] The increased risk associated with the *GSTM1*-null genotype was significant in both Chinese (OR = 1.58, 95% CI = 1.35–1.85) and other Asian ethnic groups (OR = 1.17, 95% CI = 1.01–1.36), however, not in Caucasians (OR= 1.03, 95% CI = 0.88–1.21).

Though similar studies evaluating gastric cancer susceptibility and potentially functional polymorphisms in varied candidate genes have been conducted, the results are yet inconsistent. It indicates that, in the future, well-designed large multicenter population-based studies will be needed to validate current findings and provide the rationale for identifying at-risk subpopulations for primary prevention of gastric cancer.

CONCLUSIONS

Rapid technical advances in DNA sequencing and related molecular analysis assays have disclosed somatic mutations involved in the development of GAC. A number of molecular abnormalities have been identified in GAC, including MSI, inactivation of tumor suppressor genes, activation of oncogenes, and reactivation of telomerase. Moreover, genetic susceptibility plays a role in the gastric cancer development. Although multiple molecular alterations are involved in intestinal-type GAC, the significance of these molecular changes in gastric carcinogenesis remains to be further elucidated. The diffuse-type GAC (hereditary and sporadic) is linked to defects of E-cadherin expression. Identification of E-cadherin mutations in hereditary diffuse-type GAC is critical in making decisions regarding genetic counseling including prophylactic gastrectomies. Further characterization of molecular mechanisms of the second-hit on E-cadherin inactivation should help identify potential therapeutic targets. The differential molecular alterations between intestinal- and diffuse-type gastric cancers are summarized in

Table 15-1	Differential molecular profiles of intestinal- and diffuse-type gastric cancers	
Molecular Alteration	**Intestinal-type Cancer**	**Diffuse-type Cancer**
TGFβRII gene mutation	Common	Rare
LOH of APC	Common	Uncommon
β-Catenin mutation	Common	Uncommon
TP53 gene alteration	Common	Uncommon
Her-2/neu amplification	Some	Rare
K-ras mutation	Some	Rare
B-raf mutation	Rare	Rare
E-cadherin mutation	Rare	Common
E-cadherin promoter hypermethylation	Rare	Common

Table 15-1. So far, the use of a single biomarker has been insufficient for clinical diagnosis or management of GAC. It is imperative that a battery of biomarkers be developed for aiding diagnosis and guiding clinical management of GAC.

References

1. Parkin DM, Bray F, Ferlay J, et al. Global cancer statistics, 2002. *CA Cancer J Clin.* 2005;55:74–108.
2. Laurén P. The two histological main types of gastric carcinoma: diffuse and so-called intestinal-type carcinoma: an attempt at a histo-clinical classification. *Acta Pathol Microbiol Scand* 1965;64:31–49.
3. Zheng L, Wang L, Ajani J, et al. Molecular basis of gastric cancer development and progression. *Gastric Cancer.* 2004;7:61–77.
4. Fitzgerald RC. Molecular basis of Barrett's oesophagus and oesophageal adenocarcinoma. *Gut.* 2006;55:1810–1820.
5. Correa P. Human gastric carcinogenesis: a multistep and multifactorial process—First American Cancer Society Award Lecture on cancer epidemiology and prevention. *Cancer Res.* 1992;52:6735–6740.
6. Carneiro F, Huntsman DG, Smyrk TC, et al. Model of the early development of diffuse gastric cancer in E-cadherin mutation carriers and its implications for patient screening. *J Pathol.* 2004;203:681–687.
7. Correa P, Houghton J. Carcinogenesis of *Helicobacter pylori. Gastroenterology.* 2007;133:659–672.
8. Dong CX, Deng DJ, Pan KF, et al. Promoter methylation of p16 associated with *Helicobacter pylori* infection in precancerous gastric lesions: a population-based study. *Int J Cancer.* 2009;124:434–439.
9. Murata-Kamiya N, Kurashima Y, Teishikata Y, et al. *Helicobacter pylori* CagA interacts with E-cadherin and deregulates the β-catenin signal that promotes intestinal transdifferentiation in gastric epithelial cells. *Oncogene.* 2007;26:4617–4626.
10. Zavros Y, Eaton KA, Kang W, et al. Chronic gastritis in the hypochlorhydric gastrin-deficient mouse progresses to adenocarcinoma. *Oncogene.* 2005;24:2354–2366.
11. Silberg DG, Sullivan J, Kang E, et al. Cdx2 ectopic expression induces gastric intestinal metaplasia in transgenic mice. *Gastroenterology.* 2002;122:689–696.
12. Wang LH, Choi YL, Hua XY, et al. Increased expression of sonic hedgehog and altered methylation of its promoter region in gastric cancer and its related lesions. *Mod Pathol.* 2006;19:675–683.
13. Lipkin SM, Wang V, Jacoby R, et al. MLH3: a DNA mismatch repair gene associated with mammalian microsatellite instability. *Nat Genet.* 2000;24:27–35.
14. Pinto M, Oliveira C, Machado JC, et al. MSI-L gastric carcinomas share the hMLH1 methylation status of MSI-H carcinomas but not their clinicopathological profile. *Lab Invest.* 2000;80:1915–1923.

15. Kashiwagi K, Watanabe M, Ezaki T, et al. Clinical usefulness of microsatellite instability for the prediction of gastric adenoma or adenocarcinoma in patients with chronic gastritis. *Br J Cancer*. 2000;82:1814–1818.

16. Umar A, Boland CR, Terdiman JP, et al. Revised Bethesda Guidelines for hereditary nonpolyposis colorectal cancer (Lynch syndrome) and microsatellite instability. *J Natl Cancer Inst*. 2004;96:261–268.

17. Esteller M, Corn PG, Baylin SB, et al. A gene hypermethylation profile of human cancer. *Cancer Res*. 2001;61:3225–3229.

18. Fleisher AS, Esteller M, Tamura G, et al. Hypermethylation of the hMLH1 gene promoter is associated with microsatellite instability in early human gastric neoplasia. *Oncogene*. 2001;20:329–335.

19a. Baek MJ, Kang H, Kim SE, et al. Expression of hmlh1 is inactivated in the gastric adenomas with enhanced microsatellite instability. *Br J Cancer*. 2001;85:1147–1152.

19b. Carvalho B, Pinto M, Cirnes L, et al. Concurrent hypermethylation of gene promoters is associated with a MSI-H phenotype and diploidy in gastric carcinomas. *Eur J Cancer*. 2003;39:1222–1227.

20. Ebert MP, Fei G, Kahmann S, et al. Increased beta-catenin mRNA levels and mutational alterations of the APC and beta-catenin gene are present in intestinal-type gastric cancer. *Carcinogenesis*. 2002;23:87–91.

21. Oliveira C, Seruca R, Seixas M, et al. The clinicopathological features of gastric carcinomas with microsatellite instability may be mediated by mutations of different "target genes": a study of the TGFbeta RII, IGFII R, and BAX genes. *Am J Pathol*. 1998;153:1211–1219.

22. Amendt C, Schirmacher P, Weber H, et al. Expression of a dominant negative type II TGF-beta receptor in mouse skin results in an increase in carcinoma incidence and an acceleration of carcinoma development. *Oncogene*. 1998;17:25–34.

23. Kim JJ, Baek MJ, Kim L, et al. Accumulated frameshift mutations at coding nucleotide repeats during the progression of gastric carcinoma with microsatellite instability. *Lab Invest*. 1999;79:1113–1120.

24. Kim HS, Woo DK, Bae SI, et al. Microsatellite instability in the adenoma-carcinoma sequence of the stomach. *Lab Invest*. 2000;80:57–64

25. Dennis PA, Rifkin DB. Cellular activation of latent transforming growth factor beta requires binding to the cation-independent mannose 6-phosphate/insulin-like growth factor type II receptor. *Proc Natl Acad Sci U S A*. 1991;88:580–584.

26. Falchetti M, Saieva C, Lupi R, et al. Gastric cancer with high-level microsatellite instability: target gene mutations, clinicopathologic features, and long term survival. *Hum Pathol*. 2008;39:925–932.

27. Nakatsuru S, Yanagisawa A, Ichii S, et al. Somatic mutation of the APC gene in gastric cancer: frequent mutations in very well differentiated adenocarcinoma and signet-ring cell carcinoma. *Hum Mol Genet*. 1992;1:559–563.

28. Park WS, Oh RR, Park JY, et al. Frequent somatic mutations of the beta-catenin gene in intestinal-type gastric cancer. *Cancer Res*. 1999;59:4257–4260.

29. Abraham SC, Park SJ, Lee JII, et al. Genetic alterations in gastric adenomas of intestinal and foveolar phenotypes. *Mod Pathol*. 2003;16:786–795.

30. Shiao YH, Rugge M, Correa P, et al. p53 alteration in gastric precancerous lesions. *Am J Pathol*. 1994;144:511–517.

31. Lee HS, Choi SI, Lee HK, et al. Distinct clinical features and outcomes of gastric cancers with microsatellite instability. *Mod Pathol*. 2002;15:632–640.

32. Lee JH, Abraham SC, Kim HS, et al. Inverse relationship between APC gene mutation in gastric adenomas and development of adenocarcinoma. *Am J Pathol*. 2002;161:611–618.

33. Davies H, Bignell GR, Cox C, et al. Mutations of the BRAF gene in human cancer. *Nature*. 2002;417:949–954.

34. Oliveira C, Pinto M, Duval A, et al. BRAF mutations characterize colon but not gastric cancer with mismatch repair deficiency. *Oncogene*. 2003;22:9192–9196.

35. Samuels Y, Wang Z, Bardelli A, et al. High frequency of mutations of the PIK3CA gene in human cancers. *Science*. 2004;304:554.

36. Byun DS, Cho K, Ryu BK, et al. Frequent monoallelic deletion of PTEN and its reciprocal association with PIK3CA amplification in gastric carcinoma. *Int J Cancer*. 2003;104:318–327.

37. Nakayama J, Saito M, Nakamura H, et al. TLP1: a gene encoding a protein component of mammalian telomerase is a novel member of WD repeats family. *Cell*. 1997;88:875–884.

38. Niiyama H, Mizumoto K, Sato N, et al. Quantitative analysis of hTERT mRNA expression in colorectal cancer. *Am J Gastroenterol*. 2001;96:1895–1900.

39. Park YP, Choi SC, Kim JH, et al. Up-regulation of Mac-2 binding protein by hTERT in gastric cancer. *Int J Cancer.* 2007;120:813–820.

40. Guilford P, Hopkins J, Harraway J, et al. E-Cadherin germline mutations in familial gastric cancer. *Nature.* 1998;392:402–405.

41. Oliveira C, de Bruin J, Nabais S, et al. Intragenic deletion of CDH1 as the inactivating mechanism of the wild-type allele in an HDGC tumour. *Oncogene.* 2004;23:2236–2240.

42. Carneiro F, Oliveira C, Suriano G, et al. Molecular pathology of familial gastric cancer, with an emphasis on hereditary diffuse gastric cancer. *J Clin Pathol.* 2008;61:25–30.

43. Kaurah P, MacMillan A, Boyd N, et al. Founder and recurrent CDH1 mutations in families with hereditary diffuse gastric cancer. *JAMA.* 2007;297:2360–2372.

44. Machado JC, Oliveira C, Carvalho R, et al. E-Cadherin gene (CDH1) promoter methylation as the second hit in sporadic diffuse gastric carcinoma. *Oncogene.* 2001;20:1525–1528.

45. Qian X, Karpova T, Sheppard AM, et al. E-Cadherin-mediated adhesion inhibits ligand-dependent activation of diverse receptor tyrosine kinases. *EMBO J.* 2004;23:1739–1748.

46. Mateus AR, Seruca R, Machado JC, et al. EGFR regulates RhoA-GTP dependent cell motility in E-cadherin mutant cells. *Hum Mol Genet.* 2007;16:1639–1647.

47. Yarden Y, Sliwkowski MX. Untangling the ErbB signalling network. *Nat Rev Mol Cell Biol.* 2001;2: 127–137.

48. Lynch TJ, Bell DW, Sordella R, et al. Activating mutations in the epidermal growth factor receptor underlying responsiveness of non-small-cell lung cancer to gefitinib. *N Engl J Med.* 2004;350:2129–2139.

49. Paez JG, Janne PA, Lee JC, et al. EGFR mutations in lung cancer: correlation with clinical response to gefitinib therapy. *Science.* 2004;304:1497–1500.

50. Hirashima N, Takahashi W, Yoshii S, et al. Protein overexpression and gene amplification of c-erb B-2 in pulmonary carcinomas: a comparative immunohistochemical and fluorescence in situ hybridization study. *Mod Pathol.* 2001;14:556–562.

51. Nakajima M, Sawada H, Yamada Y, et al. The prognostic significance of amplification and overexpression of c-*met* and c-*erb* B-2 in human gastric carcinomas. *Cancer.* 1999;85:1894–1902.

52. Varis A, Zaika A, Puolakkainen P, et al. Coamplified and overexpressed genes at ERBB2 locus in gastric cancer. *Int J Cancer.* 2004;109:548–553.

53. Park DI, Yun JW, Park JH, et al. HER-2/neu amplification is an independent prognostic factor in gastric cancer. *Dig Dis Sci.* 2006;51:1371–1379.

54. Bekaii-Saab TS, Roda JM, Guenterberg KD, et al. A phase I trial of paclitaxel and trastuzumab in combination with interleukin-12 in patients with HER2/neu-expressing malignancies. *Mol Cancer Ther.* 2009;8(11):2983–2991.

55. Yin M, Hu Z, Tan D, et al. Molecular epidemiology of genetic susceptibility to gastric cancer: focus on single nucleotide polymorphisms in gastric carcinogenesis. *Am J Transl Res.* 2009;1(1):44–54.

56. Bolt HM, Thier R. Relevance of the deletion polymorphisms of the glutathione S-transferases GSTT1 and GSTM1 in pharmacology and toxicology. *Curr Drug Metab.* 2006;7:613–628.

Proteomics, Morphoproteomics, and Targeted Therapy of Gastric Carcinoma

16

▶ Wei Feng
▶ Dongfeng Tan

INTRODUCTION

Gastric carcinoma has a dismal outcome due to the lack of practical screening methods and to the high percentage of cases presenting with advanced disease. Surgical resection remains the mainstay of gastric carcinoma treatment. However, the rate of local tumor recurrence and lymph node metastasis after curative surgical treatment is high (ranging from 45% to 88%, depending on the type of resection and lymph node dissection).[1] Furthermore, present standard chemotherapy regimens of cisplatin, infusional 5 fluorouracil, and epirubicin produce low and frequently short-lived response rates (20%–40%).[2]

The lack of effective treatment for gastric carcinoma has led to intensive research to identify markers for early detection, tumor resistance to drugs, and tumor aggressiveness, as well as to identify new molecular targets of therapy. These efforts have consisted of approaches from the deoxyribonucleic acid (DNA), ribonucleic acid (RNA), and protein levels. In this chapter, we highlight the therapeutic implications of studies in gastric carcinoma via proteomics (the systematic large-scale study of proteins) and morphoproteomics (the combined study of histopathology, molecular biology, and protein chemistry).

PROTEOMICS

The term "proteome" was first coined by Marc Wilkins and Keith Williams as the whole spectrum of proteins encoded in a single genome expressed under distinct conditions.[3] Following the success of the systemic human genome project, the classical study of protein chemistry has also evolved into a high-throughput and holistic science of the proteome known as proteomics. Proteomics has become an exciting field in biomedical research, as it provides an improved understanding of actual cellular functions. However, proteomics is complicated by the dynamic nature of the proteome, which is subject to posttranscriptional alterations such as alternative splicing and posttranslational modifications such as phosphorylation, glycosylation, and degradation.

Proteomic Techniques

In cancer proteomics, the protein expression profiles between cancerous tissues and corresponding noncancerous tissues are characterized, quantified, and compared. After total protein extraction from tissues, a proteomic study typically involves the concentration and separation of proteins utilizing two-dimensional gel electrophoresis (2-DE), which resolves various proteins by isoelectric point (pI) and relative molecular mass (M_r). Proteins are then subsequently identified by mass spectrometry (MS). However, these techniques are limited in the detection of low-abundance proteins by the requirement of large protein samples. At present, advancements in isolation and analysis techniques such as liquid chromatography (LC), laser capture microdissection, isotope-coded affinity tagging (ICAT), matrix-assisted laser desorption/ioinization (MALDI), surface-enhanced laser desorption/ionization (SELDI), and time-of-flight MS have allowed for a quantitatively accurate nonselective approach to analyze proteomic changes in tumor cells.

Because cancer tissue is heterogeneous and comprises neoplastic cells as well as variable numbers of fibroblasts, adipocytes, endothelial cells, lymphocytes, and histiocytes, microdissection techniques such as laser capture microdissection (LCM) have been used to sample only the targeted neoplastic cells for further proteomic analysis. LCM is, however, labor intensive and limited by the large quantity of samples required for a complete proteomic study, since up to 15 hours of LCM are needed to isolate the required number of cells per 2-DE gel analysis (approximately 250,000 cells).[4] Separation of proteins is most commonly achieved by one-dimensional (1-D) or two-dimensional gel electrophoresis (2-DE). By combining the concentrating technique of isoelectric focusing with the separation technique based on differences in molecular mass, 2-DE can resolve >10,000 different compounds. LC is another alternative method for protein separation, but in typical LC techniques the advantage of keeping the protein in solution is compromised by considerably lower separation resolution than is achieved with 2-DE.[3] The development of 2-D LC coupled with ICAT and MS has allowed for the identification of a large number of proteins, including proteins of low abundance.

After concentrating and separation steps, MS is then utilized to identify the protein/peptide composition by determining its molecular weight, chemical structure, and posttranslational modifications. The principle of MS consists of first ionizing protein/peptide compounds to generate charged molecules and then characterizing these compounds by measuring their mass-to-charge ratios (m/z). Various techniques are combined with the MS principle in proteomic applications in biomedical research. The large biomolecules, such as proteins and peptides, studied in proteomics are very fragile and tend to fragment when ionized by conventional ionization methods. This problem is overcome by MALDI, which is a soft ionization technique used in MS that combines the analyte with a solid matrix material to absorb most of the pulsed laser beam energy during the ionizing process and allows very large molecules to be preserved for further analysis. SELDI is a modified MALDI technique, with an added selective step wherein a chemically functional surface with biochemical affinity for a certain subset of proteins or peptides is used before combining the analyte with the solid matrix material.[8] MALDI or SELDI can then be combined with time of flight MS (TOF-MS), where mass spectra are determined by measuring flight times of ionized compounds accelerated by an electric field over a fixed distance.[3,5] MS data gathered are then analyzed via various online databases, such as ExPASy from the Swiss Institute of Bioinformatics or BLAST from the National Center for Biotechnology Information, to identify individual proteins.

Beyond merely identifying protein composition, a need exists to quantitatively and differentially characterize the proteome in neoplastic and normal tissues in cancer proteomics. This characterization can be achieved by difference gel electrophoresis (DIGE) or the more common ICAT procedure. In both techniques, markers are used to identify two or more samples (e.g., neoplastic and normal tissues) to allow for direct quantitative measurements between samples coresolved on the same gel electrophoresis or LC and subsequent MS analysis. DIGE utilizes fluorescent dyes (CyDyes, Cy2, Cy3, Cy5) covalently bound to protein samples, whereas ICAT utilizes isotope tags (^{12}C or ^{13}C) to label protein samples. Whereas DIGE requires separate gel electrophoresis to be performed to separate labeled samples before MS analysis, ICAT allows for direct MS analysis of the separated LC sample.[4]

Proteomic Applications in Gastric Carcinoma

Cancer proteomics have been applied to gastric carcinoma in various studies to identify particular proteins that show differential expression in cancer tissues, serum, gastric juices, and tumor cell lines. Various types of proteins, from structural cytoskeletal proteins, stress-related and chaperoning proteins, acute-phase proteins, glycolytic enzymes, enzymes involved in metabolism and cellular proliferation, tumor suppressor proteins to stomach-specific proteins, are found to be either upregulated or downregulated. Some of these proteins are potential markers for diagnosis of carcinoma or preneoplastic lesions, some are potential prognostic markers, and some are potential markers to predict therapy response.

Both small- and large-scale proteomic studies examining paired patient gastric carcinoma tumor tissues and nonneoplastic tissues using 2-DE MALDI-TOF/SELDI-TOF, LC MS, or LC tandem MS (MS/MS) have been conducted with varying results. Table 16-1 summarizes some of these studies. As with many proteomic studies, resulting data among different studies show little overlap, a finding thought to result from several issues. First, the heterogeneous nature of tissues and the underutilization of microdissection techniques cause suboptimal differential comparison between tumor cells and nonneoplastic epithelium, since other cells and connective tissues were included in the analysis. Second, the sample sizes of these studies were usually small. Even with these limitations, these studies identified many potential markers for further study. Nishigaki et al.[6] identified differential expression of proteins in gastric carcinoma, which are involved in mitotic checkpoint regulation (MAD1L1 and EB1), apoptosis (HSP27), as well as mitochondrial reduction-oxidative balance. A proteomic analysis by Zhang et al.[7] showed that there is decreased expression in MAWBP, a binding protein for MAWD, which is in turn an inhibitor of transcriptional activation mediated by transforming growth factor beta (TGF-β).

Additional proteomic studies were also performed on gastric juice and serum in attempts to identify serum markers for practical applications in early detection of gastric carcinoma. A study of patient gastric fluids from Singapore at Humphrey Oei Institute of Cancer Research showed that 106 significantly different proteomic features could be used to distinguish benign from gastric carcinoma cases with 88% sensitivity and 93% specificity.[8] Similar studies have also been performed on serum. Ren et al.[9] compared serum proteomic spectra in patients with gastric carcinoma before and after operation and showed that the serum protein profile consisting of four proteins (heat-shock protein 27, glucose-regulated protein, prohibitin, protein disulfide isomerase A3) could be used to differentiate normal from gastric carcinoma cases with 95.7% sensitivity and 92.5% specificity. These studies show that proteomics results have potential applications in early diagnosis of gastric carcinoma. However, the practicality of implementing these techniques to screen patient populations has yet to be determined.

Beyond the diagnostic implications, proteomic studies have also shed light on the carcinogenesis, metastatic potential, and drug resistance of gastric carcinoma. It is well known that the pathogenesis of gastric carcinoma starts with chronic gastritis, which then progresses to atrophy and dysplasia. One of the major causes of chronic gastritis is *Helicobacter pylori* infection, which eventually may result in clinically divergent outcomes of gastric carcinoma and duodenal ulcer.

Previous molecular studies have shown that virulence factors such as cytotoxin-associated gene A (CagA) produced increased Interleukin (IL)-8, resulting in an increased level of host inflammation, and are associated with an increased risk of gastric carcinoma.[10] Wu et al.[11] compared acid-glycine extract of *H. pylori* probed with serum samples from 15 patients with gastric carcinoma and 15 patients with duodenal ulcer. Among *H. pylori* protein antigens, which showed higher frequency in the gastric carcinoma group, cochaperonin GroES was identified as the dominant gastric carcinoma–related antigen, with significantly higher seropositivity in gastric carcinoma samples (64.2%, $n = 95$) than in gastritis (30.9%, $n = 95$) and duodenal ulcer samples (35.5%, $n = 124$). Furthermore, Wu et al.[11] also showed that GroES stimulated production of IL-8 in mononuclear inflammatory cells and induced cellular proliferation; up-regulation of c-jun, c-fos, and cyclin D1; and down-regulation of p27 (Kip1). In a proteomic study by Chan et al.,[12] the alteration in expressed proteins profile in the *H. pylori*–infected gastric epithelial AGS cell line was characterized. Eight of the proteins showing the greatest variation in *H. pylori*–infected gastric epithelial AGS cells were then shown to be more upregulated in gastric carcinoma tissues than in nonneoplastic gastric tissues (Table 16-1). These proteins include a promoter of NFκB

Table 16-1A Summary of proteomic studies in gastric cancer

Proteins categorized according to Cell Cycle and Cell Proliferation Regulation, Cell Migration and Metastasis, Cell Structure and Motility, DNA Repair Immunity Defenses, Oncoprotein, Signal Transduction, and Transcription and Translation (d: downregulated; u: upregulated)

Studies: 1. Zhang et al.[7] 2. Chen et al.[13] 3. He et al.[19] 4. Yoshihara et al.[20] 5. Nishigaski et al.[6] 6. Kon et al.[8] 7. Chan et al.[12] 8. Chen et al.[14] 9. Yang et al.[17] 10. Wang et al.[16]

		1	2	3	4	5	6	7	8	9	10
Sample size (N)		84	44	10	5	14	24	10			
Specimen type (T: tissue, J: gastric juice, C: cell line)		T	T	T	T	T	J	C/T	C	C	C
Protein	**Function**										
Cell Cycle and Cell Proliferation Regulation											
14-3-3 β/α	Regulator of cell cycle							u			
Cell division control protein 42 homologue	Regulates cadherin-mediated cell–cell adhesion								d		
Cell division kinase 6	Related to cell proliferation, tumor heterogeneity, invasion, and metastasis								u		
Foveolin precursor FOV (gastrokine-1)	Growth factor				d						
Microtubule-associated protein, RP/EB family, member 1	Regulation of cell cycle, cell proliferation, microtubule-binding, APC protein C-terminus binding							u			
Mitotic checkpoint protein isoform MAD1a	Cell proliferation, mitotic spindle checkpoint, centrosome								d		
Prohibitin	Inhibits cellular proliferation							u			
Proteasome activator PA28 b-chain	Immunoproteasome assembly and antigen processing						u				
SEPT 2 protein	Cytokinesis, mitosis					u					
S-phase kinase-associated protein 1A	Mediates the ubiquitination of proteins involved in cell cycle progression, signal transduction, and transcription								d		
T-complex protein beta	Related to p53 and activates DNA damage checkpoints								d		
Tumor RMS cell line RD specific product (CYR61)	Insulin-like growth factor binding, extracellular								d		

Cell Migration and Metastasis

Protein	Description					
Annexin I	Regulates cell proliferation, promotes membrane fusion, calcium-dependent phospholipid binding, inhibition of phospholipase A2	d			d	u
Catechol O-methyltransferase	Cancer progression and lymph node metastasis				u	
Galectin-1	Promotes cancer cell invasion and metastasis				u	
High mobility group protein 1	Interacts with transcription factors and regulates transcription related to tumor growth and invasion				u	
Laminin γ-1 chain precursor	Induces collagenase IV, matrix metalloproteinase (MMP-9)			u		
Platelet-derived endothelial cell growth factor	Angiogenesis		u			
S100 calcium-binding protein A11	Calcium-binding, actin filament bundle formation, and cell motility			u	u	
Tropomyosin (1:isoform; 2: 3/4)	Stabilizes and binds actin filaments	u	u[1]		d[2]	
Vimentin	Intermediate filament in mesenchymal cells related to migration		u		u	

Cell Structure and Motility

Protein	Description					
ACTG1 protein	Cytoskeleton	u				
Actin alpha2	Structural protein	u				
Alpha-actinin	Anchors actin to intracellular structures				u	
Cytokeratin 8	Intermediate filaments		u			
Cytokeratin 20	Intermediate filaments		d			
Cytoskeletal 5	Epidermis development, cytoskeleton organization and biogenesis, cellular morphogenesis				u	
Cytoskeletal 17	Marker of basal cell differentiation	d				

(Continued)

Table 16-1A — Summary of proteomic studies in gastric cancer (Continued)

Studies: 1. Zhang et al.[7] 2. Chen et al.[13] 3. He et al.[19] 4. Yoshihara et al.[20] 5. Nishigaski et al.[6] 6. Kon et al.[8] 7. Chan et al.[12] 8. Chen et al.[14] 9. Yang et al.[17] 10. Wang et al.[16]

Protein	Function	1	2	3	4	5	6	7	8	9	10
Sample size (N)		84	44	10	5	14	24	10			
Specimen type (T: tissue, J: gastric juice, C: cell line)		T	T	T	T	T	J	C/T	C	C	C
Tubulin alpha 6	Microtubules			u							
WDR1 protein	Induces disassembly of actin filaments			u							
DNA Repair											
Uracil DNA glycosylase	Excise uracil residues from the DNA			u							
Manganese superoxide dismutase (MnSOD)	Protection of DNA from oxidative damage			d	u						
Immunity Defenses											
α defensin	Microbicidal peptides						u				
FK506-binding protein 4 (FKBP4)	Immunoregulation, protein folding/ trafficking, binds FK506/rapamycin							u			
MHC class I antigen	Inhibits evasion of the immune system and enhances tumor growth								d		
Oncoprotein											
18-kDa Antrum mucosa protein (AMP-18)	Human stomach specific, epithelial cell mitogen				d						
Signal Transduction											
Actin filament-binding protein (frabin)	Signal transduction										u
Catenin, 120ctn	Interacts with cadherin to regulate cell adhesion properties								u		
Catenin, alpha-1	Actin crosslinking at adherens junctions								d		

Protein	Function		
Catenin, beta	Modulates of cytoskeletal dynamics and cell proliferation		u
Chloride intracellular channel protein1 (CLIC1)	Signal transduction, Ion homeostasis, cell volume regulation, transepithelial transport.	u	d
Eukaryotic translation initiation factor 5A	Signal transduction		u
Integrin alpha 6/beta 4	Cell–matrix adhesion	u	u
N-myc downstream regulated gene 1	Signal transduction		d
Peroxiredoxin 5	High antioxidant efficiency to effect cell differentiation and apoptosis		u
Raf kinase inhibitor protein	Suppresses metastasis, angiogenesis, and vascular invasion		d
Ras GTPase-activating-like protein IQGAP1	Actin cytoskeleton assembly and E-cadherin–mediated cel adhesion		d
Rho-related GTP-binding protein RhoG	Small GTPase-mediated signal transduction, positive regulation of cell proliferation, actin cytoskeleton organization		d
RMD5 homolog B (RMND5B)	Signal transduction		d
Tyrosine 3/tryptophan 5-monooxygenase activation protein	Activates protein kinase C and Ca^{2+}/calmodulin-dependent protein kinase II	u	
Vinculin	Mediates the interactions between integrins and the actin		d
Transcription and Translation			
Elongation factor 2	Transcription & translation		d
HnRNP A2	RNA trafficking, telomere maintenance	u	
HnRNP-E1	RNA-binding protein, RNA trafficking	d	
MADS box transcription enhancer factor 2, polypeptide C	Regulation of transcription, transcription from Pol II promoter, nucleus	u	
Nucleophosmin	Ribosome assembly and transport		u
Translation elongation factor EF-Tu (EF-Tu)	Translation factor, cell growth, chaperone activity	u	

Table 16-1B   Summary of proteomic studies in gastric cancer

Metabolic Proteins (d: downregulated; u: upregulated)

Studies: 1. Zhang et al.[7] 2. Chen et al.[13] 3. He et al.[19] 4. Yoshihara et al.[20] 5. Nishigaski et al.[6] 6. Melle et al.[21] 7. Lee et al.[22] 8. Kon et al.[8] 9. Chan et al.[12] 10. Chen et al.[14] 11. Yang et al.[17] 12. Wang et al.[16]

Protein	Function	1	2	3	4	5	6	7	8	9	10	11	12
Sample size (N)		84	44	10	5	14	21	30	24	10			
Specimen type (T: tissue, J: gastric juice, C: cell line)		T	T	T	T	T	T	J	J	C/T	C	C	C
Carbohydrate Metabolism													
Cytosolic malate dehydrogenase	Citric acid cycle		d										
Glyceraldehyde-3-phosphate dehydrogenase	Glycolysis		u										
Isocitrate dehydrogenase	Metabolic enzyme, citric acid cycle	d	u										
L-lactate dehydrogenase B chain	Metabolic enzyme										d		
MPI Mannose-6-phosphate isomerase	Metabolic enzyme					d							
Phosphoglycerate kinase 1 (PGK-1)	Glycolysis				u								
Phosphoglycerate mutase 1	Metabolic enzyme, glycolysis		u	u									
Pyruvate kinase (PK)	Glycolysis		u	u									
Pyruvate kinase3, isoform1	Glycolysis	d											
TPI	Glycolytic enzyme		u										
α enolase	Glycolysis, plasminogen receptor	u	u							u			
Lipid, Fatty Acid, and Steroid Metabolism													
Acyl-CoA dehydrogenase	Mitochondrial fatty acid β-oxidation	d											
ApoA-I-binding protein	Regulation of lipid transport, metabolism of HDL particles					d							

Protein	Function					
Apolipoprotein A-1 (ApoA1)/precursor	Cholesterol metabolism, acute phase protein		d			d
Fatty acid–binding protein	Transportation					d
HSDL2 protein	Steroid hormone synthesis and fatty acid metabolism	d				
Nucleic Acid Metabolism						
Bisphosphate 3′-nucleotidase	Regulation by inositol signaling pathways		u			
dUTP pyrophosphatase	Metabolism					d
GMP reductase 2 (GMPR)	Promote monocytic differentiation	d				
Protein Degradation, Metabolism and Modification						
78-kDa glucose-regulated protein	Chaperone		d			d
Acyl-CoA-binding protein (ACBP)	Protein modification					d
Alpha-1-antitrypsin (a1-AT)	Trypsin/serine protease and elastase inhibitor, acute phase protein	d	d	d		
Chaperonin containing TCP1 (CCT)	Stress related, chaperone	u				
Cathepsin B	Protein targeting, proteolysis and peptidolysis				u	
Cathepsin C	Intracellular protein degradation and turnover				u	
Cathepsin D	Elastase inhibitor, protease	u	u			
Heat-shock 27-kDa protein	Chaperone, protein folding, regulation of translational initiation, cytoplasm	u	u		u	
Heat-shock 70-kDa protein (‡ 8 isoform and 1A; † 8 isoform 1, 9B, and 1B; * 9B)	Chaperon, protein denaturation-renaturation, folding, transport translocation	u‡	u†	d*		d*

(Continued)

Table 16-1B   Summary of proteomic studies in gastric cancer (Continued)

Studies: 1. Zhang et al.[7] 2. Chen et al.[13] 3. He et al.[19] 4. Yoshihara et al.[20] 5. Nishigaski et al.[6] 6. Melle et al.[21] 7. Lee et al.[22] 8. Kon et al.[8] 9. Chan et al.[12] 10. Chen et al.[14] 11. Yang et al.[17] 12. Wang et al.[16]

		1	2	3	4	5	6	7	8	9	10	11	12
Sample size (N)		84	44	10	5	14	21	30	24	10			
Specimen type (T: tissue, J: gastric juice, C: cell line)	**Function**	T	T	T	T	T	T	T	J	C/T	C	C	C
Protein													
Protein Degradation, Metabolism and Modification													
Heat-shock cognate 71 protein (HSP70)	Chaperone, stress related			u								d	
Heat-shock protein 60	Chaperone, stress related, facilitates the correct folding of imported proteins			u							u		
Heterogeneous nuclear ribonucleoprotein F	Chaperone											d	
HSPA8 protein	Chaperone											d	
Mitochondrial matrix protein P1	Chaperon, protein denaturation-renaturation, folding, transport translocation									u			
Polypeptide N-acetylgalactosaminyltransferase 1 (pp-Gal-NAc-T1)	Protein modification												d
Protein disulfide isomerase (PDI)	Chaperone, isomerase, and redox activities			u									
Serum amyloid P component precursor	Protein folding, extracellular space, multichaperone pathway					d							

Protein	Function								
SET translocation	Chaperone		d						
T-complex protein 1	Chaperone		d	u					
Tumor rejection antigen (Gp96) 1 variant	Chaperone		d						
Valosin-containing protein	Proteasome degradation of IkBα			u					
Xenobiotic Metabolism									
3-ketoacid-coenzyme A transferase 1			d						
3-Oxoacid CoA transferase precursor	Ketone body catabolism							d	
Aldehyde dehydrogenase	Oxidative enzyme								u
Aldehyde dehydrogenase 1A1	Convert/oxidize retinaldehyde to retinoic acid, ethanol utilization							u	
Aldehyde dehydrogenase 6A1	Metabolic enzyme								d
Aldo-keto reductase family 1	Ubiquitin-dependent degradation of reactive aldehydes, apoptosis							d	d
Glutathione *S*-transferase (GST)	Drug, xenobiotic metabolism, glutathione transferase activity	d			u	d			
Nicotinamide *N*-methyltransferase	Metabolic enzyme, homocysteine, and detoxification pathway				u				
Selenium-binding protein 1 (SeBP)	Detoxification, inhibition of premalignantial cells, bind selenium; intra-Golgi protein transport						d	d	

Table 16-1C Summary of proteomic studies in gastric cancer

Miscellaneous proteins (d: downregulated; u: upregulated)

Studies: 1. Zhang et al.[7] 2. Chen et al.[13] 3. He et al.[19] 4. Yoshihara et al.[20] 5. Nishigaski et al.[6] 6. Melle et al.[21] 7. Lee et al.[22] 8. Kon et al.[8] 9. Chan et al.[12] 10. Chen et al.[14] 11. Yang et al.[17] 12. Wang et al.[16]

		1	2	3	4	5	6	7	8	9	10	11	12
Sample size (N)		84	44	10	5	14	21	30	24	10			
Specimen type (T: tissue, J: gastric juice, C: cell line)		T	T	T	T	T	T	J	J	C/T	C	C	C
Protein	**Function**												
ADCK5 protein	Unknown												u
Aspartate amino-transferase (AST)	Amino acid/α keto acid enzyme		d		d								
Alkaline phosphatase	Metabolism										d		
Annexin 5	Calcium-dependent phospholipid binding, inhibition of phospholipase A2 and protein kinase C					u						d	
Antioxidant protein 2 (acidic calcium-independent phospholipase A2)	Regulation of phospholipid turnover and protection against oxidative injury		u										
ATP-dependent proteolytic subunit E. coli homolog	Endopeptidase Clp activity, mitochondrial, peptidase activity					d							
ATP synthase	Metabolic enzyme	u											
Calponin	Calcium-binding protein	u											
Carbonic anhydrase XI (CA11 protein)	Digestion					d							
Carbonyl reductase 1	Oxidoreductases		d										

Protein	Function						
Carbonic anhydrase I and II	CO2 metabolism and pH equilibrium			d	d		d
Chain-A, thioredoxin peroxidase B	Redox regulation		u				
COX5A cytochrome c oxidase subunit Va	Cytochrome-c oxidase activity, mitochondrion, oxidoreductase activity				d		d
Creatine kinase B (CK-B)	Metabolism, proliferation transformation, energy buffering			d	d		
Cytosolic inorganic pyrophosphatase	Unknown				d		
Dihydrodiol dehydrogenase isoform DD1	Catalysis of polycyclic aromatic hydrocarbons	d					
Enoyl coenzyme A hydratase 1, mitochondrial and peroxisomal	Energy pathways, enoyl-CoA hydratase activity, fatty acid beta-oxidation, mitochondrion				d		
Ferritin, heavy chain	Intracellular iron ion storage, negative regulation of cell proliferation, plasma membrane				d		
Gastric lipase	Gastric enzyme					d	
GDP-dissociation factor 2	Regulate the GDP/GTP exchange reaction		u				
Glyoxalase I	Metabolic enzyme						u
Inorganic pyrophosphatase	Metabolic enzyme						u
MAWD-binding protein (MAWBP)	Facilitate assembling of macromolecules and TGF-β inhibition	d					
NADH dehydrogenase Fe-S protein 8	Electron transport chain	u					
NDUFV2 protein	Mitochondrial NADH oxidation	d					
Nonhistone chromosomal protein HMG-1	DNA-binding protein, chromosome structural stabilization	u					
Nucleobindin-1	Calcium binding						d

(Continued)

Table 16-1C   Summary of proteomic studies in gastric cancer (*Continued*)

Studies: 1. Zhang et al.[7] 2. Chen et al.[13] 3. He et al.[19] 4. Yoshihara et al.[20] 5. Nishigaski et al.[6] 6. Melle et al.[21] 7. Lee et al.[22] 8. Kon et al.[8] 9. Chan et al.[12] 10. Chen et al.[14] 11. Yang et al.[17] 12. Wang et al.[16]

		1	2	3	4	5	6	7	8	9	10	11	12
Sample size (N)		84	44	10	5	14	21	30	24	10			
Specimen type (T: tissue, J: gastric juice, C: cell line)		T	T	T	T	T	T	J	J	C/T	C	C	C
Protein	**Function**												
Nucleoporin SEH1-like protein (SEH1L)	Unknown												d
Pepsin A	Gastric enzyme							d	d				
Pepsin B	Gastric enzyme							d					
Pepsinogen C	Pepsin C precursor						d		d				
Reticulocalbin-1	Calcium binding											d	
SEC13-like 1, isoform b	Metabolic enzyme											d	
Serine proteinase inhibitor	Regulates proteases elastase, cathepsin G, and proteinase-3, serine-type endopeptidase inhibitor activity		d			d							
SM22	Actin-binding protein	u											
Sorcin	Calcium binding											u	
Steroidogenic acute regulatory protein (STAR)	Metabolic enzyme												u
UDP-glucuronosyl-transferase	Membrane integration, metabolism, microsome					u							

inhibitor $I_k B\alpha$ degradation and an inhibitor of apoptotic cell death, valosin-containing protein; molecular chaperones, T-complex protein 1, heat shock 70-kDa protein, and mitochondrial matrix protein P1; promoter of cell adhesion and migration, FK506-binding protein 4 (FKBP4); Laminin γ-1; enolase α; and cell cycle regulator and DNA repair protein, 14-3-3 β. These studies provide further evidence of *H. pylori*'s role in the carcinogenesis of gastric carcinoma.

Proteomic studies have also identified markers of poor prognosis in gastric carcinoma, which are associated with tumor metastasis. In a Taiwanese study using tissue samples from 56 cases of gastric carcinoma, Chen et al.[13] showed that chloride intracellular channel 1 (CLIC1) overexpression in gastric carcinoma tissues was strongly correlated with lymph node metastasis ($p = 0.001$), pathological stage ($p < 0.001$), and lymphatic invasion ($p = 0.001$). Furthermore, a proteome analysis of nonmetastatic SC-M1 and metastatic TMC-1 gastric carcinoma cell lines showed that many upregulated proteins in TMC-1 cells are involved in cancer metastasis, including cell–cell adhesion signaling (catenin-120nt, α-catenin, β-catenin, integrin α6, integrin β4, RhoG, and IQGAP1), cell metastasis and motility (cytokeratin, myosin, S100 calcium-binding protein family, and vimentin), cell cycle and proliferation (cdc42 and cell division protein kinase 6), tumor immunity and defense (galectin 1 and high mobility group protein 1), and protein degradation (cathepsin B, C).[14] A similar study examined the highly metastatic cell line MKN-45-P with almost 100% incidence of peritoneal dissemination and showed upregulated IFN-induced Mx protein, cell cycle control protein ts11, and tyrosyl- and tryptophanyl-tRMA synthetase.[15]

Multidrug resistance is a major problem in chemotherapy, since tumor cells can develop cross-resistance to several structurally unrelated chemotherapeutic drugs after exposure to only one cytotoxic drug. Proteomic studies have also found markers to identify this important subset of gastric carcinoma that does not respond to typical chemotherapy drugs to help guide treatment in this age of personalized medicine. A proteomic study by Wang et al.[16] utilized MRD gastric cell line SGC7901/VCR developed from the SGC7901 gastric cell line by selective in vitro vincristine induction. Their study used MALDI-TOF-MS to identify within the vincristine-resistant cell line the differential down-regulation of six proteins, including triosephosphate isomerase (TPI), and up-regulation of three proteins (Table 16-1). A similar study conducted by Yang et al.[17] used the same gastric cell line SGC7901/VCR to identify 30 differentially expressed proteins via MALDI-TOF-MS and enhanced chemiluminescence (ESI-Q)-TOF-MS techniques (Table 16-1). Furthermore, an additional study by Yang et al.[18] used doxorubicin (adriamycin)-resistant human gastric carcinoma cell line, SGC7901/ADR, and 2-DE in conjunction with ESI-Q-TOF-MS and identified nucleophosmin (NPM1) as an overexpressed protein related to doxorubicin chemoresistance. These studies show that multiple types of proteins, including calcium-binding proteins, chaperones, metabolic enzymes, proteins relative to signal transduction, proteins involved in transcription and translation, and transportation proteins, are all involved in gastric carcinoma MRD.

Technological advances in proteomic analysis have resulted in methodologies for identifying potential biomarkers for carcinogenesis, diagnosis, prognosis, targets of therapy, and drug resistance. However, major shortcomings still remain that limit the applicability of the biomarkers identified in proteomic studies to the clinical management of cancer patients. Because of the limited sample size in these studies, the limitation of tumor cell line studies in reflecting actual in vivo cancer biology, and the poor reproducibility of results between studies, additional studies in large cohorts of patients are needed to verify and demonstrate the clinical applicability of these identified biomarkers.

MORPHOPROTEOMICS

Thus far, the proteomic studies detailed are untargeted proteomic approaches. Clinical applications of proteomics frequently use targeted strategies, where previously known protein families and pathways are measured and quantified. This approach is familiar to anatomical pathologists in the form of immunohistochemical testing, which depends on the availability of antibodies with high affinity and specificity to bind the targeted protein of interest.

The term morphoproteomics was coined by Robert E. Brown, MD, to describe the analytical technique that combines targeted proteomics with what anatomic pathologists excel at morphology.[23] Morphoproteomics overcomes the shortfall of most conventional proteomics, where the specific localization of protein expression could not be assessed even when combined with microdissection techniques. Morphoproteomics involves the immunohistochemical assessment of the activation of metabolic pathways in neoplastic or dysplastic cells to predict susceptibility to small-molecule inhibitors, specific chemotherapeutic agents, and possibly differentiating agents. A rudimentary example of this technique utilized in current pathology is the evaluation and quantification of estrogen receptor and human epidermal growth factor receptor (EGFR) 2 (HER2/neu), c-erb-B2 expression by immunohistochemical staining. However, the established routine immunohistochemical evaluation does not always predict response to therapy. This is exemplified by the immunohistochemical evaluation of HER2/neu expression in guiding clinical application of trastuzumab therapy—even in positive (3+ staining) cases, the response rate for single-agent trastuzumab therapy is only approximately 15%. Morphoproteomics goes a step further by attempting to apply the present discoveries in proteomics and genomics clinically to better guide currently available targeted therapies. This goal is not met by merely assessing the presence of certain proteins within neoplastic cells, but is achieved in three ways. One, differential quantitative protein expression is assessed in neoplastic versus adjacent nonneoplastic cells by quantifying the intensity and/or percentage of the chromogenic signal by visual analysis or by an automated cellular-imaging system. Two, the activation state of the protein is characterized by its phosphorylative state and/or the expression of upstream regulator proteins and downstream effector proteins. Third, the activation state is further characterized by identifying the subcellular compartmentalization of proteins within the neoplastic cells, whether it is expressed in the cytoplasm, the plasma membrane, or the nucleus.[23,24]

Morphoproteomics can in retrospect explain why some drugs work in treating certain diseases and can also be used to provide insight into why certain drugs might be applicable in a particular patient's neoplasm. The choices in pharmaceutical agents and therapeutic antibodies have continued to grow. These choices include cetuximab, which targets the EGFR ectodomain; tyrosine (Tyr) kinase inhibitors such as gefitinib and erlotinib; proteasome and nuclear factor (NF)-κB pathway inhibitor: bortezomib; mammalian target of rapamycin (mTOR) inhibitors: temsirolimus and sirolimus; and differentiating agents such as histone deacetylase (HDAC) inhibitors, just to name a few.[28] However, with the rare exceptions such as BCR-ABL tyrosine kinase inhibitor, imatinib mesylate, in the specific setting of chronic myeloid leukemia, no single drug therapy has proven to have therapeutic efficacy in high percentage of clinical cancer cases. This is also the case in gastric adenocarcinoma (GAC), where even multidrug therapy regimens have poor response rates. Therefore, morphoproteomic examination of these targets of therapy can provide vital information concerning the likelihood of therapeutic efficacy of a certain drug in specific cases before these agents, which frequently have considerable side effects, are utilized.

Even with response to chemotherapeutic agents, as demonstrated in GAC, the response rate is short lived.[2] Many hypotheses exist to explain treatment refractoriness, including new mutations in the target of therapy and redundancy in many pathways such as those of the tyrosine kinase. Furthermore, increasing evidence for the presence of the cancer stem cell (CSC) provides another possible cellular mechanism for therapeutic refractoriness and dormant behavior of many neoplasms.[25] Therefore, morphoproteomics can play a role in explaining treatment refractoriness and provide possible avenues to overcome the age-old problem of the resistance to chemotherapy by examining points of convergence of multiple interconnected pathways and identifying the presence of CSCs within a specific tumor via known stem cell markers such as CD44 or CD133.

Morphoproteomic Application in Gastric Adenocarcinoma

Several main convergent and interconnected pathways involved in the plethora of molecular regulators, such as receptor tyrosine kinases (RTKs), are currently under intense investigation: the PI3 K/Akt/mTOR pathway, the Ras/Raf/extracellular signal-regulated kinase (ERK) pathway, and the NF-κB pathway.[23] In a morphoproteomic study using human gastric carcinoma, specifically

GAC tissue microarray conducted at The University of Texas Medical School at Houston and The University of Texas M. D. Anderson Cancer Center, our research group characterized the protein circuitry in signal transduction of these pathways of convergence, as well as cell cycle protein correlates in GAC tissues and nonneoplastic gastric tissues.[26]

The tissue microarray was constructed from a total of 215 total and partial gastrectomy specimens collected over the span of 20 years from the Department of Pathology tissue bank at The M. D. Anderson Cancer Center. To avoid potential confounding treatment effects, specimens from patients with preoperative treatment were not included. Immunohistochemistry with antibodies against specific protein targets and phosphospecific probes specific for phosphorylatively activated sites of a given protein target were applied to tissue microarray sections to examine the aforementioned pathways. The phosphospecific probes include antibodies directed against mTOR, p70S6K, ERK-1/2, and NF-κBp65, phosphorylated at putative sites of activation, serine (Ser) 2448, threonine (Thr) 389, Thr 202/ tyrosine (Tyr) 204, and Ser 536, respectively (Cell Signaling Technology, Inc., Beverly, Massachusetts). Other antibodies against specific protein targets included upstream stimulator of ERK and NF-κB pathways, S100P (R&D Systems, Inc., Minneapolis, Minnesota) and cell cycle–associated proteins Ki-67 (DAKO, Denmark) and S phase kinase–associated protein (Skp-2, Santa Cruz Biotechnology, Inc., Santa Cruz, California). Semi-quantitative assessment of the expression levels of protein analytes in target cells was determined using bright-field microscopy and applying a scoring system on a scale of 0–4+ as follows: 0 for no detectable chromogenic signal; 1+ for focal weak staining; 2+ for partial intermediate or focal strong target cells staining; 3+ for >50%, strong or intermediate staining, and 4+ for diffuse strong staining. The cellular compartmentalization (cytoplasmic/plasmalemmal vs. nuclear) of the protein analyte was also characterized.[26]

PI3′K/Akt/mTOR Pathway

The PI3′K/Akt/mTOR pathway (Fig. 16-1) is one of the most frequently targeted pathways in all sporadic human tumors and is known to regulate protein synthesis, cell cycle progression, metabolism, and angiogenesis.[27] The mTOR pathway is an appealing clinical target because it has an identified inhibitor, rapamycin. An analogue of rapamycin, temsirolimus, has shown promising efficacy in phase II and III clinical trials for metastatic renal cell carcinoma.[28] This pathway is regulated via sequential activation of phosphatidylinositol 3′-kinase (PI3′-K), Akt, and then phosphorylation of mTOR at serine 2448.[27] mTOR is a Ser/Thr protein kinase found in two complexes, raptor and rictor, that mediates nutrient-dependent intracellular signaling as well as extracellular signaling (growth factors) related to cell growth, proliferation, and differentiation.[29] The rapamycin-sensitive, predominantly cytoplasmic raptor mTOR protein complex (mTORC1) phosphorylatively activates its downstream effector, p70S6K, at threonine 389, resulting in an increase in mRNA translation, ribosome biogenesis, and subsequent cell growth.[27,30,31] Conversely, the relatively rapamycin-insensitive, nuclear rictor mTOR protein complex (mTORC2) activates Akt via phosphorylation of Akt at Serine 473.[23,27,31] The mTOR pathway has been shown in preclinical studies to play a role in the carcinogenesis of stomach, as well as other gastrointestinal malignancies, including pancreatic and colonic adenocarcinoma.[26,32,33] Studies involving other tumors have also demonstrated that the phosphorylative activation of p70S6K via the mTOR pathway results in increased G1 cell cycle progression, cell survival, and tumor cell proliferation.[27]

A preclinical study of human gastric carcinoma cell lines demonstrated in vitro inhibition of the mTOR pathway by rapamycin through analysis of downstream effectors such as hypoxia-inducible factor (HIF)-1α, as well as cellular proliferation rate and angiogenesis, indicating a role for the mTOR inhibitors in GAC therapy.[33] Multiple studies, including our microarray study, have confirmed the activation of the mTOR pathway in human GAC tissues.[26,34,35] Our findings are illustrated in Figure 16-2 and are summarized in Tables 16-2 and 16-3. Specifically, we found that a majority of GAC cases (88%) showed cytoplasmic/plasmalemmal expression of p-mTOR (Ser 2448), and 50.5% showed moderate to strong (>2+) cytoplasmic/plasmalemmal p-mTOR expression.[26] On the other hand, in nonneoplastic gastric mucosa (NNGM), the cytoplasmic/

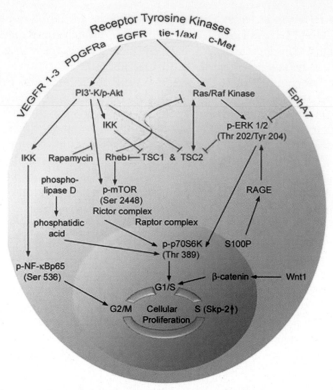

FIGURE 16-1 Morphoproteomic correlates (*) with variable expression by immunohistochemistry as demonstrated by us and others in gastric adenocarcinoma (GAC)[1,5,36–39,55,65–70,87–89] when considered in the context of signal transduction pathways of convergence illustrate the potential for: upstream signaling by tyrosine kinases to include VEGFR1-3, PDG-FR-α, EGFR, tie-1/axl, and c-Met through the PI3'-K/Akt pathway (as evidenced by p-Akt expression) and/or the Ras/Raf kinase/ERK pathway (as evidenced by p-ERK 1/2 expression and nuclear translocation)[73–82]; direct activation of ERK by the S100P/RAGE pathway[46,48,49] (again as evidenced by p-ERK-1/2 expression with nuclear translocation in some GAC cases) and of p70S6K by the product of phospholipase D catalysis, namely phosphatidic acid[19,20,51–54] (as evidenced by p-p70S6K nuclear expression that is disproportionate to p-mTOR expression, one of its putative upstream activators [see Results]); convergent signaling of the PI3'-K/Akt and Ras/Raf kinase/ERK pathways to activate the NF-kB pathway through the activation of IKK by both p-Akt and p-ERK 1/2[41–44,56,90,91] resulting in p-NF-kBp65 expression with nuclear translocation in some GAC cases; convergent signaling by p-p70S6K and p-ERK-1/2 resulting in G1 to S cell cycle progression as evidenced by Skp2 expression[60] and with a potential influence by p-NF-kB to facilitate the G2/M phase progression[21,61–63,92] leading to tumoral cell proliferation in GAC. The opportunity for complex cross-talk between the PI3'-K/Akt and Ras/Raf kinase/ERK pathways of convergence is inherent in the role of Rheb in activating the mTOR pathway,[93–95] while Rheb also interferes in the activation of ERK by inhibiting B-Raf kinase.[96–98] Similarly, there is potential interplay between the NF-kB and ERK pathways and the activation of mTOR via the respective roles of IKK in inhibiting TSC1[41–44,56,57] and p-ERK-1/2 in inhibiting TSC2,[99] the latter of which forms a complex (TSC1 + TSC2) to inhibit Rheb.[94] Such an interplay along with the variable expression of upstream tyrosine kinases including the inhibitory tyrosine kinase, EphA7[71,72] allows for variation among individual patients and speaks to the need for morphoproteomic analysis of individual tumors.

plasmalemmal expression of p-mTOR appeared to be localized to within the deep foveolar pits, isthmus, and areas of intestinal metaplasia. Thus, the overall activation of the mTOR pathway in GAC appeared to be increased compared with the nonneoplastic gastric mucosal epithelium. Moreover, the expression levels were compared in subsets of GAC cases divided according to Lauren classification of diffuse and intestinal. Moderate to strong cytoplasmic/plasmalemmal expressions of p-mTOR were seen in 58.1% of the diffuse and 46.7% of the intestinal subtypes, respectively. Similarly, moderate to strong nuclear expressions of p-p70S6K were seen in 96.9% of diffuse and 91.7% of intestinal subtypes, respectively.[26]

Various studies have shown differing evidence of the prognostic predicative potential of mTOR activation in GAC.[34,35] In a study that included 109 cases of GAC, Murayama et al. showed that cytoplasmic p-mTOR expression was associated with high tumor stage, tumor progression,

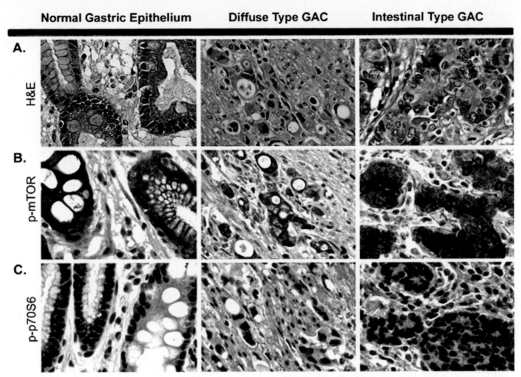

FIGURE 16-2 **A:** Hematoxylin and Eosin stain of nonneoplastic gastric mucosa (NNGM) with intestinal metaplasia (IM), diffuse and intestinal type GAC. **B:** p-mTOR (Ser2448) immunostaining showing positive expression most strongly positive within the foveolar epithelium (FE) and areas of IM in NNGM, diffuse moderate-strong cytoplasmic/plasmalemmal expression in both diffuse (4+) and intestinal (3+) type GAC. **C.** p-p70S6K (Thr389) immunostaining showing diffuse positive expression in NNGM, diffuse strong nuclear expression (4+) in both diffuse and intestinal type GAC.

and poor survival in gastric carcinoma ($n = 109$). The opposite results were shown for nuclear p-mTOR expression, indicating that the localization of p-mTOR may be critical to tumor progression and outcomes in patients with gastric carcinoma.[35] However, another study of mTOR in conjunction with p-p70S6K within 412 cases of GAC showed that the activation of the mTOR pathway was associated with lower tumor stage, less tumor progression, and favorable survival outcomes.[34] Our microarray study did not reveal statistically significant correlation of p-mTOR expression with tumor stage or survival outcomes.[26]

These conflicting data indicate that the expression patterns of the mTOR activation markers do not always coincide. For example, in our study, we uncovered a relatively poor correlation between p-mTOR (Ser 2448) and its downstream effector, p-p70S6K (Thr 389), which showed more frequent moderate to strong positive expression (93.5%) than did p-mTOR (Ser 2448) (50.5%).[26] One possible explanation for this expression discrepancy between p-mTOR and p-p70S6K is that rather than the conventional PI3′-K/Akt pathway, there are alternate p70S6K activation pathways including those mediated by phospholipase D via phosphatidic acid, guanosine triphosphatase Cdc42, and the lysophosphatidic acid pathway.[36] These alternative pathways may also explain, at least in part, the discrepant in vivo and in vitro studies utilizing rapamycin in cancer trials.[28]

Ras/Raf/ERK Pathway

The Ras/Raf pathway (Fig. 16-1), which is activated by RTK, is a well-known and important pathway in tumorigenesis.[27] The Ras/Raf pathway consists of the Ras oncogene and its direct effector in mammalian cells, Raf-1 serine/threonine kinase, which in turn activates a series of kinases including the ERK and mitogen-activated protein kinase (MAPK).[37] ERK is responsible

Table 16-2	Therapeutic agents applicable to morphoproteomics
Pharmaceutical Agent	**Molecular Targets**
Trastuzumab (Herceptin)[a]	HER2/neu (ERBB2) receptor
Gefitinib(Iressa)[b], Erlotinib (Tarceva)[a]	EGFR tyrosine kinase
Cetuximab (Erbitux)[c]	EGFR ectodomain
Imatinib mesylate (Gleevec)[d]	bcr-abl, PDGFR, and c-Kit tyrosine kinases
Statins (Lovastatin)[e]	Mevalonate/prenylation pathway and N-glycosylation of IGFR and EGFR.
Aminobisphosphonates (pamidronate,[e] zoledronate[d])	Prenylation pathway via inhibition of farnesyl diphosphate synthase
Zarnestra[e]	Prenylation pathway via inhibition of farnesyl transferase
Captopril[e] (ACE inhibitor), Losartan[e] (AT1R inhibitor)	Transactivation of PDGFR and EGFR signaling via the angiotensin system
Sirolimus[f] (rapamycin; Rapamune), Temsirolimus (CCl-779), everolimus (RAD001)	Immunophilins and mTOR pathway signaling
Bortezomib (Velcade)[e]	NF-κB signal via proteasome inhibition
Geldanamycin[f]	Hsp90 chaperon molecules
Bevacizumab (Avastin)[a]	VEGFR-A
Tamoxifen[e]	ER signaling
Nexavar[g] (BAY 43-9006)	Raf and VEGFR
Sunitinib[h] (SU11248)	VEGFR/PDGFR
HDAC inhibitors	HDAC

[a]Genetech Inc, South San Francisco, California.
[b]Astra Zeneca Pharmaceuticals LP, Wilmington, Delaware.
[c]Merck & Co, Inc, Whitehouse Station, New Jersey.
[d]Novartis, Basel, Switzerland.
[e]LCM Pharmaceuticals, Inc, Boca Raton, Florida.
[f]AG Scientific Inc, San Diego, California.
[g]Bayer Healthcare Pharmaceuticals, Wayne, New Jersey; and Onyx Pharmaceuticals, Emeryville, California.
[h]Pfizer. New York City, New York.

for phosphorylating a variety of substrates, including p70S6K, which as previously described mediates cell growth and cell cycle entry.[27,38] ERK can also activate the raptor mTOR complex via the inactivation of tuberin (TSC2).[23,26] Preclinical studies have shown increased cell survival and proliferation with respect to expression level of ERK in gastric carcinoma cell lines.[39]

Our results[26] (Fig. 16-3C and D and summarized in Tables 16-2 and 16-3) showed a small subset of GAC cases (15.2%) exhibited moderate to strong intranuclear expression of p-ERK-1/2. Moderate to strong intranuclear expression of p-ERK-1/2 was noted in 27.8% of Lauren's diffuse and 10.3% of intestinal subtypes. In most NNGM studied, the intranuclear expression of p-ERK-1/2 appeared to be present only within the foveolar pits and isthmus, with less intense staining in areas of intestinal metaplasia, but not within the gastric glands.[26]

NF-κB Pathway

The activation of transcription factor NF-κB signaling pathway is involved in the regulation of cellular proliferation, promotion of cell cycle progression at G2/M phase, apoptosis, and tumor suppression.

Table 16-3	Expression of p-mTOR, p-p70S6K, S100P, p-ERK, p-NF-kBp65, Ki-67, and Skp-2 in GACs and NNGM						
	mTOR Pathway		Ras/Raf Pathway		NF-κB Pathway	Proliferation Markers	
Immuno-histochemical Stain	p-mTOR[a]	p70S6K[b]	S100P[b]	p-ERK[b]	p-NF-κBp65[b]	Ki-67[b]	Skp-2[b]
Total positive GA cases	162 (88%)	186 (100%)	166 (90.7%)	95 (45.2%)	144 (75%)	153 (86.4%)	166 (91.2%)
Weak positive GAC cases (1–2 +)	69 (37.7%)	12 (6.5%)	18 (9.8%)	64 (30.5%)	75 (39.1%)	27 (15.3%)	43 (23.6%)
Strong positive GAC cases (>2 +)	93 (50.5%)	174 (93.5%)	148 (80.9%)	32 (15.2%)	69 (35.9%)	126 (71.2%)	123 (67.6%)
Total positive NNGM cases	16[c] (94.1%)	16 (100%)	16[d] (100%)	9[d] (64.3%)	16 (94.1%)	13[d] (86.7%)	12[d] (75%)
Weak positive NNGM cases (1–2 +)	9[c] (52.9%)	3 (18.8%)	3[d] (18.8%)	8[d] (57.1%)	8 (47.1%)	10[d] (66.7%)	10[d] (62.5%)
Strong positive NNGM cases (>2 +)	7[c] (41.2%)	13 (81.3%)	13[d] (81.3%)	1[d] (7.2%)	8 (47.1%)	3[d] (20%)	2[d] (12.5%)

[a]Cytoplasmic/plasmalemmal staining
[b]nuclear staining
[c]Positivity is the most intense at the foveolar pits and isthmus
[d]Positivity limited to the foveolar pits and isthmus

Its constitutive activation is related to progression of various cancers, including renal cell carcinoma, cervical cancer, and esophageal cancer.[40] NF-κB has been shown to be activated by the same PI3′K/Akt pathway that activates mTOR and by the Ras/Raf kinase/ERK pathway. Its role in gastric carcinoma is unclear, with conflicting reports of NF-κB expression and its prognostic significance.[41,42]

Our study showed that a subset of GAC cases (35.9%) demonstrated moderate to strong intranuclear expression of p-NF-κBp65 (Fig. 16-3E and F and summarized in Tables 16-2 and 16-3).[26] In most NNGM, the intranuclear expression of p-NF-κBp65 appeared comparable to that seen in the nuclei of GAC. When the intranuclear expression levels of this protein analyte in GAC were determined according to Lauren classification, 61.5% of cases in the diffuse and 22.2% of cases in the intestinal subtype were noted to exhibit moderate to strong intranuclear expression.[26]

Markers of Upstream Signaling and PI3′K/Akt/mTOR, Ras/Raf/ERK, and NF-κB Pathways

Multiple RTKs in GAC are variably expressed and detected by immunohistochemistry. These include the following: EphA7 RTK, cytoplasmic vascular endothelial growth factor receptors (VEGFRs) 1 to 3 and platelet-derived growth factor receptor (PDGFR) alpha, and plasmalemmal (membranous) EGFR1, receptor protein tyrosine kinases, tie-1 and axl, and c-Met.[26] Specifically, EphA7 could inhibit both basal ERK-1/2 activity and the Ras/MAPK cascade, and attenuate the activation of MAPK by other RTKs.[26] Furthermore, VEGFR, PDGFRα, EGFR, and c-Met have

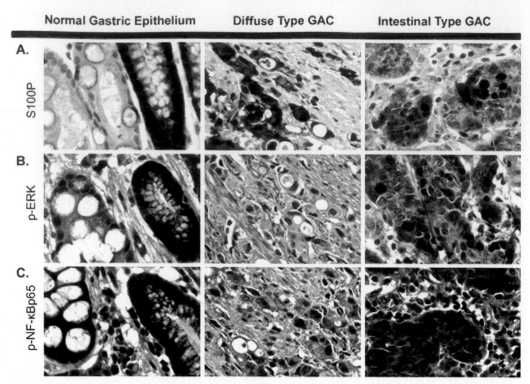

FIGURE 16-3 Nuclear staining patterns: **A:** S100P immunostaining showing positive expression limited to foveolar epithelium (FE) and focal areas of intestinal metaplasia (IM) in nonneoplastic gastric mucosa (NNGM), diffusely strong expression (4+) in diffuse type GAC and focal moderate-strong expression (2+) in intestinal type GAC. **B:** p-ERK (Thr 202/Tyr 204) immunostaining showing positive expression limited to FE and areas of IM in NNGM, focal moderate expression (2+) in both diffuse and intestinal type GAC. **C:** p-NF-kBp65 (Ser 536) immunostaining showing diffuse positive expression in NNGM, partial strong expression (2+) in diffuse type GAC and diffuse strong expression (4+) in intestinal type GAC.

been shown to activate the Akt and ERK pathways.[26] These findings demonstrate correlative expression of tyrosine kinases in GAC that occurs upstream of the Ras/Raf kinase/ERK and Akt/mTOR pathways of convergence.

S100P is a 95-amino acid Ca^{2+}-binding protein with a restricted cellular distribution that was first purified from the placenta. Its expression has been reported in GI malignancies such as colonic and pancreatic adenocarcinoma, and may have adverse prognostic significance in lung and breast cancer.[26] S100P functions in an autocrine manner via the receptor for advanced glycation end-product (RAGE) to activate ERK and NF-κB pathways and promote cell proliferation and survival.[43] Our study showed a majority of GAC cases (80.9%) exhibited moderate to strong (>2+) S100P intranuclear expression, and most NNGM showed S100P expression limited to the foveolar pits, isthmus, and areas of intestinal metaplasia but not the gastric glands (Fig. 16-3A and B and summarized in Tables 16-2 and 16-3). Moderate to strong intranuclear expression of S100P was seen in 85.1% of Lauren's diffuse and 78.1% of intestinal subtypes.[26] Along with our results, other studies also support the activation of ERK and NF-κB pathways via S100P through RAGE. Kuniyasu et al.[44] reported expression of the signal transducer of S100P stimulation, the RAGEs in gastric cancer, and that it correlates with depth of invasion and lymph node metastasis. In our series, the nuclear expression of p-ERK-1/2 in GAC was associated in most cases with concurrent expression of S100P. Furthermore, the downstream positive signaling by p-ERK-1/2 on the NF-kB pathway was supported by the expression p-NF-kBp65, with a statistically significant correlation between p-ERK-1/2 and p-NF-kBp65 ($r = 0.565$; $p < 0.0001$) and statistically greater mean levels of p-ERK-1/2 and p-NF-kBp65 in Lauren's diffuse subtype of GAC ($p = 0.001$ and $p < 0.0001$, respectively).[26]

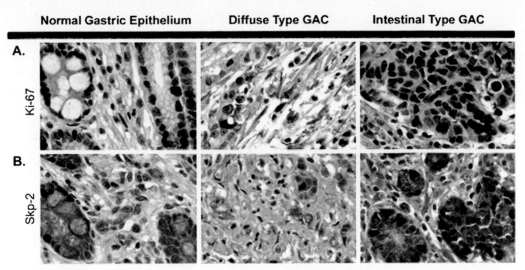

FIGURE 16-4 Nuclear staining patterns: **A:** Ki-67 immunostaining showing positive expression limited to FE and areas of IM in NNGM, focal strong expression (2+) in diffuse type GAC and partial moderate-strong expression (3+) in intestinal type GAC. **B:** Skp-2 immunostaining showing positive expression limited to FE and areas of IM in NNGM, focal weak expression (1+) in diffuse type GAC and partial moderate-strong expression (2+) in intestinal type GAC.

In summary, there is correlative morphoproteomic expression of activated markers of Ras/Raf kinase/ERK and PI3′K/Akt/mTOR pathways of convergence downstream of activating tyrosine kinases in GAC. Furthermore, there is also correlative morphoproteomic expression of activated markers of the ERK and NF-κB pathway via RAGE and S100P in GAC. These pathways are illustrated in Figure 16-1.

Markers of Cellular Proliferation: Ki-67 and Skp-2

An end result of the activation of the aforementioned three major pathways of convergence is the promotion of cell growth and proliferation. This correlation is demonstrated in our series of GAC cases in the form of the moderate to strong expression of the cell cycle–associated protein analytes, Ki-67 and Skp-2, in the majority of cases (71.2% and 67.6% for Ki-67 and Skp-2, respectively, Fig. 16-4 and Tables 16-2 and 16-3).[26] Such expressions far exceed those seen in the NNGM, where the nuclear immunopositivity was limited to the foveolar pits and the isthmus. Our observations are strengthened by the strong correlation between Ki-67 and Skp-2 expression ($r = 0.503$; $p < 0.0001$).[26]

The potential clinical importance of the Skp-2 expression lies in the association of this protein analyte with the S phase of the cell cycle.[23,24,26] Therefore, our results indicate that the majority of GAC cases are progressing from the G1 to the S phase, and such cases may be candidates for an S phase active chemotherapeutic agent. Moreover, this progression has been shown to be promoted by the PI3′K/Akt/mTOR and Ras/Raf/ERK pathways, which are also demonstrated to be activated in GAC.[27,45] It is of potential clinical importance that the mTOR inhibitor, rapamycin, has been shown in a cancer cell line study to significantly decrease Skp-2 mRNA and protein levels in a dose- and time-dependent fashion, which in turn is followed by cell growth arrest at G1.

Markers of Cancer Stem Cells

CSCs are a unique subpopulation that possesses the capacity to repopulate tumors, drive malignant progression, and mediate radio/chemoresistance. Some of the CSC markers reported in the literature include CD44, CD133, EpCAM, and CD24.[25] Recent studies suggest that CD44-expressing gastric carcinoma cells show increased resistance to chemotherapy or radiation-induced cell death.[46]

Table 16-4	Percentage of cases with respect to level of expression of p-mTOR, p-p70S6K, S100P, p-ERK, p-NF-κBp65, Ki-67, and Skp-2 in diffuse and intestinal subtypes of GACs

Immunohistochemical Stain	mTOR Pathway				Ras/Raf Pathway				NF-κB Pathway		Proliferation Markers			
	p-mTOR*		p70S6K†		S100P†		p-ERK†		p-NF-κBp65†		Ki-67†		Skp-2†	
	+	++	+	++	+	++	+	++	+	++	+	++	+	++
Lauren classification														
Diffuse (*n* = 77)	32.3	58.1	3.1	96.9	7.5	85.1	34.4	27.8	26.2	61.5	16.9	66.1	29.5	65.6
Intestinal (*n* = 133)	40	46.7	8.3	91.7	11.3	78.3	25	10.3	46	22.2	14.5	73.5	20.8	69.3

+: 1–2 + staining.
++: >2 + staining.
*Cytoplasmic/plasmalemmal staining.
†Nuclear staining.

Preliminary results from our study also confirm the expression of CD44 in GAC. Specifically, membranous CD44 expression was identified in 52% (79/151) cases of GAC. In contrast, adjacent NNGM showed expression of CD44 in 24% (10/41) cases.[47]

Another known CSC marker in the gastrointestinal tract is CD133 (prominin-1). In a gastric carcinoma cell line study, Matsumoto et al.[48] showed that the inhibition of mTOR signaling under normoxic conditions upregulated CD133 expression, whereas HIF-1a induction under hypoxic conditions downregulated CD133. These findings suggest that the CSC may play a role in GAC carcinogenesis and progression and that aforementioned pathways such as mTOR may be involved in the modulation of CSCs.

Therapeutic Implications

The aforementioned findings in gastric carcinoma have important potential roles to better predict the therapeutic efficacy of a certain treatment and to overcome the obstacles of treatment refractoriness.

At present, the pathologic classification or phenotype of a neoplasm is routinely characterized, and this information is used to select the agents that have shown historical treatment efficacy. Many of the chemotherapy agents utilized today are cytotoxic agents. In order to predict their efficacy in a specific neoplasm, the neoplastic cell's stage in the cell cycle must be characterized, since a specific cytotoxic agent may be most effective in the G1, S, G2/M, or mitotic phase. By utilizing Ki-67 immunohistochemical staining, we can identify whether the neoplastic cells have entered the cell cycle (G1, S, G2, and M phases). Similarly, Skp-2 can be used to identify if the neoplastic cells are in the S phase of the cell cycle. As shown in our study,[26] a majority of GAC cases have positive Ki-67 and Skp-2 expression and therefore are in the S-phase of the cell cycle.

The finding of PI3′K/Akt/mTOR and pathway activation in the majority of GAC cases and NF-κB pathway activation in a significant subset of GAC cases indicate that the mTOR pathway inhibitor, rapamycin, and the NF-κB pathway inhibitor, bortezomib, may be used in combinatorial therapy to treat patients with GAC. Specifically, rapamycin may be utilized first to synchronize the entrance of tumor cells into the cell cycle to maximize the efficacy of subsequent cytotoxic therapy.[49,50]

These above findings demonstrates that morphoproteomic profiling of an individual patient's tumor may be necessary to uncover potential targets in signal transduction pathways that may contribute to the tumor's proliferative capacity, invasive potential, and chemo/radioresistance. Such profiling may allow for the development of personalized medicine, which utilizes combinatorial therapeutic regimens that incorporate signal transduction pathway inhibitors and cell cycle–specific cytotoxic therapies appropriate to an individual patient's GAC.

References

1. Gunderson LL, Sosin H. Adenocarcinoma of the stomach: areas of failure in a re-operation series (second or symptomatic look) clinicopathologic correlation and implications for adjuvant therapy. *Int J Radiat Oncol Biol Phys.* 1982;8:1–11.
2. Rivera F, Vega-Villegas ME, Lopez-Brea MF. Chemotherapy of advanced gastric cancer. *Cancer Treat Rev.* 2007;33:315–324.
3. Reinders J, Sickmann A. *Proteomics: methods and protocols.* Dordrecht, NY: Humana Press; 2009.
4. Kuramitsu Y, Nakamura K. Proteomic analysis of cancer tissues: shedding light on carcinogenesis and possible biomarkers. *Proteomics.* 2006;6:5650–5661.
5. Herrmann K, Walch A, Baluff B, et al. Proteomic and metabolic prediction of response to therapy in gastrointestinal cancers. *Nat Clin Pract Gastroenterol Hepatol.* 2009;6:170–183.
6. Nishigaki R, Osaki M, Hiratsuka M, et al. Proteomic identification of differentially-expressed genes in human gastric carcinomas. *Proteomics.* 2005;5:3205–3213.

7. Zhang J, Kang B, Tan X, et al. Comparative analysis of the protein profiles from primary gastric tumors and their adjacent regions: MAWBP could be a new protein candidate involved in gastric cancer. *J Proteome Res*. 2007;6:4423–4432.

8. Kon OL, Yip TT, Ho MF, et al. The distinctive gastric fluid proteome in gastric cancer reveals a multibiomarker diagnostic profile. *BMC Med Genomics*. 2008;1:54.

9. Ren H, Du N, Liu G, et al. Analysis of variabilities of serum proteomic spectra in patients with gastric cancer before and after operation. *World J Gastroenterol*. 2006;12:2789–2792.

10. Gologan A, Graham DY, Sepulveda AR. Molecular markers in Helicobacter pylori-associated gastric carcinogenesis. *Clin Lab Med*. 2005;25:197–222.

11. Wu MS, Chow LP, Lin JT, et al. Proteomic identification of biomarkers related to Helicobacter pylori-associated gastroduodenal disease: challenges and opportunities. *J Gastroenterol Hepatol*. 2008;23: 1657–1661.

12. Chan CH, Ko CC, Chang JG, et al. Subcellular and functional proteomic analysis of the cellular responses induced by Helicobacter pylori. *Mol Cell Proteomics*. 2006;5:702–713.

13. Chen CD, Wang CS, Huang H, et al. Overexpression of CLIC1 in human gastric carcinoma and its clinicopathological significance. *Proteomics*. 2007;7:155–167.

14. Chen YR, et al. Quantitative proteomic and genomic profiling reveals metastasis-related protein expression patterns in gastric cancer cells. *J Proteome Res*. 2006;5:2727–2742.

15. Takikawa M, Akiyama Y, Maruyama K, et al. Proteomic analysis of a highly metastatic gastric cancer cell line using two-dimensional differential gel electrophoresis. *Oncol Rep*. 2006;16:705–711.

16. Wang X, Lu Y, Yang J, et al. Identification of triosephosphate isomerase as an anti-drug resistance agent in human gastric cancer cells using functional proteomic analysis. *J Cancer Res Clin Oncol*. 2008;134: 995–1003.

17. Yang YX, Chen ZC, Zhang GY, et al. A subcellular proteomic investigation into vincristine-resistant gastric cancer cell line. *J Cell Biochem*. 2008;104:1010–1021.

18. Yang YX, Hu HD, Zhang DZ, et al. Identification of proteins responsible for the development of adriamycin resistance in human gastric cancer cells using comparative proteomics analysis. *J Biochem Mol Biol*. 2007;40:853–860.

19. He QY, Cheung YH, Leung SY, et al. Diverse proteomic alterations in gastric adenocarcinoma. *Proteomics*. 2004;4:3276–3287.

20. Yoshihara T, et al. Proteomic alteration in gastric adenocarcinomas from Japanese patients. *Mol Cancer*. 2006;5:75.

21. Melle C, Ernst G, Schimmel B, et al. Characterization of pepsinogen C as a potential biomarker for gastric cancer using a histo-proteomic approach. *J Proteome Res*. 2005;4:1799–1804.

22. Lee K, Kye M, Jang JS, et al. Proteomic analysis revealed a strong association of a high level of alpha1-antitrypsin in gastric juice with gastric cancer. *Proteomics*. 2004;4:3343–3352.

23. Brown RE. Morphoproteomics: exposing protein circuitries in tumors to identify potential therapeutic targets in cancer patients. *Expert Rev Proteomics*. 2005;2:337–348.

24. Brown RE. Morphogenomics and morphoproteomics: a role for anatomic pathology in personalized medicine. *Arch Pathol Lab Med*. 2009;133:568–579.

25. Visvader JE, Lindeman GJ. Cancer stem cells in solid tumours: accumulating evidence and unresolved questions. *Nat Rev Cancer*. 2008;8:755–768.

26. Feng W, Brown RE, Trung CD, et al. Morphoproteomic profile of mTOR, Ras/Raf kinase/ERK, and NF-kappaB pathways in human gastric adenocarcinoma. *Ann Clin Lab Sci*. 2008;38:195–209.

27. Shaw RJ, Cantley LC. Ras, PI(3)K and mTOR signalling controls tumour cell growth. *Nature*. 2006;441:424–430.

28. Hudes A. Phase III, randomized, 3 arm study of temsirolinus (TEMSR) or interferon-alpha (IFN) or the combination of TEMSR + IFN in the treatment of first-line, poor risk patients with advanced renal cell carcinoma. *Proc Am Soc Clin Oncol*. 2006;24:2S.

29. Rosner M, Siegel N, Valli A, et al. mTOR phosphorylated at S2448 binds to raptor and rictor. *Amino Acids*. 2010;38:223–228.

30. Dennis PB, Pullen N, Kozma SC, et al. The principal rapamycin-sensitive p70(s6k) phosphorylation sites, T-229 and T-389, are differentially regulated by rapamycin-insensitive kinase kinases. *Mol Cell Biol*. 1996;16:6242–6251.

31. Rosner M, Hengstschlager M. Cytoplasmic and nuclear distribution of the protein complexes mTORC1 and mTORC2: rapamycin triggers dephosphorylation and delocalization of the mTORC2 components rictor and sin1. *Hum Mol Genet*. 2008;17:2934–2948.

32. Xu G, Zhang W, Bertram P, et al. Pharmacogenomic profiling of the PI3K/PTEN-AKT-mTOR pathway in common human tumors. *Int J Oncol.* 2004;24:893–900.

33. Lang SA, Gaumann A, Koeh GE, et al. Mammalian target of rapamycin is activated in human gastric cancer and serves as a target for therapy in an experimental model. *Int J Cancer.* 2007;120:1803–1810.

34. Xiao L, Wang YC, Li WS, et al. The role of mTOR and phospho-p70S6K in pathogenesis and progression of gastric carcinomas: an immunohistochemical study on tissue microarray. *J Exp Clin Cancer Res.* 2009;28:152.

35. Murayama T, Inokuchi M, Takagi Y, et al. Relation between outcomes and localisation of p-mTOR expression in gastric cancer. *Br J Cancer.* 2009;100:782–788.

36. Chen J, Fang Y. A novel pathway regulating the mammalian target of rapamycin (mTOR) signaling. *Biochem Pharmacol.* 2002;64:1071–1077.

37. Adnane L, Trail PA, Taylor I, et al. Sorafenib (BAY 43–9006, Nexavar), a dual-action inhibitor that targets RAF/MEK/ERK pathway in tumor cells and tyrosine kinases VEGFR/PDGFR in tumor vasculature. *Methods Enzymol.* 2006;407:597–612.

38. Roux PP, Blenis J. ERK and p38 MAPK-activated protein kinases: a family of protein kinases with diverse biological functions. *Microbiol Mol Biol Rev.* 2004;68:320–344.

39. Verma A, Atten MJ, Attar BM, et al. Selenomethionine stimulates MAPK (ERK) phosphorylation, protein oxidation, and DNA synthesis in gastric cancer cells. *Nutr Cancer.* 2004;49:184–190.

40. Gilmore TD, Koedood M, Piffat KA, et al. Rel/NF-kappaB/IkappaB proteins and cancer. *Oncogene.* 1996;13:1367–1378.

41. Lee BL, Lee HS, Jung J, et al. Nuclear factor-kappaB activation correlates with better prognosis and Akt activation in human gastric cancer. *Clin Cancer Res.* 2005;11:2518–2525.

42. Sasaki N, Morisaki T, Hashizume K, et al. Nuclear factor-kappaB p65 (RelA) transcription factor is constitutively activated in human gastric carcinoma tissue. *Clin Cancer Res.* 2001;7:4136–4142.

43. Arumugam T, Simeone DM, Schmidt AM, et al. S100P stimulates cell proliferation and survival via receptor for activated glycation end products (RAGE). *J Biol Chem.* 2004;279:5059–5065.

44. Kuniyasu H, Oue N, Wakikawa H, et al. Expression of receptors for advanced glycation end-products (RAGE) is closely associated with the invasive and metastatic activity of gastric cancer. *J Pathol.* 2002;196:163–170.

45. Meloche S, Pouyssegur J. The ERK1/2 mitogen-activated protein kinase pathway as a master regulator of the G1- to S-phase transition. *Oncogene.* 2007;26:3227–3239.

46. Ghaffarzadehgan K, Jafarzadeh M, Raziee HR, et al. Expression of cell adhesion molecule CD44 in gastric adenocarcinoma and its prognostic importance. *World J Gastroenterol.* 2008;14:6376–6381.

47. Dhingra S, Feng W, Zhou D, et al. Expression of stem cell markers in human gastric adenocarcinoma and non-neoplastic gastric mucosa, a study of 209 cases. *Mod Pathol.* 2010;23:143A.

48. Matsumoto K, Arao T, Tanaka K, et al. mTOR signal and hypoxia-inducible factor-1 alpha regulate CD133 expression in cancer cells. *Cancer Res.* 2009;69:7160–7164.

49. Matsuzaki T, Yashiro M, Kaizaki R, et al. Synergistic antiproliferative effect of mTOR inhibitors in combination with 5-fluorouracil in scirrhous gastric cancer. *Cancer Sci.* 2009;100:2402–2410.

50. Shigematsu H, Yoshida K, Sanada Y, et al. Rapamycin enhances chemotherapy-induced cytotoxicity by inhibiting the expressions of TS and ERK in gastric cancer cells. *Int J Cancer.* 2009;126:2716–2725.

17 Molecular Prognostic Markers of Gastric Cancer

▶ Mahmoud Goodarzi
▶ Dongfeng Tan

INTRODUCTION

According to a recent global estimate of cancer incidence, stomach cancer is the second most frequent cancer-related cause of death after lung cancer. Although the worldwide incidence of gastric cancer has been declining in recent years, its mortality rate in China is the highest among all tumors and represents 25% of gastric cancer mortalities worldwide.[1] Though advances in diagnosis and treatment have provided significantly improved long-term overall survival (OS) rates for early gastric cancer, the prognosis for advanced gastric cancer still remains poor.

Many factors are associated with gastric cancer prognosis, including the location of the tumor in the stomach, histological grade, and lymphovascular tumor invasion. For instance, Asian race, female sex, and younger age are predictive of a better outcome, while signet ring cell carcinoma of the stomach is reported as a major and independent predictor of poor prognosis due to specific characteristics such as more infiltrating tumors showing affinity for lymphatic tissue accompanied by a higher rate of peritoneal carcinomatosis.[2]

Nevertheless, among all factors, regional lymphatic spread and disease stage are probably the most powerful prognostic factors determining the survival, management, and prognosis of patients with stomach cancer. Currently, surgical resection remains the most reasonable treatment option for stomach cancer; tumor node metastasis (TNM) stage (by AJCC Cancer Staging Manual, see Chapter 18), which is assessed after tumor resection, is used as the main prognostic factor,[3] with 5-year survival rates of 58% to 78% and 34% for stage I and II disease, respectively.[1] However, it is not rare that stomach cancer patients with the same TNM stage, receiving the same integrated treatments, have different clinical outcomes. Therefore, new prognostic determinants capable of selecting patients at high risk of treatment resistance in conjunction with the TNM-staging information are required.

Extensive research in past 2 decades has increased our understanding of the biological mechanisms of tumor invasion and metastasis, which are critical determinants of clinical behavior of cancer. Tumor invasion and metastasis is a very complicated process, involving a multistep progression through a series of sequential selective events.[3] It has been documented that metastatic process involves many related steps, including tumor cell detachment, local invasion, motility, vascular invasion and neoangiogenesis, access to and survival in circulation, adhesion to endothelial cells, extravasation, settlement and regrowth in different organs.[3] At the molecular level, multiple genes regulating these events contribute to the metastatic process, including cell cycle regulators, cell adhesion molecules, protein catabolic enzymes, and various angiogenic and growth factors, which are often used as prognostic factors.[1,3] Better knowledge of the molecular basis for tumor metastasis will lead to new paradigms and possible improvements in diagnostic and therapeutic approaches. This chapter describes changes in genes and molecules that can be used as prognostic markers of gastric cancer and their potential application in the clinical setting.

MOLECULAR PROGNOSTIC MARKERS OF GASTRIC CANCER

Tumor-infiltrating Lymphocytes in Gastric Cancer

Cell-mediated adaptive immunity is thought to play a major role in antitumor immunity. In mouse models using transgenic or knockout mice or applying monoclonal antibodies specific for distinct immunologic components, adaptive immunity has been demonstrated to protect murine hosts against the development of both chemically induced and spontaneous tumors.[4] Several types of tumor-infiltrating lymphocytes (TILs) have been shown to be associated with better outcomes for different human cancers, such as melanoma and colorectal cancer.[4] This study demonstrated that high numbers of CD3[+], CD8[+], or CD45RO[+] T cells in tumor tissue are significantly correlated with lower frequencies of lymph node metastasis or disease recurrence and improved patient survival. Lee et al.[4] have shown that the type and density of TILs correlate with clinical outcome after gastrectomy in stomach cancer patients. A high density of CD3[+], CD8[+], or CD45RO[+] tumor-infiltrating total T lymphocytes (cytotoxic T cells and memory T cells) was found to be an independent predictor of lymph node metastasis and an independent prognostic factor for patients' OS by multivariate analyses, suggesting that adaptive immunity does act to prevent tumor progression and helps predict clinical outcome.[4]

EBV (Epstein-Barr virus)-associated gastric cancer (EBVAGA, see Chapter 4) is frequently seen in medullary type or lymphoepithelial type of gastric cancer, with dense lymphocyte infiltration.[5] EBVAGA is also seen in other types of gastric cancer, including intestinal type gastric adeno carcinoma. Nevertheless, one of the main clinical features is that EBVAGA is associated with a favorable clinical outcome. Though it is still not quite clear the underlying mechanism(s), infiltrating lymphocytes, particularly T lymphocytes, seem to play a role in limiting the spread of cancer cells.[6] An intestinal-type EBVAGA with intratumoral T lymphocytes is illustrated in Figure 17-1.

Cell Cycle Regulators

Gastric carcinoma is characterized by numerous genetic and epigenetic alterations that may influence cell cycle progression and apoptosis.[7] Abnormal expression of cell cycle regulatory proteins that control the G1-S phase transition, a critical rate-limiting step in cell cycle progression, is frequently observed in tumorigenesis.[8] These proteins include three D-type cyclins (D_1, D_2, and D_3) that bind to one of two cyclin-dependent protein kinase (CDK) subunits, CDK_4 and CDK_6, as well as the E-type cyclins, which control the activity of CDK_2.[8] It has been shown that the *cyclin E* gene is amplified in 15% to 20% of gastric cancers and overexpression of cyclin E correlates with the aggressiveness of the tumor.[3]

The *P21* and *P27* tumor-suppressor genes produce proteins that are activated by P53 and induce cell cycle arrest by inhibiting the kinase activity of the cyclin/CDK complexes regulating cell cycle progression.[9] A reduction in the expression of P27[Kip1] is frequently associated with advanced gastric cancers and is also significantly correlated with deep tumor invasion and lymph node metastasis.[3] Furthermore, it has been demonstrated that P21 expression, alone or in combination with P27, is associated with a favorable prognosis and is an independent predictor of patient survival in gastric cancer.[7] Moreover, the tumor suppressor gene *P53* encodes a nuclear protein that plays a key role in tumor progression by regulating DNA repair, cell division, and apoptosis. P53 induces the expression of P21, which promotes cell cycle arrest by inhibiting the phosphorylation of the CDK complexes and blocking cell cycle progression to the S-phase.[10]

The prognostic usefulness of P53 in gastric cancer has been controversial; most studies show an association of P53 with patient survival, while other investigations do not support these

FIGURE 17-1 **A:** Intratumoral lymphocytes, along with eosinophils, are notice-
able in this EBV associated gastric
adenocarcinoma. **B:** In-situ hybridization
of EBV probe highlights the viral infected
tumor cells (*large black dots*); the intratumoral lymphocytes and inflammatory
cells are negative.

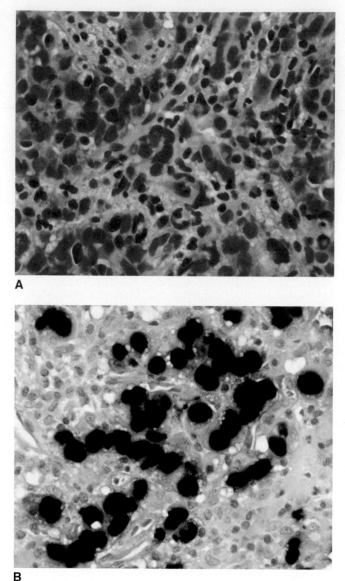

findings.[7] These conflicting reports may be explained in part by the investigators' use of different techniques and antibodies in the studies.[9] Fondevila et al.[11] found that P53 expression is an
independent prognostic factor for both disease-free survival and OS in patients with curatively
resected gastric cancer, and when tumor cells express P53, the therapeutic efficacy of adjuvant
chemotherapy is lost.

   Despite the controversy regarding the usefulness of P53 as a prognostic marker for gastric
cancer, the combined P53/P21 status may be a useful prognostic marker for survival in patients
with surgically resected gastric cancer.[10] In fact, expression of P21 in combination with a lack of
P53 expression was significantly associated with longer survival.[7,10] In addition, Liu et al.[12] suggested that the combined examination of P27, P21, and P53 expression allows the precise prediction of prognosis in patients with gastric cancer. Therefore, the simultaneous evaluation of the
expression of P53, P21, and P27 may be a useful diagnostic tool for predicting clinical prognosis
in patients with stomach cancer.[7,10]

The Rb Pathway

The retinoblastoma tumor suppressor *(Rb-1)*, *P16* (CDKN2/MTS1), and cyclin D1 genes are components of the Rb pathway, which controls the G1/S checkpoint of the cell cycle.[13] The active hypophosphorylated form of the Rb protein binds to and blocks the action of the transcription factor E_2F, inhibiting the progression of the cell cycle from the G_1 phase to the S phase. Cyclins D_1 and E, in association with their cyclin-dependent kinase partners, are responsible for the phosphorylation of Rb.[3,13] P16 binds to CDK4 and CDK6, blocking their association with D-type cyclins. Thus, inactivating mutations or deletion of *Rb* or *P16* with loss of protein expression or overexpression of cyclin D_1 or cyclin E can activate E_2F and promote cellular proliferation.[14] Survival studies suggest that most gastric adenocarcinomas exhibit abnormal expression of at least one of the *pRb*, *P16*, or *cyclin D_1* genes, raising the possibility that most gastric cancers harbor Rb pathway abnormalities.[13] Univariate and multivariate survival analyses have revealed that reduced expression of Rb is associated with worse OS.[13,14] Furthermore, it has been shown that Rb expression is lower in lymph node metastases than in the corresponding primary tumors. However, P16 and cyclin D_1 overexpression had no prognostic value for gastric cancers in those studies.[13]

Cell Adhesion Molecules

E-cadherin, which is encoded by the *CDH1* gene, is a 120-kDa transmembrane glycoprotein that is responsible for calcium-dependent homotypic intercellular adhesion,[15] cell polarity, and mucosal architecture.[16] Loss of E-cadherin expression has been found in many sporadic cancers; however, germline *CDH1* mutations are found only rarely in most cancers.[10]

Several studies have shown that *CDH1* promoter methylation or polymorphisms lead to the transcriptional down-regulation of the gene.[10] *CDH1* gene mutations have been associated with familial gastric cancers.[16] Moreover, E-cadherin has been implicated in gastric carcinogenesis.[15] Multivariate analyses of E-cadherin expression in cancer patients have revealed that reduced E-cadherin expression is an independent prognostic factor in gastric cancer patients.[3] The soluble form of E-cadherin has been shown to be elevated in the serum of patients with gastric cancer, and patients with a high serum concentration of E-cadherin were more likely to have palliative/conservative treatment than operable cancers.[17] Interestingly, gastric carcinomas with secondary E-cadherin loss during metastasis were found to be associated with a worse outcome than those with E-cadherin expression at both the primary and the metastatic sites.[18a]

Functional cadherin-dependent epithelial cell adhesion requires the formation of complexes between E-cadherin and cytoplasmic proteins known as the catenins (e.g., β-catenin).[15] β-catenin, a 92-kDa protein, plays a multifunctional role in the cell. β-catenin is a component of the cell adhesion complex, and it acts as a coactivator of a transcription factor involved in the Wnt signaling pathway. Dysfunction of the Wnt regulatory pathway may lead to the accumulation of a hypophosphorylated stable form of β-catenin in the cytoplasm, where it translocates to the nucleus and binds to the high mobility group–domain factors Tcf/LEF and stimulates the transcription of target genes such as *c-myc* and cyclin D_1.[15] Zhou et al. found abnormal expression of E-cadherin and β-catenin in 46% and 44% of gastric carcinomas, respectively. Moreover, these alterations occurred more frequently in the diffuse type of gastric carcinoma than in the intestinal type.[18b] In another study, Jung et al.[15] showed that combined β-catenin nuclear accumulation and E-cadherin alteration in gastric carcinoma is associated with poor patient survival. Impairment of one or more components of the E-cadherin/β-catenin complex is associated with poor differentiation, a dysfunction in intercellular adhesion, and the increased invasiveness of carcinomas, as well as tumor progression and metastasis.[16]

CD24

CD24, a small glycosylphosphatidylinositol-anchored cell surface sialoprotein, is a ligand of P-selection, an adhesive molecule on activated endothelial cells and platelets. Expression of CD24 facilitates the P-selection-mediated rolling of the tumor cells on the surface of the endothelium, prompting the dissemination of CD24-expressing cancer cells.[19] Chou et al. found that cytoplasmic CD24 expression in gastric adenocarcinoma correlated with tumors of a higher stage (stages III–IV), serosal invasion, lymphovascular invasion, and a lower 10-year survival rate. Moreover, patients with diffuse-type gastric adenocarcinoma who had cytoplasmic CD24 expression had a significantly lower 10-year survival rate than those without cytoplasmic CD24 expression.[19]

CD44

CD44 is a highly glycosylated cell-surface molecule, and its variants, which are generated by alternative splicing of ten exons, recognize hyaluronate and mediate diverse functions such as cell-cell and cell-matrix adhesion, lymphocyte homing, and metastasis.[20] There is a significant survival advantage in patients with low mRNA levels of CD44 isoforms with the exon variant 6 (CD44v6) compared with patients with high expression of these variants.[20] Interestingly, this survival advantage is observed only in patients with early-stage tumors.[21] Therefore, assessment of CD44v6 mRNA expression in preoperative biopsy specimens may be useful as a preoperative indicator of future distant metastasis.[21,22] Furthermore, the serum concentration of soluble isoforms of CD44v6 before surgical treatment is an indicator of tumor progression and prognosis in patients with diffuse-type gastric carcinoma.[20] CD44 expression is significantly associated with distant metastases at the time of diagnosis. CD44 expression is also associated with tumor recurrence and increased mortality rates among curatively resected patients.

One of the main features of CD44 is that it has been identified as a cancer stem cell (CSC) biomarker (see Chapter 1). CSCs are a unique subpopulation that possesses the capacity to repopulate tumors, drive malignant progression, and mediate chemoresistance.[23–25] A number of factors have been reported to regulate CD44 expression and eventually determine tumor progression and prognosis.[26,27] Y-box binding protein-1 (YB-1), an oncogenic transcription/translation factor, has been found promotes cancer cell growth and drug resistance through its induction of CD44 and CD49f.[27]

Integrin αvβ6

Among the various families of cell adhesion molecules, integrin expression patterns are implicated in cancer progression. It has been shown that αvβ6 is expressed in 36% of gastric carcinomas, and a striking difference was seen in the median survival time between patients with αvβ6-negative and -positive carcinomas, especially in early-stage tumors, suggesting that positive expression of αvβ6 may be a prognostic indicator of poor survival in patients with gastric carcinoma.[28]

Protocadherin

Epigenetic disruption of protocadherin 10 (PCDH10), a gene that encodes a protocadherin, as other cadherins, including E-cadherin (CDH-1), R-cadherin (CDH4), and H-cadherin (CDH13) has been observed in gastric cancer.[24] Yu et al. showed that methylation of the *PCDH10* promoter, which leads to gene silencing, is a frequent event in gastric cancers and their adjacent nontumor tissues. Furthermore, multivariate analysis of PCDH10 changes in gastric cancer revealed that stage I to III gastric cancer patients with *PCDH10* methylation in adjacent nontumor areas have significantly reduced OS. PCDH10 acts as a tumor suppressor by inducing apoptosis, controlling cell growth, and inhibiting cell invasion and metastasis.[29]

Matrix Metalloproteinase and COX-2

A balance between the matrix metalloproteinase (MMP) family and their tissue inhibition factors plays an important role in the degradation of the extracellular matrix, which is one of the initial steps in tumor invasion, angiogenesis, and metastasis.[30] The MMP gene family is composed of at least 16 metalloproteinases, which are produced by tumor cells and/or stromal cells and can degrade the extracellular matrix and basal membrane. In addition to these proteinases, the tissue inhibitors of metalloproteinase (TIMPs) play a role in extracellular matrix degradation.[31] Among the various MMPs expressed in gastric carcinomas, MMP-7 is reported to be selectively expressed by carcinoma cells, especially those of the intestinal type, and its expression correlates with vascular/lymphatic invasion and metastasis.[32] The prognosis of patients with MMP-1–positive tumors has been shown to be worse than that of patients with MMP-1–negative tumors,[3] and enhanced production and activation of pro-MMP-2 correlate with the degree of local tumor invasion and lymphatic permeation.[32] Furthermore, epithelial MMP-2 expression is associated with higher tumor stage, noncurative surgery, and poor survival, but multivariate analysis shows no independent prognostic value for this marker.[30,33]

The concentration of tissue inhibitor of metalloproteinase-1 (TIMP-1) in tumor extracts has been suggested to be a useful prognostic marker for disease-free survival and recurrence and serves as an independent prognostic factor for OS.[33] The finding that a high level of TIMP-1 correlates with better patient prognosis is counterintuitive, given that TIMP-1 inhibits MMPs, which play a major role in tumor cell–induced tissue degradation. However, additional functions of TIMP-1 have been reported, including tissue growth, growth stimulation, and inhibition of apoptosis.[29] Moreover, immunohistochemical staining of gastric carcinoma tissue samples for TIMP-2 shows that tissue from infiltrative poorly differentiated cancers has lower expression of TIMP-2, and tissue samples from gastric cancers with distant metastases show significantly less TIMP-2 expression compared with tissues from nonmetastatic cancers.[33] These studies indicate TIMPs are not monofunctional, but biofunctional or multifunctional, depending on the growth phase and microenvironment of the tumor.

Cyclooxygenase-2

COX-2 is one of the rate-limiting enzymes involved in the synthesis of prostaglandin from arachidonic acid. In humans, COX-2 is overexpressed in noninvasive gastric dysplasia and in gastric cancer tissue. Furthermore, COX-2–derived prostanoids may induce the production of MMPs such as MMP-2.[30] In addition, overexpression of COX-2 is associated with lymph node metastasis, depth of invasion, and poor prognosis.[34] Furthermore, COX-2 has been shown to be an independent prognostic factor in gastric cancer.[30] Thus, selective inhibitors of COX-2, such as celecoxib and other nonsteroidal anti-inflammatory drugs (NSAIDs), could provide additional treatment options for gastric cancer patients.

Cell Growth Factors

Gastric cancer cells express a variety of growth factors and their receptors, which are part of several autocrine and paracrine loops. The type I human epidermal growth factor receptor (HER) family consists of four members: HER-1/ErbB1 (also known as EGFR), HER-2/ErbB2, HER-3/ErbB3, and HER-4/ErbB4. All share a common structure, which is composed of an extracellular ligand binding domain, a transmembrane domain, and an intracytoplasmic tyrosine kinase domain.[35] The binding of different ligands to the receptor's extracellular domain initiates a signal transduction cascade that can influence cell proliferation, apoptosis, differentiation, angiogenesis, and cell adhesion and migration.[3]

The *Her-2/neu* gene located in chromosomal region 17q21 encodes a 185-kDa transmembrane protein with tyrosine kinase activity that acts as an oncogene.[36] Park et al. detected *Her-2/neu* amplification in 3.8% of gastric cancer patients studied and showed by fluorescence in situ hybridization or immunohistochemical staining that patients with tumors with *Her-2/neu* amplification had poor mean survival rates. A gastric cancer with *Her-2/neu* gene amplification is illustrated in Figure 17-2. Moreover, intestinal-type cancers show higher rates of *Her-2/neu* gene amplification than diffuse-type cancers. In addition, *Her-2/neu* amplification is independently related to survival and, thus, HER-2 may be a potential target for new adjuvant therapies involving humanized monoclonal antibodies,[36] which are in fact currently used in management of gastric cancer patients with *Her-2/neu* amplification.

Expression of another HER family member, HER-3, is significantly associated with clinicopathological factors involved in tumor progression, including depth of tumor invasion, lymph node and distant metastasis, and recurrent disease. HER-1 expression is also associated with depth of tumor invasion, lymph node metastasis, and recurrent disease, but not distant metastases.[35] Moreover, in curatively treated patients, EGFR expression has been shown to be correlated with worse survival in both univariate and multivariate analyses.[37] HER-3 overexpression was

FIGURE 17-2 Her-2 *neu* gene amplification in gastric carcinoma. Notice, the *pink dots* (labeled and probed Her-2 *neu* gene) are five times more than the *green dots* (labeled and probed centromeres of chromosome 17).

also associated with worse survival and was an independent prognostic factor in a multivariate analysis.[35]

In a series study of 260 gastric cancer tissue samples, HER-2 expression was an independent prognostic factor, and the intensity of HER-2 staining was correlated with tumor size, serosal invasion, and lymph node metastasis.[38] In a retrospective study of 108 cases, patients with HER-2 overexpression were associated with a poorer 10-year survival rate than those without HER-2 overexpression. Interestingly, HER-2 overexpression and/or amplification are more common in gastroesophageal-junction cancers than in gastric tumors (25% vs. 9.5%, respectively).[38]

Microsatellite Instability

Microsatellite instability (MSI) caused by dysfunction of the DNA mismatch repair system leads to the accumulation of tandem oligonucleotide repeats in the genome. Cancers with MSI can be categorized as MSI-stable (MSS), MSI-High(MSI-H), and MSI-Low(MSI-L). It has been reported that MSI-H cancers have clinicopathologic characteristics and genetic alterations that are distinct from MSI-L and MSS cancers.[39] In gastric cancer, the frequency of MSI varies between 15% and 38%, depending on the number of loci investigated.[40] The subset of sporadic gastric cancers with MSI-H phenotypes shows clinicopathologic and genetic profiles that are distinct from those with MSI-L phenotypes. MSI-H gastric cancers have been reported to be frequently found in an antral location and in older patients and are frequently intestinal type and seropositive for *H. pylori*. In addition, MSI-H gastric cancers have a lower prevalence of lymph node metastasis in some reports.[10,41] Moreover, these tumors more frequently display frameshift mutations of the *TGFβR11, BAX,* and *hMSH3* genes but a lower rate of *P53* mutations.[10]

Univariate analysis of the patients with different microsatellite types showed that patients with tumors of all stages with MSI-H or loss of heterozygosity-low (LOH-L) had favorable survival rate, and those with LOH-high, or LOH-nondetectable had poor survival rate. In sporadic gastric cancers, MSI was closely associated with CpG island hypermethylation (CIMP) of *hMLH1*, leading to loss of the hMLH1 protein. In addition, the concordant methylation of multiple genes (CIMP-H) was associated with better survival but was not an independent predictor of prognosis in patients with resected gastric cancer.[42] However, other studies indicate that MSI status is associated with tumor stage, and the difference in the 5-year survival rates of the MSS and MSI gastric cancers was significant only for patients with stage II tumors.[43] The overall clinicopathological characteristics of gastric cancer with MSI abnormalities are summarized in Table 17-1.

Table 17-1	Clinicopathological characteristics of MSI-H gastric cancer
Anatomic location	Frequently in antrum
H. pylori infection	Frequently
Patient age	More in older patients (>65)
Histological type	More intestinal type
Node metastasis	Infrequent
Genetic changes	Associated with *TGFpR11*, *BAX*, and *hMSH3* gene mutation
Epigenetic changes	Associated with CpG island hypermethylation (CIMP) of *hMLH1*
Overall survival	Favorable

In conclusion, increased evidence has demonstrated that tumor underlying molecular abnormalities have significant impacts on tumor progression and prognosis. In the near future, the tumoral expression of specific molecules, for example, *Her-2/neu* overexpression, DNA MSI, or CSC biomarker CD44, may be proven to be associated either with prognosis or response to therapy that is independent of TNM stage or histology type.

References

1. Zhao ZS, Wang YY, Ye ZY, et al. Prognostic value of tumor-related molecular expression in gastric carcinoma. *Pathol Oncol Res.* 2009;15:589–596.
2. Piessen G, Messager M, Leteurtre E, et al. Signet ring cell histology is an independent predictor of poor prognosis in gastric adenocarcinoma regardless of tumoral clinical presentation. *Ann Surg.* 2009;250(6):878–887.
3. Yasui W, Oue N, Aung PP, et al. Molecular-pathological prognostic factors of gastric cancer: a review. *Gastric Cancer.* 2005;8:86–94.
4. Lee HE, Chae SW, Lee YJ, et al. Prognostic implications of type and density of tumor-infiltrating lymphocytes in gastric cancer. *Br J Cancer.* 2008;99:1704–1711.
5. Truong CD, Feng W, Li W, et al. Characteristics of Epstein-Barr virus-associated gastric cancer: a study of 235 cases at a comprehensive cancer center in U.S.A. *J Exp Clin Cancer Res.* 2009;28:14.
6. Osato T, Imai S. Epstein-Barr virus and gastric carcinoma. *Semin Cancer Biol.* 1996;7(4):175–182.
7. Gamboa-Dominguez A, Seidl S, Reyes-Gutierrez E, et al. Prognostic significance of p21[WAF1/CIP1], P27 [Kip1], p53 and E-cadherin expression in gastric cancer. *J Clin Pathol.* 2007;60:756–761.
8. Lee KH, Lee HE, Cho SJ, et al. Immunohistochemical analysis of cell cycle related molecules in gastric carcinoma: prognostic significance, correlation with clinicopathological parameters, proliferation and apoptosis. *Pathobiology.* 2008;75:364–372.
9. Al-Moundhri MS, Nirmala V, Al-Hadabi I, et al. The prognostic significance of p53, p27 [kip1], p21 [warfl], Her-2/neu, and Ki67 proteins expression in gastric cancer: a clinicopathological and immunohistochemical study of 121 Arab patients. *J Surg Oncol.* 2005;91:243–252.
10. Scartozzi M, Galizia E, Freddari F, et al. Molecular biology of sporadic gastric cancer: prognostic indicators and novel therapeutic approaches. *Cancer Treat Rev.* 2004;30:451–459.
11. Fondevila C, Metges JP, Fuster J, et al. p53 and VEGF expression are independent predictors of tumor recurrence and survival following curative resection of gastric cancer. *Br J Cancer.* 2004;90:206–215.
12. Liu XP, Kawauchi S, Oga A, et al. Combined examination of p27[kip1], p21[wafl/Cip1] and p53 expression allows precise estimation of prognosis in patients with gastric carcinoma. *Histopathology.* 2001;39:603–610.

13. Feakins RM, Nickols CD, Walton SJ. Abnormal expression of pRb, p16, and Cyclin D1 in gastric adenocarcinoma and its lymph node metastases: relationship with pathological features and survival. *Hum Pathol*. 2003;34:1276–1282.

14. Kouraklis G, Katsoulis IE, Theocharis S, et al. Does the expression of Cyclin E, pRb, and P21 correlate with prognosis in gastric adenocarcinoma. *Dig Dis Sci*. 2009;54:1015–1020.

15. Jung IM, Chung JK, Kim YA, et al. Epstein-Barr virus, Beta-Catenin, and E-cadherin in gastric carcinomas. *J Korean Med Sci*. 2007;22:855–861.

16. Sliva EM, Begnami M, Fregnani JH, et al. Cadherin-catenin adhesion system and mucin expression: a comparison between young and older patients with gastric carcinoma. *Gastric Cancer*. 2008;11: 149–159.

17. Chan AOO, Lam SK, Chu KM, et al. Soluble E-cadherin is a valid prognostic marker in gastric carcinoma. *Gut*. 2001;48:808–811.

18a. Kim JH, Kim MA, Lee HS, et al. Comparative analysis of protein expression in primary and metastatic gastric carcinomas. *Hum Pathol*. 2009;40:314–322.

18b. Zhou YN, Xu CP, Han B, et al. Expression of E-cadherin and beta-catenin in gastric carcinoma and its correlation with the clinicopathological features and patient survival. *World J Gastroenterol*. 2002; 8:987–993.

19. Chou YY, Jeng YM, Lee TT, et al. Cytoplasmic CD24 expression is a novel prognostic factor in diffuse-type gastric adenocarcinoma. *Ann Surg Oncol*. 2007;14(10):2748–2758.

20. Saito H, Tsujitani S, Katano K, et al. Serum concentration of CD44 variant 6 and its relation to prognosis in patients with gastric carcinoma. *Cancer*. 1998;83:1094–1101.

21. Yamamichi K, Uehara Y, Kitamura N, et al. Increased expression of CD44v6 mRNA significantly correlates with distant metastasis and poor prognosis in gastric cancer. *Int J Cancer*. 1998;79:256–262.

22. Mayer B, Jauch KW, Gunthert U, et al. De-novo expression of CD44 and survival in gastric cancer. *Lancet*. 1993;342:1019–1022.

23. Miyoshi N, Ishii H, Nagai K, et al. Defined factors induce reprogramming of gastrointestinal cancer cells. *Proc Natl Acad Sci U S A*. 2010;107(1):40–45.

24. Okumura T, Wang SS, Takaishi S, et al. Identification of a bone marrow-derived mesenchymal progenitor cell subset that can contribute to the gastric epithelium. *Lab Invest*. 2009;89(12):1410–1422.

25. Barker N, Huch M, Kujala P, et al. Lgr5(+ve) stem cells drive self-renewal in the stomach and build long-lived gastric units in vitro. *Cell Stem Cell*. 2010;6(1):25–36.

26. Ishimoto T, Oshima H, Oshima M, et al. CD44(+) slow-cycling tumor cell expansion is triggered by cooperative actions of Wnt and prostaglandin E(2) in gastric tumorigenesis. *Cancer Sci*. 2010;101(3): 673–678.

27. To K, Fotovati A, Reipas KM, et al. Y-box binding protein-1 induces the expression of CD44 and CD49f leading to enhanced self-renewal, mammosphere growth, and drug resistance. *Cancer Res*. 2010;70:2840–2851.

28. Zhang ZY, Xu KS, Wang JS, et al. Integrin $\alpha v \beta 6$ acts as a prognostic indicator in gastric carcinoma. *Clin Oncol*. 2008;20:61–66.

29. Yu J, Cheng YY, Tao Q, et al. Methylation of protocadherin 10, a novel tumor suppressor, is associated with poor prognosis in patients with gastric cancer. *Gastroenterology*. 2009;136:640–651.

30. Mrena J, Wiksten JP, Nordling S, et al. MMP-2 but not MMP-9 associated with COX-2 and survival in gastric cancer. *J Clin Pathol*. 2006;59:618–623.

31. Yoshikawa T, Tsuburaya A, Kobayashi O, et al. Protein levels of tissue inhibitor of metalloproteinase in tumor extracts as a marker for prognosis and recurrence in patients with gastric cancer. *Gastric Cancer*. 2006;9:106–113.

32. Yamashita K, Azumano I, Mai M, et al. Expression and tissue localization of matrix metalloproteinase 7 (Matrilysin) in human gastric carcinomas: implications for vessel invasion and metastasis. *Int J Cancer*. 1998;79:187–194.

33. Alakus H, Grass G, Hennecken JK, et al. Clinicopathological significance of MMP-2 and its specific inhibitor TIMP-2 in gastric cancer. *Histol Histopathol*. 2008;23:917–923.

34. Li M, Liu W, Zhu YF, et al. Correlation of COX-2 and K-ras expression to clinical outcome in gastric cancer. *Acta Oncologica*. 2006;45:1115–1119.

35. Hayashi M, Inokuchi M, Takagi Y, et al. High expression of HER3 is associated with a decreased survival in gastric cancer. *Clin Cancer Res*. 2008;14(23):7843–7849.

36. Park D, Yun JW, Park JH, et al. HER-2/neu amplification is an independent prognostic factor in gastric cancer. *Dig Dis Sci*. 2006;51:1371–1379.

37. Lieto E, Ferraraccio F, Orditura M, et al. Expression of Vascular endothelial growth factor (VEGF) and epidermal growth factor receptor (EGFR) is an independent prognostic indicator of worse outcome in gastric cancer patients. *Ann Surg Oncol.* 2008;15(1):69–79.
38. Gravalos C, Jimeno A. HER2 in gastric cancer: a new prognostic factor and a novel therapeutic target. *Ann Oncol.* 2008;19:1523–1529.
39. Seo HM, Chang YS, Joo SH, et al. Clinicopathologic characteristic and outcomes of gastric cancers with the MSI-H phenotype. *J Surg Oncol.* 2009;99:143–147.
40. Wirtz HC, Muller W, Nogochi T, et al. Prognostic value and clinicopathological profile of microsatellite instability in gastric cancer. *Clin Cancer Res.* 1998;4:1749–1754.
41. An C, Choi IS, Yao JC, et al. Prognostic significance of CpG island methylator phenotype and microsatellite instability in gastric carcinoma. *Clin Cancer Res.* 2005;11:656–663.
42. Choi SW, Choi JR, Chung YJ, et al. Prognostic implications of microsatellite genotypes in gastric carcinoma. *Int J Cancer.* 2000;89:378–383.
43. Beghelli S, Manzoni G, Barbi S, et al. Microsatellite instability in gastric cancer is associated with better prognosis in only stage II cancers. *Surgery.* 2006;139:347–356.

Staging

TNM and Concerns in the Staging of Gastric Cancer

18

▶ Dongfeng Tan

INTRODUCTION

Properly staging cancer allows the clinician to choose the appropriate treatment modalities, reliably evaluate and predict outcomes of disease management, and uniformly document cancer cases worldwide. Although there are several classification systems for gastric cancer, the *Cancer Staging Manual* developed by the American Joint Committee on Cancer (AJCC) with support from International Union for Cancer Control (UICC), the American Cancer Society, American College of Surgeons, American Society of Clinical Oncology, and International Union against Cancer is the generally accepted classification system.[1–3] The cancer-staging criteria have been continually refined since 1959, with the combined efforts of medical community, and multiple medical and oncology organizations. The latest edition (7th edition) of the *AJCC Cancer Staging Manual* was published in early 2010.[1] In the new edition, the AJCC and UICC used large datasets and emerging evidence to support changes in the cancer-staging criteria in general, and they used datasets from Asia, Europe, and the United States for the gastric cancer-staging systems in particular.

Because gastric cancer is a heterogeneous disease, attempts have been made to subclassify gastric cancers within a given tumor stage.[4–10] A recent study of 1,056 patients with stage IV gastric cancer (diagnosed on the basis of the 6th edition of the *Cancer Staging Manual*) divided patients into three groups on the basis of the tumor, node, metastasis (TNM) stage of their disease: group 1 (T4 N1-3 M0), group 2 (T1-3 N3 M0), and group 3 (T[any] N[any] M1).[11] The clinicopathological characteristics, recurrence patterns, and survival rates of the three groups were compared. After R0 resection, locoregional recurrence (40.9%) followed by peritoneal recurrence (27.3%) was most common in group 1, whereas distant (30.2%) and peritoneal (26.7%) recurrence were most common in group 2. The 5-year survival rates in groups 1, 2, and 3 were 18.3%, 27.1%, and 9.3%, respectively ($p < 0.001$). Multivariate analysis showed that each subgroup had different clinical outcomes, including histological behavior, recurrence pattern, survival rates, and prognostic factors. Therefore, subclassification of stage IV gastric cancer into subgroups IVA (T1-3 N3 M0), IVB (T4 N1-3 M0), and IVM (T[any] N[any] M1) may provide a more accurate prediction of prognosis and selection of appropriate therapeutic options.[11] This study was among the data supporting the reclassification of the advanced gastric cancer, regrouping the IVA (T1-3 N3 M0) and IVB (T4 N1-3 M0) subgroups into stages IIB and III, respectively, leaving only the T[any] N[any] M1 subgroup in stage IV.

Since the past couple of decades, there are more gastric cancers in the proximal stomach now than there used to be.[12] Tumors of the esophagogastric junction (EGJ) may be difficult to stage as either a gastric or an esophageal primary tumor, especially as there is an increased incidence of adenocarcinoma in the esophagus. The arbitrary 10-cm segment encompassing the distal 5 cm of the esophagus and proximal 5 cm of the stomach (cardia), with the EGJ in the middle, is an area of contention. Cancers arising in this segment have been variably staged as esophageal or gastric tumors, depending on the discretion of the treating physician.[13] In the new edition of the *AJCC Staging Manual*, tumors arising at the EGJ, or arising within the proximal 5 cm of the stomach (cardia) that extends into the EGJ or esophagus, are staged using the TNM system for adenocarcinoma of the esophagus. All other cancers with a midpoint in the stomach lying >5 cm distal to the EGJ, or those within 5 cm of the EGJ but not extending into the EGJ or esophagus, are staged using the gastric cancer-staging system.

DEFINITIONS OF TNM

TNM staging describes three major anatomic characteristics of cancer: (a) the location and extension of the primary tumor, (b) the presence or absence of lymph node involvement, and (c) the presence or absence of distant tumor metastasis. These features can be evaluated by physical examination, imaging studies, and histopathologic evaluation. All cancers, though, should be confirmed histologically.

Clinical Staging and Pathologic Staging

Clinical staging, designated cTNM, is relied on evidence of the extent of disease before definitive treatment is started. Clinical staging includes physical examination, imaging, endoscopy, biopsy, and laboratory findings, which all establish the baseline stage. Imaging studies and endoscopy are most valuable tools in assessing clinical staging of gastric cancers (see Chapters 6 and 19).[14-17]

Before pathologic staging, efforts should be made to differentiate primary gastric cancer from metastatic disease, which is not an uncommon event (see Chapters 5 and 8). After the primary gastric cancer is established, gastric cancer should be classified. Majority of gastric cancer is adenocarcinoma. The histological subtypes of gastric cancer are listed in Table 18-1 (also refer to Chapter 5 for details).

Pathologically, the extent of the tumor needs to be carefully assessed. Pathologic staging depends on data acquired clinically together with findings on subsequent gross and microscopic examination of the surgically resected specimen.

Of note, the TNM-staging recommendations apply only to carcinomas. Lymphomas, sarcomas, and carcinoid tumors (well-differentiated neuroendocrine tumors) are excluded. Mixed glandular/neuroendocrine carcinomas should be staged using the gastric carcinoma–staging system for well-differentiated gastrointestinal neuroendocrine tumors.

Table 18-1	The histological subtypes of gastric cancer
Adenocarcinoma (>90%)	
Adenosquamous carcinoma	
Mucinous adenocarcinoma	
Papillary adenocarcinoma	
Signet ring cell carcinoma	
Squamous cell carcinoma	
Tubular adenocarcinoma	
Undifferentiated carcinoma	

Table 18-2	Primary tumor (T) of gastric cancer
TX	Primary tumor cannot be assessed
T0	No evidence of primary tumor
Tis	Carcinoma in situ: intraepithelial tumor without invasion of the lamina propria
T1	Tumor invades lamina propria, muscularis mucosae, or submucosa
	T1a Tumor invades lamina propria or muscularis mucosae
	T1b Tumor invades submucosa
T2	Tumor invades muscularis propria
T3	Tumor penetrates subserosal connective tissue without invasion of visceral peritoneum or adjacent structures[a]
T4	Tumor invades serosa (visceral peritoneum) or adjacent structures[a]
	T4a Tumor invades serosa (visceral peritoneum)
	T4b Tumor invades adjacent structures

[a]The adjacent structures of the stomach include the spleen, transverse colon, liver, diaphragm, pancreas, abdominal wall, adrenal gland, kidney, small intestine, and retroperitoneum.

Designation of Primary Gastric Cancer Status

Staging of primary gastric adenocarcinoma is dependent on the extension and depth of penetration of the primary tumor. Histologically, the wall of the stomach has five layers: mucosa, submucosa, muscular propria, subserosal connective tissue, and serosal surface (see Chapter 1).

One of the major changes to the T designation for gastric cancer in the 7th edition of the *AJCC Cancer Staging Manual* is that the T categories have been modified to correspond to the T categories for cancers of the esophagus and small and large intestines. Specifically, T1 lesions have been subdivided into T1a and T1b, which are defined as tumor invades muscularis mucosae and tumor invades submucosa, respectively; T2 is defined as a tumor that invades the muscularis propria; T3 is defined as a tumor that invades the subserosal connective tissue (formerly T2b in *AJCC Cancer Staging Manual*, 6th edition); and T4 is defined as a tumor that invades the serosa (visceral peritoneum, formerly T3 in *AJCC Cancer Staging Manual*, 6th edition) or adjacent structures.[18] The T (primary tumor) designation of gastric cancer is listed in Table 18-2.

Designation of Regional Lymph Node Status

The regional lymph nodes of the stomach are roughly divided into two major groups: (a) the perigastric nodes, which include nodes in the greater curvature of the stomach and nodes in the lesser curvature of the stomach and (b) the local nodes in the pancreatic and splenic area (see Chapter 6).

Adequate dissection of these regional nodal areas is important to ensure the appropriate pN designations and final staging. For pathologic assessment, the regional lymph nodes are removed and examined histologically to evaluate the total number of lymph nodes as well as the number that contain metastatic tumors. N categories have been modified in the new *AJCC Staging Manual*, with N1 = 1–2 positive regional lymph nodes, N2 = 3–6 positive regional lymph nodes (N1 in the 6th edition of *AJCC Staging Manual*), and N3 = 7 or more positive regional lymph nodes. In addition, metastatic nodules in the fat adjacent to a gastric carcinoma, without evidence of residual lymph node tissue, are considered regional lymph node metastases. Although it has been suggested that pathologists assess at least 16 regional lymph nodes, a pN determination may be assigned on the basis of the actual number of nodes evaluated microscopically. The N (regional lymph node) designation of gastric cancer is listed in Table 18-3.

Table 18-3	Regional lymph nodes (N) of gastric cancer
NX	Regional lymph node(s) cannot be assessed
N0	No regional lymph node metastasis[a]
N1	Metastasis in 1–2 regional lymph nodes
N2	Metastasis in 3–6 regional lymph nodes
N3	Metastasis in 7 or more regional lymph nodes
	N3a Metastasis in 7–15 regional lymph nodes
	N3b Metastasis in 16 or more regional lymph nodes

[a]*Note*: A designation of pN0 should be used if all examined lymph nodes are negative, regardless of the total number removed and examined.

Designation of Distant Metastasis Status

Two designations of metastatic status are included in the 7th edition of the *AJCC Cancer Staging Manual*, namely, M0: No distant metastasis, and M1: Distant metastasis. Of note, no Mx designation was mentioned in the 7th edition of the *AJCC Cancer Staging Manual*.

Distant metastasis means that the tumor has disseminated to distant lymph nodes or a distant organ system. The distant lymph nodes of gastric cancer include retropancreatic, hepatoduodenal, para-aortic, portal, retroperitoneal, and mesenteric. Involvement of these intra-abdominal lymph nodes is classified as distant metastasis. Other metastatic sites include distant organs (liver, lungs, and central nervous system) and peritoneal surfaces (tumor implants). Positive peritoneal cytology is now classified as metastatic disease (M1). A summary of designation of distal metastatic tumor is listed in Table 18-4.

Table 18-4	Designation of distal metastatic tumor (M1)
Metastatic carcinoma in distant lymph nodes	
Hepatoduodenal	
Mesenteric	
Para-aortic	
Portal	
Retropancreatic	
Retroperitoneal	
Metastatic carcinoma in distant organs	
Liver	
Lungs	
CNS	
Other less common organ sites	
Metastatic carcinoma in peritoneal surfaces	
Metastatic carcinoma in peritoneal cytology	

DESIGNATION OF ANATOMIC STAGE

The final grouping (staging) of gastric cancer is dependent on the appropriate designations of T, N, and M. The anatomic stage, based on the current *AJCC Cancer Staging Manual*, is listed in Table 18-5. Of note, if there is uncertainty concerning the appropriate T, N, or M designation, the lower (less advanced) category should be assigned, in accordance with the general rules of staging.

CONCERNS IN THE STAGING OF GASTRIC CANCER

Gastric Cancer or Esophageal Cancer?

First of all, it is important to determine a tumor of the upper gastrointestinal tract as gastric cancer or esophageal cancer. Though attempts have been made to uniformly report tumor location in the upper gastrointestinal tract, cancers arising in the neighborhood of the EGJ have been variably classified as either esophageal or gastric cancers. Tumors within the proximal 5 cm of the stomach that extend into the EGJ are staged using the TNM system for esophageal cancer in the 7th edition of the *AJCC Cancer Staging Manual*. This designation seems arbitrary, as there is no strong evidence, for example, that a 6-cm tumor arising within the proximal 5 cm of the stomach

Table 18-5	Anatomic stage of gastric cancer		
Stage 0	Tis	N0	M0
Stage IA	T1	N0	M0
Stage IB	T2	N0	M0
	T1	N1	M0
Stage IIA	T3	N0	M0
	T2	N1	M0
	T1	N2	M0
Stage IIB	T4a	N0	M0
	T3	N1	M0
	T2	N2	M0
	T1	N3	M0
Stage IIIA	T4a	N1	M0
	T3	N2	M0
	T2	N3	M0
Stage IIIB	T4b	N0	M0
	T4b	N1	M0
	T4a	N2	M0
	T3	N3	M0
Stage IIIC	T4b	N2	M0
	T4b	N3	M0
	T4a	N3	M0
Stage IV	Any T	Any N	M1

Source: Used with permission from the *AJCC Cancer Staging Manual,* 7th edition.

that extends and passes 1 cm from the EGJ is an esophageal cancer rather than gastric cancer. In this regard, the prior designation using the EGJ as an anatomic border to determine primary tumor location seems logical.[19]

Does the Size of Gastric Cancer Matter?

In some solid cancers, such as breast, lung, and pancreatic cancers, tumor size is included in the classification of disease stage.[20,21] However, tumor size is not considered in the staging of gastric cancer, since its clinical significance in gastric cancer remains elusive. Nevertheless, a recent study of a large cohort of gastric cancer patients ($n = 1,473$) found that the size of a gastric tumor has prognostic significance.[22] The authors found that the threshold for the size of tumor that affects patient survival was 8 cm, because the small-size (SSG = tumor size < 8 cm) and large-size groups (LSG = tumor size ≥ 8 cm) had different clinical outcomes. The prognosis of LSG patients was significantly worse than that of SSG patients. Multivariate analysis showed that tumor size was an independent prognostic factor, along with depth of invasion, lymph node metastasis, and lymphatic invasion. Furthermore, the disease recurrence patterns differed between the two groups. Peritoneal recurrence was observed in the LSG patients more frequently than in the SSG patients ($p < 0.001$), whereas hematogenous recurrence was observed in the SSG patients more frequently than in the LSG patients ($p < 0.05$). The survival rates of LSG patients with stages II, IIIa, and IIIb disease were almost the same as those for SSG patients with stages IIIa, IIIb, and IV disease, respectively. These data indicate that tumor size plays a role in determining the overall clinical outcome of gastric cancer and, therefore, should be considered when the progress and stage of gastric cancer are assessed.[22]

Surgical Procedures Affect Lymph Node Assignment and Staging

One of the challenges to TNM staging is assessing the status of lymph nodes. Staging lymph node status depends on the type of surgery performed, type of healthcare facilities where the surgery and pathology analysis were performed, and preoperative treatment, among other things. Different surgical procedures of gastric cancer produce different number and type of lymph nodes. In Japan, lymph nodes of the stomach are classified into four compartments.[23] Compartment I includes perigastric lymph nodes, while Compartment II consists of left gastric artery, common hepatic artery, and splenic artery lymph nodes. Compartment III includes lymph nodes along the hepatoduodenal ligament, posterior to the head of the pancreas, and at the root of the mesentery, whereas Compartment IV consists of those along the middle colic vessels and para-aortic region. Radical gastrectomy and dissection of lymph nodes in Compartment I-II and beyond are widely used in Asia, particularly in Japan and Korea, yielding more lymph nodes than procedures done in the West countries, including the United States, where the procedures are more conservative.[24,25] Studies have also shown that gastrectomies performed in major teaching medical centers yield more lymph nodes than those done in small hospitals.[26]

Imaging Studies Affect Clinical TNM Staging

Imaging studies predict different clinical staging values.[27,28] One recent study compared the performance of helical computed tomography (CT) and endoscopic ultrasonography (US) for the preoperative staging of gastric cancer.[29] The report showed that helical CT focused on the stomach provides valuable results regarding T and N staging in patients with gastric cancer. Fifty-one consecutive patients with a primary malignant gastric tumor (stage T2-4) were preoperatively evaluated with both imaging methods, and each tumor was staged using both modalities. The results of CT and endoscopic US were compared with the pathologic staging of tumor. In comparison with the histological results, CT resulted in the correct T staging in 39 patients (76%) and the correct N staging in 35 patients (70%). The endoscopic US resulted in the correct T staging in 44 patients (86%) and the correct N staging in 45 patients (90%). There was no significant difference between the accuracy of the imaging methods for T staging ($p = 0.55$) or N staging ($p > 0.99$). Because it is challenging to detect stomach[28] wall layers with CT and endoscopic US, these methods did not differentiate between the T2 and T3 lesions very well.

Preoperative Treatment Affects TNM Staging

Preoperative neoadjuvant chemotherapy has been frequently applied to patients for possible subsequent surgical resection.[30,31] Preoperative chemoradiation for localized gastric cancer can modify the baseline stage (defined by imaging studies and laparoscopy). Among clinical TNM staging, staging of nodal (N) disease is probably most challenging, even with the current advances in imaging technology. The shortcoming of N staging using imaging studies is its inability to detect microscopic metastases. Even newer technology such as PET-CT is limited by poor resolution.[32,33] In one recent study, patients first received induction chemotherapy for up to 2 months followed by chemoradiation (45 Gy) and surgery.[34] The correlation between overall survival and pretreatment and posttreatment parameters, including surgical pathology stage, was assessed. Sixty-nine patients had surgery. Nineteen patients (26%) had a pathologic complete response and fifty-five (81%) had a curative (R0) resection. None of the pretreatment parameters correlated with overall survival; however, analysis of the data using a multivariate Cox model showed that the pathologic stage and R0 resection were independent prognostic factors for overall survival. Therefore, when a preoperative chemoradiation strategy was employed for gastric cancer, the surgical pathology stage, a reflection of the cancer's biologic heterogeneity, was a better predictor of overall survival than the baseline clinical stage.

Similarly, preoperative treatment, chemoradiation in particular, influences the *pathological* assessment of lymph nodes in daily practice. On the one hand, lymph nodes get smaller or disappear owing to the treatment effect. On the other hand, treatment also makes the evaluation of lymph nodes more difficult. Oftentimes, additional evaluations, including more level examination of histology slides and immunohistochemical staining, are needed to determine whether metastatic disease is present in the lymph nodes (Figs. 18-1 and 18-2). Furthermore, the designation and significance of rare single atypical cells (cytokeratin positive cells) in the lymph nodes of gastric cancer patients are not clear.

Role of Molecular Prognostic Factors

TNM is important for predicting the outcome of gastric cancer. Increased depth of tumor invasion into the gastric wall (T) correlates with reduced survival, and lymph node metastasis is one of the most powerful prognostic factors. However, patients (age-adjusted) with same TNM frequently have different clinical outcome, indicating that underlying tumor biology play a role. With better understanding of cancer biology, molecular stratification and molecular staging of gastric cancer hold a great promise (see Chapters 13 and 17).[35–38]

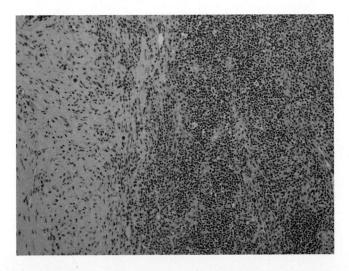

FIGURE 18-1 H&E slide shows rare degenerative cells in one lymph node with treatment effect.

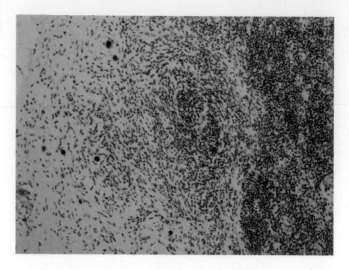

FIGURE 18-2 Cytokeratin immunostain confirms that the epithelial nature of the rare metastatic cells.

Last but not least, it is not clear why the designation of Mx (distant metastasis cannot be assessed) is omitted in the new edition of the *AJCC Cancer Staging Manual*, though the designation of Nx—regional lymph node(s) cannot be assessed—still remains unchanged.

In conclusion, though no classification and staging system for gastric cancer is perfect, the new edition of the *AJCC Cancer Staging Manual* provides a collection of standardized data to support clinical care and future evaluation and refinement of gastric cancer staging. In addition, in the near future, the discovery of new biomarkers will make it necessary to include these parameters in the staging of gastric cancer and will likely require the development of novel strategies beyond the current staging and grouping scheme, which is mainly based on the anatomical aspects of the tumor.

References

1. Edge SB. *AJCC cancer staging manual.* 7 ed. New York, NY: Springer-Verlag; 2010.
2. Hamilton SR, Aaltonen LA, eds. *World Health Organization classification of tumors. Pathology and genetics of tumor of the digestive system.* Lyon: IARC; 2000.
3. Schlemper RJ, Riddell RH, Kato Y, et al. The Vienna classification of gastrointestinal epithelial neoplasia. *Gut.* 2000;47(2):251–255.
4. Fotia G, Marrelli D, De Stefano A, et al. Factors influencing outcome in gastric cancer involving muscularis and subserosal layer. *Eur J Surg Oncol.* 2004;30:930–934.
5. Sasako M, Sano T, Yamamoto S, et al. D2 lymphadenectomy alone or with para-aortic nodal dissection for gastric cancer. *N Eng J Med.* 2008;359:453–462.
6. Kooby DA, Suriawinata A, Klimstra DS, et al. Biologic predictors of survival in node-negative gastric cancer. *Ann Surg.* 2003;237:828–835.
7. Sarela AI, Turnbull AD, Coit DG, et al. Accurate lymph node staging is of greater prognostic importance than subclassification of the T2 category for gastric adenocarcinoma. *Ann Surg Oncol.* 2003;10: 783–791.
8. Komatsu S, Ichikawa D, Kurioka H, et al. Prognostic and clinical evaluation of patients with T2 gastric cancer. *Hepatogastroenterology.* 2005;52:965–968.
9. Wu CW, Hsiung CA, Lo SS, et al. Stage migration influences on stage-specific survival comparison between D1 and D3 gastric cancer surgeries. *Eur J Surg Oncol.* 2005;31:153–157.
10. Shen JY, Kim S, Cheong JH, et al. The impact of total retrieved lymph nodes on staging and survival of patients with pT3 gastric cancer. *Cancer.* 2007;110:745–751.

11. An JY, Ha TK, Noh JH, et al. Proposal to subclassify stage IV gastric cancer into IVA, IVB, and IVM. *Arch Surg.* 2009;144(1):38–45.

12. Dicken BJ, Bigam DL, Cass C, et al. Gastric adenocarcinoma: review and considerations for future directions. *Ann Surg.* 2005;241:27–39.

13. Abbas SM, Booth MW. Correlation between the current TNM staging and long-term survival after curative D1 lymphadenectomy for stomach cancer. *Langenbecks Arch Surg.* 2005;390:294–299.

14. Horton KM, Fishman EK. Current role of CT in imaging of the stomach. *Radiographics.* 2003;23:75–87.

15. Takao M, Fukuda T, Iwanaga S, et al. Gastric cancer: evaluation of triphasic spiral CT and radiologic-pathologic correlation. *J Comput Assist Tomogr.* 1998;22:288–294.

16. Chen CY, Hsu JS, Wu DC, et al. Gastric cancer: preoperative local staging with 3D multi-detector row CT—correlation with surgical and histopathologic results. *Radiology.* 2007;242:472–482.

17. Sohn KM, Lee JM, Lee SY, et al. Comparing MR imaging and CT in the staging of gastric carcinoma. *Am J Roentgenol.* 2000;174:1551–1557.

18. Green FL. *AJCC cancer staging manual.* 6 ed. New York, NY: Springer-Velrag; 2002.

19. Talamonti MS, Kim SP, Yao KA, et al. Surgical outcomes of patients with gastric carcinoma: importance of primary tumor location and microvessel invasion. *Surgery.* 2003;134:720–727.

20. Ball DL, Fisher R, Burmeister B, et al. Stage is not a reliable indicator of tumor volume in non-small cell lung cancer: a preliminary analysis of the Trans-Tasman Radiation Oncology Group 99-05 database. *J Thorac Oncol.* 2006;7:667–672.

21. Iqbal N, Lovegrove RE, Tilney HS, et al. A comparison of pancreaticoduodenectomy with extended pancreaticoduodenectomy: a meta-analysis of 1909 patients. *Eur J Surg Oncol.* 2009;35(1):79–86.

22. Saito H, Osaki T, Murakami D, et al. Macroscopic tumor size as a simple prognostic indicator in patients with gastric cancer. *Am J Surg.* 2006;192(3):296–300.

23. Lim JS, Yun MJ, Kim MJ, et al. CT and PET in stomach cancer: preoperative staging and monitoring of response to therapy. *Radiographics.* 2006;26:143–156.

24. Bonenkamp JJ, Hermans J, Sasako M, et al. Extended lymph-node dissection for gastric cancer. *N Engl J Med.* 1999;340:908–914.

25. Cuschieri A, Weeden S, Fielding J, et al. Patient survival after D1 and D2 resections for gastric cancer: long-term results of the MRC randomized surgical trial. Surgical Co-operative Group. *Br J Cancer.* 1999;79:1522–1530.

26. Baxter NN, Tuttle TM. Inadequacy of lymph node staging in gastric cancer patients: a population-based study. *Ann Surg Oncol.* 2005;12:981–987.

27. Iyer R, Dubrow R. Imaging upper gastrointestinal malignancy. *Semin Roentgenol.* 2006;41:105–112.

28. Hargunani R, Maclachlan J, Kaniyur S, et al. Cross-sectional imaging of gastric neoplasia. *Clin Radiol.* 2009;64:420–429.

29. Habermann CR, Weiss F, Riecken R, et al. Preoperative staging of gastric adenocarcinoma: comparison of helical CT and endoscopic US. *Radiology.* 2004;230(2):465–471.

30. Kinoshita T, Sasako M, Sano T, et al. Phase II trial of S-1 for neoadjuvant chemotherapy against scirrhous gastric cancer (JCOG 0002). *Gastric Cancer.* 2009;12(1):37–42.

31. Mezhir JJ, Tang LH, Coit DG. Neoadjuvant therapy of locally advanced gastric cancer. *J Surg Oncol.* 2010;101(4):305–314.

32. Mawlawi O, Podoloff DA, Kohlmyer S, et al. Performance characteristics of a newly developed PET/CT scanner using NEMA standards in 2D and 3D modes. *J Nucl Med.* 2004;45:1734–1742.

33. Monig SP, Zirbes TK, Schroder W, et al. Staging of gastric cancer: correlation of lymph node size and metastatic infiltration. *Am J Roentgenol.* 1999;173:365–367.

34. Rohatgi PR, Mansfield PF, Crane CH, et al. Surgical pathology stage by American Joint Commission on Cancer criteria predicts patient survival after preoperative chemoradiation for localized gastric carcinoma. *Cancer.* 2006;107(7):1475–1482.

35. Ren T, Jiang B, Xing X, et al. Prognostic significance of phosphatase of regenerating liver-3 expression in ovarian cancer. *Pathol Oncol Res.* 2009;15:555–560.

36. Xing X, Peng L, Qu L, et al. Prognostic value of PRL-3 overexpression in early stages of colonic cancer. *Histopathology.* 2009;54:309–318.

37. Okayama H, Kumamoto K, Saitou K, et al. CD44v6, MMP-7 and nuclear Cdx2 are significant biomarkers for prediction of lymph node metastasis in primary gastric cancer. *Oncol Rep.* 2009;22:745–755.

38. Lee J, Kang WK, Park JO, et al. Expression of activated signal transducer and activator of transcription 3 predicts poor clinical outcome in gastric adenocarcinoma. *APMIS.* 2009;117:598–606.

19

New Staging System for Gastric Cancer

▶ Madhavi Patnana

▶ Raghunandan Vikram

INTRODUCTION

Various imaging techniques, including double-contrast upper gastrointestinal barium examinations, multidetector computed tomography (MDCT), magnetic resonance imaging (MRI), positron emission tomography-computed tomography (PET-CT), and endoscopic ultrasound (EUS), can be used in the diagnosis and staging of gastric cancer.

In the past decade, upper gastrointestinal endoscopy had almost entirely replaced double-contrast barium studies for diagnosis of gastric cancer, but double-contrast barium studies may still have a role in the diagnosis of diffuse infiltrative gastric cancer, in which the endoscopic view may be deceiving. Imaging of gastric cancer is currently used predominantly to detect nodal involvement and distant metastases. In most institutions, the T (tumor) staging of gastric cancer is performed by endoscopic ultrasound. However, recent advances in MDCT and gradient echo MRI have resulted in promising new developments, particularly in T staging of gastric cancer.

In this chapter, we discuss the different imaging modalities used in gastric cancer evaluation—their strengths and weaknesses, and the role of each in preoperative staging, treatment monitoring, and surveillance of gastric cancer.

RELEVANT ISSUES IN STAGING AND IMAGING OF GASTRIC CANCER

Anatomy

It is important to understand the anatomy of the stomach (in terms of vascular supply, lymphatic drainage, and ligaments) and to be able to recognize these details on cross-sectional imaging, as they constitute important potential pathways of direct spread of gastric cancer.

The primitive foregut from which the stomach develops is connected to the dorsal and ventral abdominal walls via the dorsal and ventral mesogastrium in the embryo.[1,2] During the stomach's development, the greater curvature and the dorsal mesogastrium grow at a relatively accelerated pace compared with the lesser curvature. This growth and a 180-degree rotation of the bowel along its axis are responsible for the formation of various peritoneal reflections and for the shape of the adult stomach. Embryology of the stomach is described in more detail in Chapter 1. The gastrohepatic and hepatoduodenal ligaments (lesser omentum) are formed from the ventral mesogastrium. The gastrosplenic and splenorenal ligaments and the greater omentum are derived from the dorsal mesogastrium (Table 19-1 and Fig. 19-1).[1,2]

Since the stomach develops from the primitive foregut, the blood supply to the stomach is derived predominantly from the branches of the celiac trunk.[3] The arterial supply of the stomach is best visualized on dual-phase computed tomography (CT) imaging of the stomach and consists of the left gastric, right gastric, right gastroepiploic, and left gastroepiploic and short gastric

Table 19-1	Peritoneal ligaments[1,2]	
Ligament	**Relation to Organs**	**Vascular Landmarks**
Gastrohepatic	Lesser curvature of the stomach to the liver	Left and right gastric arteries
Hepatoduodenal	From the duodenum to the hepatic fissure	Proper hepatic artery, portal vein
Gastrocolic	Greater curvature of the stomach to the transverse colon	Left and right gastroepiploic arteries and vein
Gastrosplenic	From the left side, greater curvature of the stomach to the splenic hilum	Left gastroepiploic vessels

Sources: Meyers MA. *Dynamic radiology of the abdomen.* 5 ed. New York, NY: Springer-Velrag; 2000; Vikram R, Balachandran A, Bhosale PR, et al. Pancreas: peritoneal reflections, ligamentous connections, and pathways of disease spread. *Radiographics.* 2009;29:e34.

branches. Recognizing the blood vessels enables the identification of the peritoneal reflections and ligamentous attachments to the stomach.[2] The left gastric artery is a branch of the celiac axis and travels along the gastrohepatic ligament or lesser omentum supplying the lesser curvature of the stomach.[3] The right gastric artery arises from the common hepatic artery and also travels along the gastrohepatic ligament along the distal lesser curvature of the stomach to anastomose

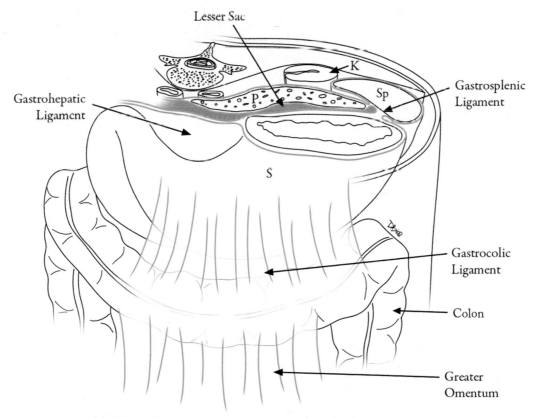

FIGURE 19-1 Gastric Peritoneal Ligaments. The gastrosplenic and splenorenal ligaments and the greater omentum are derived from the dorsal mesogastrium. The gastrohepatic ligament (lesser omentum) and hepatoduodenal ligament (not shown in the diagram) evolve from the ventral mesogastrium. These anatomic locations are important to know for paths of gastric carcinoma spread.

FIGURE 19-2 Axial CT image of the abdomen after the administration of oral and intravenous contrast in a patient with metastatic gastric cancer. Nodal metastasis to the left gastric nodal station is seen (*large arrow*) along with infiltrative tumor involving the lesser curvature of the stomach with extension into the gastrohepatic ligament (*small arrow*). Incidental note is made of old oral barium from a prior leak in the fundus of the stomach (*arrowhead*). Numerous hepatic metastases are also seen.

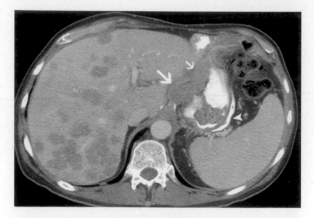

FIGURE 19-3 Axial CT image of the abdomen after the administration of oral and intravenous contrast in a patient with metastatic gastric cancer. Nodal metastasis is seen posterior to the head of the pancreas, compartment III (*small arrowhead*). Multiple enlarged lymph nodes are seen in the retroperitoneum in the para-aortic region, compartment IV (*large arrowhead*).

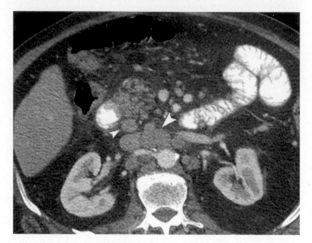

with the left gastric artery. The greater curvature of the stomach is supplied by the right and the left gastroepiploic arteries. The right gastroepiploic artery arises from the gastroduodenal artery and traverses the gastrocolic ligament, after briefly traversing the transverse mesocolon. The left gastroepiploic artery arises from the splenic artery and traverses the gastrosplenic and gastrocolic ligaments. The body and the fundus of the stomach are also supplied by short gastric arteries, which are branches of the splenic artery.[3]

Venous drainage of the stomach accompanies the main arteries. The right gastroepiploic vein drains into the superior mesenteric vein and then into the portal vein. The left gastroepiploic vein drains into the splenic vein and then into the portal vein. The left and right gastric veins drain directly into the portal vein.[3] The shape and position of the stomach vary depending on the volume of gastric contents.

Lymphatic Drainage and Staging Relevance

Lymphatics are numerous and follow the arterial supply of the stomach.[3] The tumor, node, metastasis (TNM) staging as described by the American Joint Committee for Cancer (AJCC) is explained in detail in Chapter 6 and is based on the number of tumor-involved lymph nodes.[4] N1 disease indicates involvement of 1 to 6 nodes, N2 indicates involvement of 7 to 15 nodes, and N3 disease indicates involvement of >15 nodes.[4,5]

The Japanese Research Society for Gastric Cancer has classified the regional lymph nodes of the stomach into four major compartments.[6] Compartment I includes perigastric lymph nodes. Compartment II includes left gastric artery, common hepatic artery, and splenic artery lymph nodes (Fig. 19-2). Lymph nodes along the hepatoduodenal ligament, posterior to the head of the pancreas, and at the root of the mesentery comprise compartment III (Fig. 19-3). Compartment

Table 19-2	Lymphatic nodal stations
D1	Right paracardiac
	Left paracardiac
	Greater curvature
	Lesser curvature
	Suprapyloric
	Infrapyloric
D2	Left gastric
	Common hepatic
	Celiac axis
	Splenic hilum
	Splenic artery
D3	Hepatoduodenal ligament
	Posterior to head of pancreas
	Root of mesentery
D4	Transverse mesocolon
	Para-aortic

IV includes lymph nodes along the middle colic vessels and para-aortic lymph nodes (Fig. 19-3). The D classification or description of extent of lymphadenectomy is based on the extent of nodal dissection (D1–D4) (Table 19-2).[7]

A D1 lymph node dissection includes removal of all lymph nodes from compartment I. A D2 dissection includes removal of lymph nodes from compartments I and II, and a D3 dissection includes a D2 dissection and removal of lymph nodes from compartment III. A D4 dissection includes resection of all four compartments.[7]

The extent of lymph node dissection is a controversial topic.[8] In general, a more extensive dissection is performed in the East such as Japan and Korea. A more conservative approach is followed in the West where studies have shown no increase in survival and instead have seen increased morbidity and mortality associated with extensive lymphatic dissections.[9,10] However, a subgroup analysis showed that in stage 2 and stage 3 gastric cancers, a D2 lymphadenectomy was associated with improved survival when compared with limited D1 lymph node dissection.[10] Patients with D1 dissection also experienced a higher chance of recurrence than did patients with a D2 dissection.[9–11] Cuschieri et al.[10] determined that inclusion of splenectomy and partial pancreatectomy was the main reason for the increased postsurgical morbidity and mortality associated with traditional D2 dissection. D3 and D4 lymphadenectomy are practiced mainly in the East, but recent studies have shown no survival benefit in those patients who undergo a more radical dissection.[12] Thus, D2 dissection that spares the spleen and pancreas is currently the accepted standard in several institutions, including The University of Texas M. D. Anderson Cancer Center.[13] Therefore, recognition of suspicious lymph nodes in compartments III and IV is very important in the staging of gastric cancer and may have a profound effect on which treatment strategies are used.

RADIOLOGIC EVALUATION

T Staging

The radiographic appearance of early gastric cancers on double-contrast examination can vary, since lesions can exhibit various morphologies. Lesions may be polypoid, nodular, or plaque-like; double-contrast examination may reveal areas of ulceration and advanced lesions may also be polypoid and/or ulcerated.[14] However, an infiltrating type of advanced gastric cancer can be seen in scirrhous-type lesions (linitis plastica). Polypoid lesions can present as irregular filling defects when surrounded by barium or as lobulated shadows on double-contrast examination (Fig. 19-4). Ulcerative lesions have irregular eccentrically located depressions or craters.[14] The infiltrating-type tumor produces a narrowed stomach that is poorly distensible secondary to tumor-induced fibrosis, also known as the "leather bottle" appearance.[15]

Endoscopic ultrasound is the modality of choice in differentiating the gastric wall layers, which appear as a five-layer structure with alternating hyperechoic and hypoechoic bands: serosa, muscularis propria, submucosa, deep mucosa, and superficial mucosa (Fig. 19-5).[16] Endoscopic ultrasound is the most accurate method for T staging of gastric cancer, with a diagnostic rate of 78% to 94%.[17,18] T1 tumors involve the lamina propria or submucosa, and T2 tumors extend to the muscularis propria or subserosa. Tumors that extend through the serosa are classified as T3, and T4 tumors demonstrate direct invasion of adjacent organs. Gastric cancers on EUS are typically hypoechoic masses that interrupt the normal five-layer gastric wall pattern. An example of a T3 lesion is a lobulated hypoechoic mass invading the serosa (Fig. 19-6). Findings of diffuse gastric wall thickening can be seen in linitis plastica.[17,18]

Cross-sectional imaging is used in patients with a known diagnosis of gastric cancer to stage the disease and determine surgical resectability. Cross-sectional imaging is also used for postchemotherapy follow-up. Understanding the anatomy and pattern of spread of gastric cancer is important for appropriate staging. CT is useful for identifying the tumor's location; gastric wall invasion, with extension into the perigastric fat and ligaments; and regional or distant adenopathy and metastases.

FIGURE 19-4 Image from a double contrast upper gastrointestinal series demonstrates a polypoid lesion in the gastric antrum. The barium outlines the lobulated appearance of the tumor.

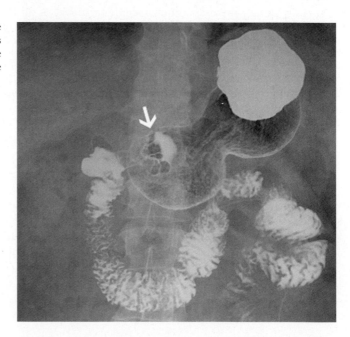

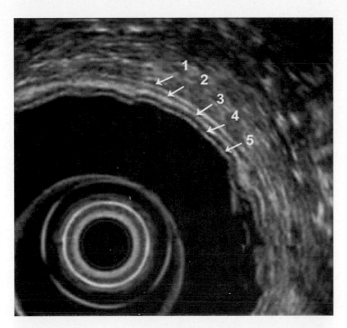

FIGURE 19-5 Endoscopic ultrasound image of the normal gastric wall. The endoscope is in the gastric lumen. The layers of the stomach wall appear as alternating hyperechoic and hypoechoic bands. *1*, serosal; *2*, muscularis propria; *3*, submucosa; *4*, muscularis mucosa; *5*, mucosa. (Courtesy of Dr. Manoop Bhutani, M.D.)

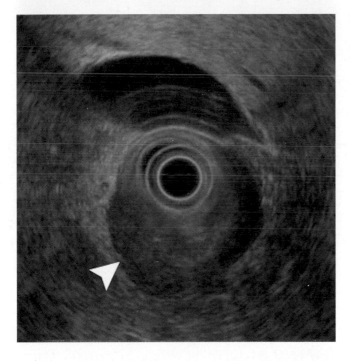

FIGURE 19-6 Endoscopic ultrasound image showing the loss of the normal gastric layers caused by the gastric tumor which appears as a hypoechoic mass (*arrowhead*). Here the tumor is seen infiltrating through the serosa, a T3 lesion. (Courtesy of Dr. Manoop Bhutani M.D.)

Optimal gastric luminal distention should ideally be achieved for CT staging.[19,20] Choosing the appropriate CT oral contrast agent is important, especially for detection of small-volume disease. High-density (positive) oral contrast agents are typically used for opacification of the gastrointestinal tract. Since the gastric wall can demonstrate intense enhancement after intravenous contrast, the high attenuation of the high-density contrast agent may mask or miss small-volume disease.[19,20] Even though these agents are safe and result in adequate gastric distention, there may be uneven mixing with gastric contents resulting in a pseudotumor (an abnormality that resembles a tumor).[20] Thus, a negative-contrast agent such as water can be used to prevent this potential pitfall. Water is well tolerated, inexpensive, and provides adequate gastric distention

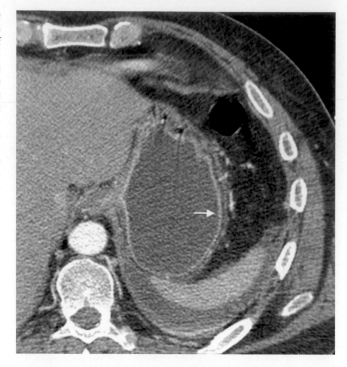

FIGURE 19-7 Axial CT image of the abdomen demonstrates the normal layers of the stomach after the administration of intravenous contrast. Water (low attenuation material) within the stomach was administered for oral contrast. A three layered normal gastric wall is seen. The layer with the most intense enhancement (*arrow*) is the mucosal layer. The submucosal layer is seen as a low attenuation stripe adjacent to the mucosa. The outermost layer demonstrates intermediate enhancement which represents the muscularis propria and serosal layer. Incidental note is made of perisplenic ascites.

while allowing proper visualization of the areas of high attenuation enhancement in the gastric wall.[20,21] Intravenous contrast should then be given with subsequent acquisition of CT images.

Recent development and refinement of MDCT have enabled identification of three distinct layers in the normal gastric wall.[1] The normal gastric wall typically has an enhancing inner layer (mucosa), a middle low-attenuating band comprising the submucosa, and an outer enhancing layer comprising the muscularis and the serosa (Fig. 19-7).[16] This finding of three distinct layers has prompted several small studies to attempt to identify the T stage of early gastric cancers.

When previously compared with EUS, CT was considered inadequate for T staging of gastric tumors. However, optimization of gastric distention, negative oral contrast, and dynamic contrast-enhanced CT with multiplanar reconstructions appears to have improved CT's potential to stage gastric tumors.[16]

Mani et al.[22] reported that the early phase of multiphase dynamic imaging after administering intravenous contrast was helpful in determining depth of tumor invasion of advanced gastric cancers as well as defining the vascular anatomy of the stomach. Mani et al.[22] also found that delayed phase images (performed at 3 minutes postcontrast) did not provide any additional information. In a different study, Takao et al.[23] studied 108 patients with gastric cancer identified by CT: 53 of these patients had early gastric cancer and 55 had advanced disease. Takao et al. also found that early cancers were best depicted on the arterial-dominant or parenchymal phase. However, the advanced cancers were best seen in the equilibrium phase owing to tumor-induced fibrosis, since most of the tumors in their study group were scirrhous-type tumors. Takao et al.'s accuracy rate for CT tumor detection and T staging was 98% and 82%, respectively. For early gastric cancers, the accuracy was much lower; accuracy of tumor detection and T staging was 23% and 15%, respectively.[23]

If available, the scanning protocol for CT can be performed on a 16- or a 64-slice multidetector row CT scanner for faster image acquisition, instead of on a single detector row CT scanner. Water is used for oral contrast and approximately 125 mL of nonionic intravenous contrast (e.g., Optiray 350; Mallinckrodt Medical Inc, St. Louis, Missouri) is injected at a rate of 4 to 5 mL/s. It is also important that the patient receive additional water just prior to the CT scan so that the stomach is well filled and distended. Sections at 2.5-mm thickness are generally acquired for routine imaging. Dual-phase imaging may be performed with the arterial phase obtained approximately 25 seconds after the start of the injection and the venous phase obtained approximately 50 seconds postinjection.

Several institutions have equipment allowing the ability to reconstruct images into the coronal and sagittal planes to be obtained in conjunction with the acquired axial images from the CT scanner.[20] Otherwise these images, referred to as two-dimensional multiplanar reformatted (MPR) images, can be constructed using a separate workstation or software. An abnormality in one plane can be localized to the other planes, thus increasing diagnostic characterization of lesions.[20] Kim et al.[24] studied the value of MPR images in the coronal and sagittal planes and found them helpful for distinguishing T3 from T4 tumors and showing adjacent organ involvement. Chen et al.[25] also reported improvement of T staging with MDCT MPR images (89%) compared with using axial images alone (73%). To improve the quality of three-dimensional (3-D) imaging, thinner slices (1.25-mm thickness) can be obtained on CT scan.[20] 3-D volume-rendered images increase the depth perception of the region of interest, and the images can be rotated to achieve an optimal viewing plane of the lesion in question. The images also can be rendered by changing the window width and level or by eliminating certain tissues and thereby accentuating certain tissues or vessels. Images can also be reconstructed with volume rendering to produce an endoscopic-type image (virtual gastroscopy) to accentuate gastric rugae or lesions.[20]

Gastric cancer on CT can present as focal thickening, diffuse wall thickening (linitis plastica) (Fig. 19-8), or polypoid or lobulated masses with or without ulceration. T1 and T2 lesions are confined to the gastric wall, and T3 lesions invade the serosa and may demonstrate some alteration of the serosal contour with stranding of the perigastric fat.[7] CT and EUS are limited in their

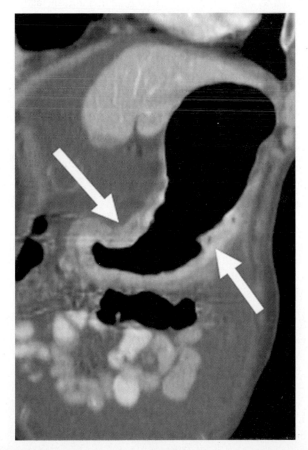

FIGURE 19-8 Coronal reformatted CT image after the administration of oral and intravenous contrast demonstrates diffuse wall thickening of the distal body and antrum of the stomach from linitis plastica (*arrows*). Incidental note is made of diffuse abdominal and pelvic ascites.

ability to distinguish between T2 and T3 lesions.[17,26] However, T4 lesions on CT can be identified by ligamentous spread and invasion into adjacent structures.[7]

The usefulness of MRI in gastric cancer staging is controversial. MRI has not been as widely used for gastric cancer staging owing to limitations including peristalsis, respiratory and cardiac motion artifacts, lack of adequate oral contrast medium, and high cost.[27] However, MRI does have some advantages, including no ionizing radiation, soft-tissue contrast, and multiplanar capability. Faster imaging techniques along with breath-hold sequences have decreased acquisition time, resulting in fewer motion artifacts. Other improvements include the use of phased array coils to increase the signal-to-noise ratio and spatial resolution.[27] Sohn et al.[28] studied 31 patients with gastric cancer who underwent preoperative MRI and CT imaging and reported that MRI was comparable with CT in T and N staging of gastric cancer, with a T-staging accuracy of 73.3%. Oi et al.[29] studied 37 patients with gastric cancer using postdynamic gadolinium spoiled gradient echo (SGE) MRI sequences and reported a T-staging accuracy of 81%, which showed the utility of dynamic gadolinium enhancement for identifying tumor invasion into adjacent organs. Though such promising research is available, MRI has not had widespread use owing to the increased cost, limited availability, and associated technical challenges.

Normal gastric mucosa accumulates fluorodeoxyglucose F-18 (FDG), and thus FDG PET is not useful in T staging of gastric cancer.[30] Moreover, certain cell types such as mucin-producing tumors and signet cells and poorly differentiated cancer are not particularly FDG avid making it challenging to use PET-CT for staging and detection of gastric cancer.[31]

N Staging

Staging of nodal (N) disease is challenging, even with the current advances in imaging technology. The shortcoming of N staging is its inability to detect microscopic metastases based on non-invasive methods. Even newer technology such as PET-CT is limited by poor resolution.[32] The problem with size and metastases in a lymph node is described by a study by Monig et al.[33] Monig et al. reported in a prospective study of patients with gastric cancer that the mean diameter of regional lymph nodes not involved with tumor was 4.1 mm, whereas those lymph nodes involved with tumor had a mean diameter of 6 mm. Of the lymph nodes that were tumor free, 80% were <5 mm and 55% of the lymph nodes that contained tumor measured <5 mm.[33]

EUS has the ability to examine lymph nodes in the immediate vicinity of the stomach but has limited ability to visualize and thus characterize other regional lymph nodes in the draining nodal stations.[16] When using EUS, metastatic lymph nodes are suspected based on their location, morphology (rounded), and echotexture (hypoechoic). EUS not only can assess local tumor infiltration but also can assess regional lymph node involvement (such as perigastric lymph nodes) with pathological diagnosis obtainable by EUS-guided fine-needle aspiration.[16] Distant nodal stations, however, cannot be evaluated and sampled via EUS. It should be noted that EUS is an invasive technique, is operator dependent, and is not readily available in all institutions.

For N staging on CT, size is predominantly used as a measure of metastatic disease. Upper limits of a normal lymph node are 8 to 10 mm in short axis. Using size as a criterion is not always accurate, since enlarged lymph nodes may be from inflammation and normal-sized lymph nodes may have tumor involvement.[33] There are no accurate criteria for determining lymph node involvement on CT.[34,35] However, characteristics other than size (such as shape, heterogeneity, peripheral enhancement, or central necrosis) are considered when evaluating for metastatic involvement.[36,37]

Some studies have shown EUS and CT to be similar in N-staging accuracy. Bhandari et al.[17] studied 63 patients and showed the accuracy of nodal staging to be 75% for MDCT and 79% for EUS. In a different study, Davies et al.[38] reported a CT sensitivity ranging from 24% to 43% for N1 and N2 nodal disease and a specificity of 100%. In a study by Chen et al.,[25] MDCT MPR images showed improved N stage detection and increased accuracy with the addition of orthogonal planes for MDCT MPR images (78% vs. 71% with MDCT axial images alone). With more advanced disease, the accuracy of N staging increases. A study by Yang et al.[39] showed accuracies of lymph node involvement to be 71% in early gastric cancer and 90% in advanced disease.

MRI shares with CT the same challenge of size when staging lymph nodes.[40] This challenge may be further compounded by the movement artifact seen in MRI caused by peristalsis and breathing. Kim et al.[41] showed that N staging was 65% accurate using MRI versus 73% accurate using CT, whereas Sohn et al.[28] reported N staging that was 55% accurate using MRI and 59% accurate using CT. Tatsumi et al.[42] studied lymph nodes in patients with late stages of gastric cancer using lymphotrophic ultrasmall superparamagnetic iron oxide (USPIO) particles-feru-moxtran-10 for detecting metastatic lymph nodes. Tatsumi et al. found that nodes in the retro-peritoneal and para-aortic regions were more easily identified than were those in the perigastric region, secondary to motion artifacts. The presence or absence of metastatic disease was based on enhancement patterns. On T2-weighted images, normal lymph nodes were hypointense (dark signal intensity) secondary to macrophages within the lymph nodes phagocytosing the iron oxide particles. Nodes were considered metastatic if they demonstrated partial high signal intensity from partial uptake or if they did not decrease in T2 signal due to lack of iron oxide particle uptake, with a sensitivity of 100% and a specificity of 92.6%.[42] USPIO is currently not commercially available in the United States, which has limited testing and clinical application of USPIO.

The role of PET in detecting locoregional nodal metastases is limited. PET is not helpful in detecting station I and II lymph nodes due to proximity to the primary tumor and PET's utility for detecting station III and IV lymph nodes is still unknown.[7] However, PET-CT is again limited by size, with the resolution of lymph nodes on commercially available PET-CT being approximately 1.2 cm.[32] Thus, there is little likelihood of this modality improving N staging, unless there is widespread availability of high-resolution PET-CT scanners.

M Staging

Gastric cancer can extend locally through the gastric layers into the surrounding fat and infiltrate along the various ligaments by direct invasion. Gastric cancer can also spread via lymphatic, hematogenous routes or peritoneal seeding. Demonstrating metastatic disease may obviate the need for surgical intervention with curative intent.

Even though EUS can potentially detect mediastinal adenopathy, liver metastases, and peritoneal disease, EUS is limited because it is not the modality of choice for identifying distant metastatic disease outside of its field of view.[16]

CT is used widely for detecting metastatic disease. Gastric cancer commonly metastasizes to the liver, and the lesions are typically more hypovascular than the surrounding liver parenchyma (Figs. 19-2 and 19-11). Davis et al.[43] showed that CT had a sensitivity of 76% for detecting direct spread of gastric cancer to the mesocolon and the colon.[43] The sensitivity for identifying pancreatic involvement, hepatic involvement, and peritoneal spread was shown to be 50%, 71%, and 71%, respectively.

Peritoneal carcinomatosis is common in gastric cancer and is associated with advanced disease. Diagnosis of early peritoneal involvement is difficult with CT, and therefore diagnostic laparoscopy is commonly used as an adjunct to cross-sectional imaging to determine surgical resectability. Presence of ascites is considered an ominous sign, with high specificity for peritoneal carcinomatosis.[44]

With CT, peritoneal spread appears as areas of soft tissue nodularity, thickening, and stranding or even as soft tissue masses within the peritoneal cavity or omentum (Fig. 19-9).[7] Metastases to the ovaries or Krukenberg tumors are suspected when the ovaries are enlarged. Imaging findings are nonspecific and range in appearance from predominantly solid to a mixture of cystic and solid areas, which can often mimic primary ovarian tumors. Other sites of disease include metastatic disease to the umbilicus (Sister Mary Joseph nodule) or metastatic disease to the rectovesical pouch (Blumer shelf). Distant metastases can also occur outside of the abdomen. Metastatic adenopathy can occur in the left supraclavicular region, also known as Virchow node.[45] The lymphatic drainage from the abdomen is via the thoracic duct, with the end node of the thoracic duct located at the left jugulo-subclavian venous junction. Metastatic disease is caused by lymph reflux from the thoracic duct into the cervical nodes in this region.[45] Lung metastases can also occur but are rare.

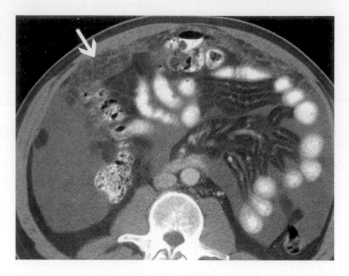

FIGURE 19-9 Axial CT image of the abdomen after the administration of oral and intravenous contrast demonstrates diffuse abdominal ascites. There are areas of stranding and nodularity within the omentum (*white arrow*) secondary to peritoneal carcinomatosis in this patient with gastric cancer.

MRI has been considered superior to CT in detection of liver metastases in patients with gastric cancer because of greater soft tissue contrast resolution, greater sensitivity to contrast enhancement, and newly developed hepatobiliary agents such as gadolinium benzyloxypropionictetraacetate (Gd-BOPTA) and gadolinium ethoxybenzyl-diethylenetriaminepentaacetic acid (Gd-EOB-DTPA).[40] MRI is also more useful in detecting liver metastases in a fatty infiltrated liver than CT.

A review by Motohara and Semelka[40]. concluded that MRI's role in staging of gastric cancer is useful in detecting liver metastases. The same study found that like CT, MRI is not accurate in detecting small tumors in a nondistended stomach but does have increased utility in evaluating gastric wall invasion and peritoneal spread. However, laparoscopy is still superior to both CT and MRI for detecting peritoneal spread. Bone involvement from metastatic gastric cancer is also uncommon, but MRI is better at detecting early bone disease than CT.[40] MRI appearances of Krukenberg tumors include bilateral complex masses with T2 hypointense solid components from dense stromal reaction and internal T2 hyperintensity from mucin. Intratumoral cysts can sometimes be seen in Krukenberg tumors, demonstrating strong contrast enhancement of the cyst wall.[46] An example of a Krukenberg tumor involving the left ovary is seen in Figure 19-10 and is exhibited as a solid mass on T2 weighted images.

PET-CT can be useful for detecting distant metastases and can decrease the need for unnecessary surgery by detecting distant metastatic disease not diagnosed with conventional imaging.[7] PET-CT can help detect distant nodal metastases, such as Virchow node. Metastatic disease to the liver, adrenal glands, and ovaries can be detected easily with PET. Some researchers have shown that PET has a greater sensitivity for detecting peritoneal metastases than does CT.[47,48]

TREATMENT AND RECURRENCE

Treatment for gastric cancer depends on disease staging at diagnosis. For localized disease, surgical resection may be considered. A combination of radiation therapy, chemotherapy, and/or surgery may be options for treating advanced disease. Preoperative neoadjuvant chemotherapy has been used to downstage a patient for possible resection.[49] CT is the primary modality used to evaluate suspected recurrence, since there are no reliable tumor markers for suspected recurrent disease. CT, however, was not found to be accurate in assessing locoregional disease post chemotherapy, since it is often difficult to differentiate posttreatment changes from tumor recurrence.[7,49] Imaging of early recurrence may appear initially as an area of focal thickening, but often can be indistinguishable from postsurgical and/or posttherapy changes. On follow-up examination, if an area of previous focal thickening has become more mass-like or infiltrative in appearance,

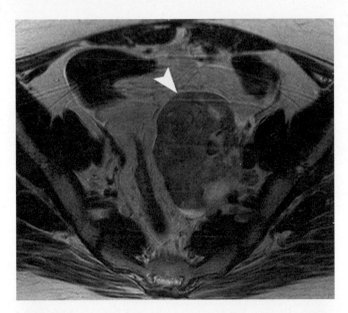

FIGURE 19-10 Axial T2-weighted MRI image of the pelvis in a women with gastric cancer. There is a solid heterogenous predominantly intermediate signal intensity mass involving the left adnexa (*arrowhead*). This mass grew over serial MRI examinations. Her right ovary was previously removed revealing metastatic disease from gastric cancer.

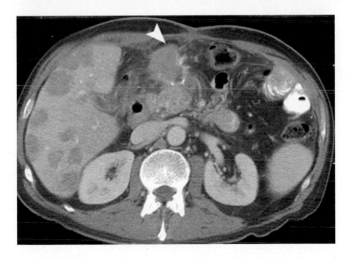

FIGURE 19-11 Axial CT image of the abdomen after the administration of oral and intravenous contrast in a patient with metastatic gastric cancer. Multiple low attenuation lesions are seen in the liver from metastatic disease. A soft tissue mass from recurrence (*arrowhead*) is seen along the duodenal stump in this patient status post subtotal gastrectomy for gastric cancer.

recurrence should be suspected. A study by Ikeda et al.[47] found that 42% of patients had recurrences within the first 2 years after curative resection. In some patients, recurrence can occur at the postsurgical anastomoses or duodenal stump (Fig. 19-11).[50] PET-CT may be useful in differentiating tumor recurrence from postsurgical or treatment changes. In patients undergoing chemotherapy, response to treatment based on size measurements on CT can potentially be inaccurate, since a majority of gastric tumors are not measurable.[7] PET-CT may also be helpful in evaluating tumor response to treatment by demonstrating decreased FDG uptake.

CONCLUSIONS

To accurately stage and manage gastric cancer, it is important to understand cross-sectional anatomy including nodal stations, ligamentous attachments, and patterns of disease spread locally and distally. As discussed, several modalities are currently combined to accurately stage gastric cancer. Using CT MPR images has increased the diagnostic accuracy of staging in CT imaging. Endoscopic ultrasound still remains the modality of choice for visualizing the gastric wall layers and for T staging. Both CT and MRI are useful methods to identify peritoneal spread, with MRI being more sensitive for liver metastases detection.

References

1. Meyers MA. *Dynamic radiology of the abdomen.* 5 ed. New York, NY: Springer-Velrag; 2000.
2. Vikram R, Balachandran A, Bhosale PR, et al. Pancreas: peritoneal reflections, ligamentous connections, and pathways of disease spread. *Radiographics.* 2009;29:e34.
3. Gray H. *Anatomy of the human body.* 20th ed. Philadelphia, PA: Lea & Febiger; 1918.
4. Green FL. *AJCC cancer staging manual.* 6 ed. New York, NY: Springer-Velrag; 2002.
5. Miller FH, Kochman ML, Talamonti MS, et al. Gastric cancer: radiologic staging. *Radiol Clin North Am.* 1997;35:331–349.
6. Nishi M OY, Miwa K. Japanese Research Society for Gastric Cancer (JRSGC): Japanese classification of gastric carcinoma. In: Nishi M OY, Miwa K, ed. Tokyo, Japan; 1995:6–15.
7. Lim JS, Yun MJ, Kim MJ, et al. CT and PET in stomach cancer: preoperative staging and monitoring of response to therapy. *Radiographics.* 2006;26:143–156.
8. Dicken BJ, Bigam DL, Cass C, et al. Gastric adenocarcinoma: review and considerations for future directions. *Ann Surg.* 2005;241:27–39.
9. Bonenkamp JJ, Hermans J, Sasako M, et al. Extended lymph-node dissection for gastric cancer. *N EnglJ Med.* 1999;340:908–914.
10. Cuschieri A, Weeden S, Fielding J, et al. Patient survival after D1 and D2 resections for gastric cancer: long-term results of the MRC randomized surgical trial. Surgical Co-operative Group. *Br J Cancer.* 1999;79:1522–1530.
11. Hundahl SA, Phillips JL, Menck HR. The National Cancer Data Base Report on poor survival of U.S. gastric carcinoma patients treated with gastrectomy: Fifth Edition American Joint Committee on Cancer staging, proximal disease, and the "different disease" hypothesis. *Cancer.* 2000;88:921–932.
12. Sasako M, Sano T, Yamamoto S, et al. D2 lymphadenectomy alone or with para-aortic nodal dissection for gastric cancer. *N Engl J Med.* 2008;359:453–462.
13. Al-Refaie WB, Abdalla EK, Ahmad SA, et al. Gastric cancer. In: Feig BW, Berger DH, Fuhrman GM, eds. *The MD Anderson surgical oncology handbook.* Philadelphia, PA: Lippincott Williams & Wilkins; 2006; 205–240.
14. Iyer R, Dubrow R. Imaging upper gastrointestinal malignancy. *Semin Roentgenol.* 2006;41:105–112.
15. Gore RM, Levine MS, Ghahremani GG, et al. Gastric cancer: radiologic diagnosis. *Radiol Clin N Am.* 1997;35:311–329.
16. Hargunani R, Maclachlan J, Kaniyur S, et al. Cross-sectional imaging of gastric neoplasia. *Clin Radiol.* 2009;64:420–429.
17. Bhandari S, Shim CS, Kim JH, et al. Usefulness of three-dimensional, multidetector row CT (virtual gastroscopy and multiplanar reconstruction) in the evaluation of gastric cancer: a comparison with conventional endoscopy, EUS, and histopathology. *Gastrointestinal endoscopy* 2004;59:619–626.
18. Kelly S, Harris KM, Berry E, et al. A systematic review of the staging performance of endoscopic ultrasound in gastro-oesophageal carcinoma. *Gut.* 2001;49:534–539.
19. Horton KM, Eng J, Fishman EK. Normal enhancement of the small bowel: evaluation with spiral CT. *J Comptr Assist Tomogr.* 2000;24:67–71.
20. Horton KM, Fishman EK. Current role of CT in imaging of the stomach. *Radiographics.* 2003;23:75–87.
21. Winter TC, Ager JD, Nghiem HV, et al. Upper gastrointestinal tract and abdomen: water as an orally administered contrast agent for helical CT. *Radiology.* 1996;201:365–370.
22. Mani NB, Suri S, Gupta S, et al. Two-phase dynamic contrast-enhanced computed tomography with water-filling method for staging of gastric carcinoma. *Clin Imag.* 2001;25:38–43.
23. Takao M, Fukuda T, Iwanaga S, et al. Gastric cancer: evaluation of triphasic spiral CT and radiologic-pathologic correlation. *J Comp Assis Tomogr.* 1998;22:288–294.
24. Kim YH, Lee KH, Park SH, et al. Staging of T3 and T4 gastric carcinoma with multidetector CT: added value of multiplanar reformations for prediction of adjacent organ invasion. *Radiology.* 2009;250: 767–775.

25. Chen CY, Hsu JS, Wu DC, et al. Gastric cancer: preoperative local staging with 3D multi-detector row CT—correlation with surgical and histopathologic results. *Radiology*. 2007;242:472–482.

26. Habermann CR, Weiss F, Riecken R, et al. Preoperative staging of gastric adenocarcinoma: comparison of helical CT and endoscopic US. *Radiology*. 2004;230:465–471.

27. Campeau NG, Johnson CD, Felmlee JP, et al. MR imaging of the abdomen with a phased-array multicoil: prospective clinical evaluation. *Radiology*. 1995;195:769–776.

28. Sohn KM, Lee JM, Lee SY, et al. Comparing MR imaging and CT in the staging of gastric carcinoma. *Am J Roentgenol*. 2000;174:1551–1557.

29. Oi H, Matsushita M, Murakami T, et al. Dynamic MR imaging for extraserosal invasion of advanced gastric cancer. *Abdom Imag*. 1997;22:35–40.

30. Cook GJ, Fogelman I, Maisey MN. Normal physiological and benign pathological variants of 18-fluoro-2-deoxyglucose positron-emission tomography scanning: potential for error in interpretation. *Semin Nucl Med*. 1996;26:308–314.

31. Yoshioka T, Yamaguchi K, Kubota K, et al. Evaluation of 18F-FDG PET in patients with a, metastatic, or recurrent gastric cancer. *J Nucl Med*. 2003;44:690–699.

32. Mawlawi O, Podoloff DA, Kohlmyer S, et al. Performance characteristics of a newly developed PET/CT scanner using NEMA standards in 2D and 3D modes. *J Nucl Med*. 2004;45:1734–1742.

33. Monig SP, Zirbes TK, Schroder W, et al. Staging of gastric cancer: correlation of lymph node size and metastatic infiltration. *Am J Roentgenol*. 1999;173:365–367.

34. Dorfman RE, Alpern MB, Gross BH, et al. Upper abdominal lymph nodes: criteria for normal size determined with CT. *Radiology*. 1991;180:319–322.

35. Harisinghani MG, Saini S, Weissleder R, et al. MR lymphangiography using ultrasmall superparamagnetic iron oxide in patients with primary abdominal and pelvic malignancies: radiographic-pathologic correlation. *Am J Roentgenol*. 1999;172:1347–1351.

36. D'Elia F, Zingarelli A, Palli D, et al. Hydro-dynamic CT preoperative staging of gastric cancer: correlation with pathological findings: a prospective study of 107 cases. *Eur Radiol*. 2000;10:1877–1885.

37. Fukuya T, Honda H, Hayashi T, et al. Lymph-node metastases: efficacy for detection with helical CT in patients with gastric cancer. *Radiology*. 1995;197:705–711.

38. Davies J, Chalmers AG, Sue-Ling HM, et al. Spiral computed tomography and operative staging of gastric carcinoma: a comparison with histopathological staging. *Gut*. 1997;41:314–319.

39. Yang DM, Kim HC, Jin W, et al. 64 multidetector-row computed tomography for preoperative evaluation of gastric cancer: histological correlation. *J Comp Assist Tomogr*. 2007;31:98–103.

40. Motohara T, Semelka RC. MRI in staging of gastric cancer. *Abdom Imag*. 2002;27:376–383.

41. Kim AY, Han JK, Seong CK, et al. MRI in staging advanced gastric cancer: is it useful compared with spiral CT? *J Comp Assist Tomogr*. 2000;24:389–394.

42. Tatsumi Y, Tanigawa N, Nishimura H, et al. Preoperative diagnosis of lymph node metastases in gastric cancer by magnetic resonance imaging with ferumoxtran-10. *Gastric Cancer*. 2006;9:120–128.

43. Davis PA, Sano T. The difference in gastric cancer between Japan, USA and Europe: what are the facts? what are the suggestions? *Crit Rev Oncol Hematol*. 2001;40:77–94.

44. Yajima K, Kanda T, Ohashi M, et al. Clinical and diagnostic significance of preoperative computed tomography findings of ascites in patients with advanced gastric cancer. *Am J Surg*. 2006;192:185–190.

45. Negus D, Edwards JM, Kinmonth JB. Filling of cervical and mediastinal nodes from the thoracic duct and the physiology of Virchow's node—studies by lymphography. *Br J Surg*. 1970;57:267–271.

46. Kim SH, Kim WH, Park KJ, et al. CT and MR findings of Krukenberg tumors: comparison with primary ovarian tumors. *J Comp Assist Tomogr*. 1996;20:393–398.

47. Ikeda Y, Saku M, Kishihara F, et al. Effective follow-up for recurrence or a second primary cancer in patients with early gastric cancer. *Br J Surg*. 2005;92:235–239.

48. Turlakow A, Yeung HW, Salmon AS, et al. Peritoneal carcinomatosis: role of (18)F-FDG PET. *J Nucl Med*. 2003;44:1407–1412.

49. Ng CS, Husband JE, MacVicar AD, et al. Correlation of CT with histopathological findings in patients with gastric and gastro-oesophageal carcinomas following neoadjuvant chemotherapy. *Clin Radiol*. 1998;53:422–427.

50. Ha HK, Kim HH, Kim HS, et al. Local recurrence after surgery for gastric carcinoma: CT findings. *Am J Roentgenol*. 1993;161:975–977.

Preneoplastic and Preinvasive Lesions

Chronic Gastritis and Gastric Precancerous Conditions

20

▶ Massimo Rugge
▶ Donato Nitti
▶ Gregory Y. Lauwers
▶ David Y. Graham

INTRODUCTION

This chapter describes the basic clinical context, natural history, and histological phenotypes of gastric precancerous conditions (particularly chronic gastritis); it also addresses the clinicobiological relationship between these diseases and the natural history of gastric cancer. Information is also provided to support the biological rationale for follow-up and preventive therapeutic strategies.

Within gastric mucosa, as in other regions of the gastrointestinal tract, full-blown cancer is the final event of a multistep pathway, usually triggered by (multifactorial) inflammation (Table 20-1).[1,2] This link between inflammation and cancer is mediated by a progressive accumulation of genotypic changes associated with dedifferentiation of the native epithelial phenotype. The cascade of biological events results in a new, neoplastic cell capable of infiltrating the surrounding stroma and metastasizing. It has recently been demonstrated that either resident or bone marrow–derived stem cells may be involved in the onset of cancer.[3–5] This oncogenic pathway is defined as "environmental" because the etiologic agents responsible for inflammatory diseases are of environmental origin, as opposed to the pathway resulting mainly from (host-related) genetic syndromes.

Less than 10% of stomach cancers are hereditary.[6] While most of the genetic factors involved in familial gastric cancers are unknown, specific mutations have been well characterized as being responsible for a minor subset of gastric epithelial malignancies. Families harboring germline truncating *E-cadherin* mutations (with an autosomal dominant pattern of inheritance) have a high prevalence of diffuse-type gastric cancer.[7,8] Other hereditary conditions predisposing to gastric cancer include familial adenomatous polyposis (FAP), hereditary nonpolyposis colorectal cancer (HNPCC), and the Li-Fraumeni and Peutz-Jeghers syndromes.[6]

The natural history of sporadic gastric cancer involves a multistage oncogenic cascade. This chapter will specifically address the "inflammatory step" along this biological pathway.[1]

In the stomach, a distinction has been established between precancerous *conditions* and precancerous *lesions*. Precancerous conditions are clinicopathological situations due to hereditary syndromes and environmental etiologies that are associated with an increased risk of cancer, while precancerous lesions are histological abnormalities in the cell substrate that can lead to cancer.[9]

Table 20-1	Long-standing inflammatory conditions potentially leading to cancer in the gastrointestinal tract	
Anatomical Site	**Etiology of Disease**	**Inflammatory Disease > Malignancy**
Esophagus	Gastroesophageal reflux	Barrett mucosa > adenocarcinoma
Stomach	Gastritis (*H. pylori* associated) Immunomediated	Atrophic gastritis > adenocarcinoma
Small bowel	Immunomediated	Celiac enteritis > lymphomas
Small and large bowel	Immunomediated	Crohn disease > adenocarcinoma
Large bowel	Immunomediated	Inflammatory bowel disease > adenocarcinoma
Liver	Viral, metabolic, toxic	Cirrhosis > hepatocellular cancer
Pancreas	Toxic, immunomediated	Chronic pancreatitis > adenocarcinoma

NONHEREDITARY PRECANCEROUS CONDITIONS

The risk of gastric cancer increases significantly for patients with (a) gastritis, (b) gastric ulcer disease, and (c) gastric mucosa hyperplasia (be it diffuse or focal/polypoid). None of these conditions are primarily hereditary, though a genetic predisposition has been claimed for some, and gene polymorphisms leading to a stronger inflammatory response may increase the risk of onset.[10]

Gastritis

Gastritis is defined as histologically proven inflammation of the gastric mucosa. Worldwide, the primary cause of gastritis is *Helicobacter pylori* infection. Approximately 50% of the world's population is infected, the prevalence being higher in developing and disadvantaged countries, since the prevalence of *H. pylori* is inversely related to socioeconomic status.[11]

The etiology of gastritis is established from clinical examination, serology (pepsinogens and antibodies against infectious agents and/or autoantigens), endoscopy (which should include biopsy), and histology. From a clinical standpoint, gastritis may be acute or chronic, though no clear cutoff in duration of disease has been established to distinguish them. In practice, the best way to separate them is by histological examination of gastric mucosal biopsies.

There are robust criteria for classifying gastritis by etiology, and strong correlations have been established between etiology and clinical course. Table 20-2 lists the most common agents responsible for inflammatory conditions of the gastric mucosa and also indicates those most frequently associated with a prolonged (chronic) clinical course.

Gastritis: Basic Morphology

Histology identifies two main histological variants of the disease, that is, nonatrophic and atrophic gastritis.[12,13]

Nonatrophic gastritis is basically characterized by the presence of inflammatory cells within the lamina propria (lymphocytes, monocytes, polymorphs, and granulocytes), with no loss of the gland units normally present. However, inflammation may coexist with visible alterations, such as columnar epithelia hyperplasia, fibrosis of the lamina propria, and smooth muscle hyperplasia.

Atrophic gastritis is characterized by loss of appropriate glandular units.[12] The distinction between atrophic and nonatrophic gastritis is important because there is a well-established clinicobiological relationship between gastric atrophy and adenocarcinoma. The loss of appropriate

Table 20-2	Etiological classification of gastritis			
Etiological Category	**Agents**	**Specific Etiology**	**Clinical Presentation**	**Notes (Prevalence: High***, Low**, Very Low*)**
Infectious Agents	Virus	Cytomegalovirus	Acute	Nonatrophic**
		Herpes virus	Acute	Nonatrophic**
		H. pylori	Acute or chronic	Nonatrophic and atrophic, type B***
	Bacteria	*Mycobacterium tuberculosis*	Acute (?)	Nonatrophic*
		Mycobacterium avium complex	Acute(?)	Nonatrophic*
		Mycobacterium diphtheriae	Acute	Nonatrophic*
		Actinomyces	Acute	Nonatrophic*
		Spirochaeta	Acute	Nonatrophic**
	Fungi	Cardida	Acute	Nonatrophic*
		Histoplasma	Acute	Nonatrophic*
		Phycomycosis	Acute	Nonatrophic*
		Cryptosporidium	Acute	Nonatrophic*
	Parasites	Strongyloides	Acute	Nonatrophic*
		Anisakis	Acute	Nonatrophic*
		Ascaris lumbricoides	Acute	Nonatrophic*

(Continued)

Table 20-2	Etiological classification of gastritis *(Continued)*			
Etiological Category	**Agents**	**Specific Etiology**	**Clinical Presentation**	**Notes (Prevalence: High***, Low**, Very Low*)**
Chemical Agents (with Low Inflammatory Trait)	Environment (dietary and drug related)	Dietary factors	Chronic	Nonatrophic and atrophic***
		Drugs: NSAIDs, ticlopidine	Acute or chronic	Nonatrophic; type C***
		Alcohol	Acute	Nonatrophic; type C**
		Cocaine	Acute	Nonatrophic; type C*
		Bile (reflux)	Acute or chronic	Nonatrophic; type C***
Physical Agents	Radiation		Acute or chronic	Nonatrophic and atrophic*
		Autoimmune	Chronic	Atrophic (corpus); type A**
		Drugs (ticlopidine)	Acute	
Immunomediated	Various pathogenesis (mostly unknown)	?Gluten	Chronic	Lymphocytic gastritis**
		Food sensitivity	Acute or chronic	Eosinophilic gastritis**
		H. pylori (autoimmune component)	Chronic	Nonatrophic and atrophic
		GVHD	Acute or chronic	Nonatrophic and atrophic*
		Crohn disease	Chronic (?)	Nonatrophic/focal atrophy**
		Sarcoidosis	Chronic (?)	Nonatrophic or focal atrophy*
		Wegener granulomatosis	Chronic (?)	Nonatrophic or focal atrophy*
Idiopathic		Collagenous gastritis	Chronic	Nonatrophic*
		Idiopathic "isolated" gastritis	Acute or chronic	Nonatrophic and atrophic

(?): Not confirmed.

glands may coexist with the histological (inflammatory and/or hyperplastic) changes that also occur in nonatrophic gastritis.

The Inflammatory Infiltrate

The inflammatory infiltrate mainly consists of lymphocytes, plasma cells, histiocytes, and granulocytes within the lamina propria and, less commonly, within the single glandular units. Lymphocytes may be either dispersed or packed in follicular lymphoid structures; lymphoid follicles are usually seen in *H. pylori* infections. Visual analog scales (VASs) have been developed to improve interobserver consistency in scoring the mononuclear infiltrate.[14]

The term *lymphocytic gastritis* is applied when a prominent lymphocyte infiltrate is detected within the glandular gastric epithelia. Different cutoff values have been suggested for assessing lymphocytic gastritis, ranging from about 20 to 25 inflammatory cells per 100 epithelial cells. Lymphocytic gastritis is suggestive of, but not diagnostic for, an immunomediated component in the inflammatory disease. An association has also been suggested between lymphocytic gastritis and celiac disease.[15-18] A more severe (nodular) lymphocytic intraglandular infiltrate that destroys or partially replaces the glandular structures (i.e., "lymphoepithelial lesion") is almost pathognomonic of primary gastric B-cell lymphoma, which is almost always associated with *H. pylori* infection.

Active inflammation of the gastric mucosa is defined as the presence of neutrophils within the lamina propria and/or in the glandular lumen. Activity is scored on a VAS according to the intensity of the neutrophilic infiltrate. Inflammatory activity suggests *H. pylori* infection, the presence of which in cases of chronic inflammation should suggest the presence of an active infection; otherwise, the activity score is clinically of no prognostic value. Active inflammation also is seen in association with any mucosal erosion, as in NSAID-related gastritis, for instance (see below). Intramucosal eosinophilic infiltrate is prominent in eosinophilic gastritis, though the cutoff for its histological assessment (the number of eosinophils per high-power microscopic field) has not been firmly established. The etiopathogenesis and clinical significance of this histological category remain to be clarified.[17]

Accessory Lesions

These include mucosal erosions, fibrosis of the lamina propria, smooth muscle hyperplasia, and columnar cell hyperplasia.

Mucosal erosions are commonly seen at endoscopy and histology; they can be due to infectious (*H. pylori*) or chemical (NSAIDs, drugs, bile) agents. Gastric epithelia adjacent to the erosion may undergo reactive hyperplastic changes (see below).

Expansion of the collagen tissue of the lamina propria (fibrosis), coupled with loss of glandular units, is defined as mucosal atrophy. Fibrosis of the lamina propria also may be focal, as seen in scars from prior peptic ulcers.

Hyperplasia of the *muscularis mucosae* may result from long-term proton pump inhibitor therapy; smooth muscle fascicle hyperplasia may push the glandular coils apart, expanding the interglandular spaces and giving rise to a pseudoatrophic pattern.

All inflammatory conditions of the gastric mucosa are associated with some degree of regenerative epithelial changes (regenerative hyperplasia), and this is generally seen associated topographically with erosions and peptic ulcers.[19] Chemicals (NSAIDs, bile reflux) or infectious stimuli increase the cell turnover by expanding the proliferative compartment of the glands (*neck region*), resulting in hyperplastic *foveolae* (Fig. 20-1). Atypical regeneration of the glandular neck may be difficult to differentiate from dysplastic lesions (lesions "indefinite for noninvasive neoplasia").[17,20]

Changes occurring in the oxyntic epithelia as a result of proton pump inhibitor (PPI) are sometimes considered hyperplastic changes, but they may simply represent a remodeling of the epithelial structure due to cytoskeletal rearrangements.[21]

FIGURE 20-1 Foveolar hyperplasia in antral mucosa (hyperplastic foveolae indicated by *arrows*) (hematoxylin & eosin [H&E], original magnification 25×).

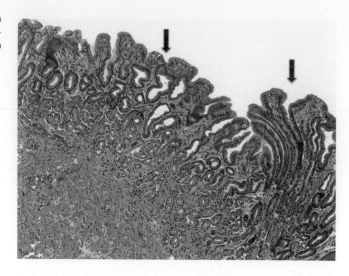

Atrophic Gastritis

Atrophic gastritis is a long-standing (and non–self-limiting) mucosal inflammatory process resulting in the loss of appropriate glands. All the histological lesions seen in nonatrophic disease may be encountered in atrophic gastritis as well. The epidemiological, clinical, and biological relationship between gastric atrophy and adenocarcinoma provides the rationale for distinguishing nonatrophic from atrophic mucosa. Gastric mucosa atrophy is seen as the "field cancerization" for the development of gastric cancer. In atrophic gastritis, (metaplastic) glands are prone to neoplastic transformation (i.e., dysplasia, noninvasive or intraepithelial neoplasia; acronyms: NiN and IEN), which may evolve into invasive adenocarcinoma.[5,22,23]

Atrophy Etiology: Environmental and Host Related

Gastric atrophy may result from both environmental and host-related factors, and the two etiologic pathways may coexist; host-related factors may modulate the atrophy risk triggered by environmental agents.[10]

Atrophy most commonly derives from *H. pylori* infection, frequently coexisting with other environmental factors (e.g., a salt-rich diet, low fruit intake, etc.).[2] At both population and individual patient levels, the risk of atrophy is modulated by interactions among bacterial factors, host-related factors, and environmental factors.

The second most incident etiology of atrophy is primarily host related and is represented by autoimmune gastritis. Autoimmune gastritis is due to immunomediated selective destruction of parietal cells, so "autoimmune atrophy" is restricted to the specialized (oxyntic) mucosa. The antibodies that destroy chief and parietal cells (which are the source of intrinsic factor) may eventually cause pernicious anemia. Pernicious anemia also may result from *H. pylori*–associated gastritis, but the two conditions can be distinguished histologically, because autoimmune gastritis spares the antrum, while it is always involved in *H. pylori* infections. Adenocarcinoma risk is largely associated with *H. pylori* infection, whereas autoimmune gastritis is predominantly associated with Type 1 neuroendocrine tumors (i.e., *carcinoid*) and much less with adenocarcinoma.

Atrophy Assessment: Noninvasive Tests

The gold standard for assessing gastric mucosal atrophy is histology. However, several serological tests (pepsinogen I [PGI], pepsinogen II [PGII], gastrin-17) are also good markers of mucosal atrophy. PGI is secreted by chief and mucous neck cells, while PGII is secreted by the same cells but also by pyloric and Brunner glands. Therefore, PG levels reflect the functional and morphological status of the stomach and the topography of the atrophic and metaplastic mucosa. Consequently, a number of studies on different ethnic populations have consistently shown that PGI or the PGI/PGII ratio is sensitive and a specific indicator of the extent of atrophic gastritis (involving the oxyntic mucosa).[24–29]

In the stomach, the gastrin-secreting cells are normally located in the antrum, so severe atrophy, whether restricted to the antrum or pan-gastric, can coincide with low plasma levels of gastrin-17. On the other hand, low gastric-17 levels are also found in acid hypersecretion, and most cases with atrophy in the corpus have hypergastrinemia due to the constantly high intragastric pH. As a result, gastrin-17 levels are clinically less useful than PGI levels or the PGI/PGII ratio for identifying atrophic gastritis. Noninvasive testing for assessing atrophy from pepsinogen levels is probably an efficient and cost-effective method to screen candidates for endoscopy in populations at high risk for gastric cancer, to confirm the presence of atrophy and the absence of noninvasive or invasive neoplasia, as well as to determine whether endoscopy surveillance is needed.[24,30,31]

Atrophy Assessment: Endoscopy and Biopsy Sampling Protocols

Except in expert (i.e., Japanese) hands, the endoscopic assessment of atrophic changes in the gastric mucosa is inconsistent, so atrophy assessment should be based on histology. A reliable assessment demands the use of a validated endoscopic biopsy sampling protocol. Based on the assumption that differing extent and topographical distribution of atrophy expresses different clinicobiological situations associated with different cancer risks, the Houston-updated Sydney System recommends taking biopsy samples from the different mucosal compartments.[14] Although various biopsy sampling protocols have been suggested, they all recommend sampling both the oxyntic and the antral mucosa (Fig. 20-2). The *incisura angularis* is the site of earliest onset of atrophic-metaplastic changes.[32]

In theory, the assessment of the extent and severity of the atrophy will be all the more reliable, the greater the number of tissue samples considered. The Sydney System and its updated 1996 Houston version recommend taking five biopsy samples representative of the oxyntic (two

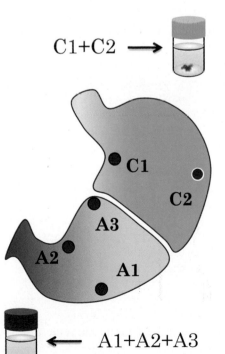

FIGURE 20-2 Biopsy sampling protocol of gastric mucosa. Biopsy sampling protocol includes two distal (antral) biopsies (A1 and A2), one biopsy obtained from the incisura angularis (A3), and two biopsy samples obtained from the corpus mucosa (C1 and C2). Biopsy samples obtained from A1, A2, and A3 can be submitted in the same vial; a distinct container should be used for the C1 and C2 biopsy samples.

C1+C2 →

A1+A2+A3

samples, one from the lesser and one from the greater curvature), antral (two samples), and incisura angularis mucosa. Unfortunately, in clinical practice, the Sydney protocol is frequently not followed. However, a more extensive sampling of the gastric mucosa may result in a more sensitive assessment of atrophy, as demonstrated in the Houston proposal).[24,25] The five-biopsy protocol is considered sufficient for routine cases, while more extensive biopsy sampling is recommended for research purposes, or to follow-up patients whose previous endoscopy disclosed the need for an "extended" histological exploration due to advanced precancerous lesions such as intraepithelial neoplasia. Additional specimens should always be obtained from any endoscopically visible focal lesions.

Finally, the manner in which biopsy samples are submitted is important, because pyloric metaplasia (mucus metaplasia) of the oxyntic mucosa can easily be confused with native antral mucosa. So, while biopsy samples obtained from the antrum and *incisura angularis* can be collected in one vial, the two oxyntic mucosa samples should be specifically identified and submitted in a separate container. The clinicopathological importance of such a distinction will be further addressed below, in the section on the histological assessment of gastric atrophy (Fig. 20-2).

Atrophy Assessment: Histology

Normal gastric biopsy samples feature different populations of glands (mucos secreting or oxyntic) that are appropriate for the functional compartment (antrum or corpus) where the specimen was obtained (i.e., they are "appropriate glands").[12] Minuscule foci of metaplastic (goblet) cells may occasionally be encountered in the foveolar epithelium (called "foveolar-restricted intestinal metaplasia"), but the overall density of appropriate glands is unaffected.

The current definition of gastric atrophy is "loss of appropriate glands." Different phenotypes may be encountered[33]:

1. Shrinkage or complete disappearance of glandular units, replaced by expanded (fibrotic) lamina propria. This situation results in a reduced glandular mass but does not imply any modification of the original cell phenotype (Figs. 20-3 and 20-4). Severe inflammation sometimes obscures the gland population (particularly in *H. pylori*–associated gastritis), making it impossible to assess atrophy reliably. Such cases should be labeled temporarily as "indefinite for atrophy" or, better still, as "inflammation precluding assessment of atrophy," and the final judgment deferred until the inflammation has regressed (e.g., after eradicating the *H. pylori* infection).
2. Replacement of the native glands by others featuring a new commitment (i.e., intestinal and/or pseudopyloric metaplasia) (Fig. 20-3). The number of glands does not necessarily decrease, but the metaplastic replacement of native glands results in a reduction of the number of glandular structures appropriate for the (antral or oxyntic) compartment considered. This condition is consistent with the definition of "loss of appropriate glands" (Fig. 20-3).

Metaplasia means the transformation of the native commitment of a cell (never associated with dedifferentiation). Any metaplastic transformation of the native gastric glands implies a reduction of the population of appropriate glandular units (i.e., atrophy). There are two main types of gastric gland metaplasia, pseudopyloric and intestinal. A third variant is so-called pseudopancreatic metaplasia, which consists of small groups of pancreatic-like glandular structures usually encountered in biopsy samples obtained from the proximal stomach. Since it has no clinical impact, "pseudopancreatic metaplasia" is considered no more than an anatomical curiosity, and it will not be further addressed here.

Pseudopyloric metaplasia (also termed spasmolytic polypeptide–expressing metaplasia or SPEM) is associated with atrophy of the oxyntic mucosa and is characterized by expression of TTF2 (Fig. 20-3). The pseudopyloric transformation may be due to an autoimmune disease

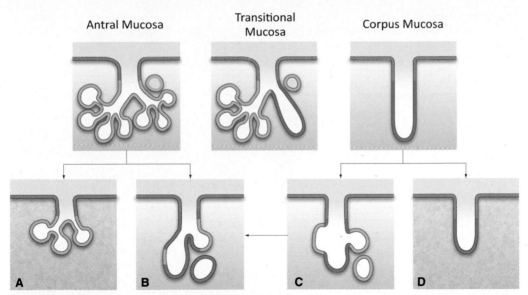

FIGURE 20-3 The cartoon shows the different types of gastric native mucosa (*yellow line* indicates mucos-secreting antral glands; *green line* indicates oxyntic glands; in between, the transitional mucosa shows both mucos-secreting and oxyntic phenotypes). Atrophic changes occurring in the different types of gastric mucosa are also shown: (**A**) Shrinkage of an antral glandular unit, partially replaced by expanded (fibrotic) lamina propria; (**B**) Metaplastic intestinalization of antral (mucos-secreting) gland (IM is indicated as *blue line*); (**C**) Metaplastic "antralization" of oxyntic gland (pseudopyloric metaplasia = *yellow line*); and (**D**) Shrinkage of an oxyntic glandular unit, partially replaced by expanded (fibrotic) lamina propria. Pseudopyloric metaplastic glands may further undergo intestinalization (**C → B**).

targeting parietal cells (corpus-restricted atrophy), to host-related factors (atrophic corpus gastritis in long-standing *H. pylori* infection), or to a combination of the two. Autoimmune corpus gastritis is the most typical setting for pseudopyloric metaplasia, which may coexist with the disappearance of glandular units, replaced by fibrosis (the nonmetaplastic atrophy variant) or intestinal metaplasia (IM). In such a setting, IM is believed to arise in oxyntic glands that were previously antralized as a result of pseudopyloric metaplasia (see below). The endoscopist should always identify the site from which the biopsy specimens are obtained, or else the pathologist is likely to overlook the fact that the antral-appearing mucosa is metaplastic. The original oxyntic

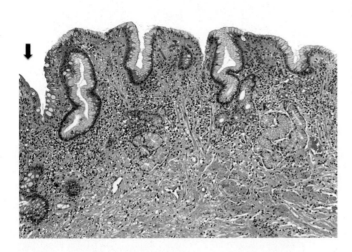

FIGURE 20-4 Atrophic gastritis: gastric biopsy (stained by H&E) shows loss of appropriate glands. The biopsy specimen shows evident reduction of glandular coils; a fibrotic expansion of the lamina propria replaces the native gland population. The *arrow* indicates a focus of coexisting intestinal metaplasia (original magnification 20×).

FIGURE 20-5 Atrophic gastritis: gastric biopsy
obtained form the oxyntic mucosa shows diffuse
pseudopyloric metaplasia. The native oxyntic
commitment of the glands is revealed by immunostain (*brown*) for PgI. No native oxyntic glands
are recognizable (= severe metaplastic [pseudopy-
loric] atrophy) (original magnification 20×).

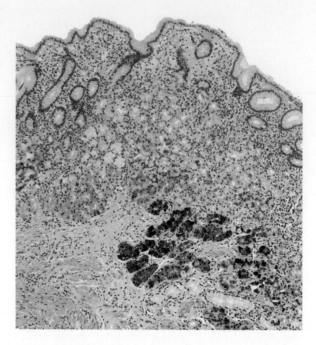

commitment of pseudopyloric epithelium can be revealed by its immunostain for pepsinogen I
(typically found in the oxyntic mucosa) (Fig. 20-5) or by a negative gastrin immunostain revealing, therefore, that the biopsy is not of antral origin.

IM (Fig. 20-6) may arise in either native mucos-secreting (antral) epithelia or previously
antralized oxyntic glands (pseudopyloric metaplasia)[34,35] (Fig. 20-3). Different subtypes of IM

FIGURE 20-6 Atrophic gastritis: gastric biopsy
obtained form the antral mucosa shows diffuse
intestinal metaplasia. No native antral glands are
recognizable (=severe metaplastic [intestinal]
atrophy (H&E, original magnification 25×).

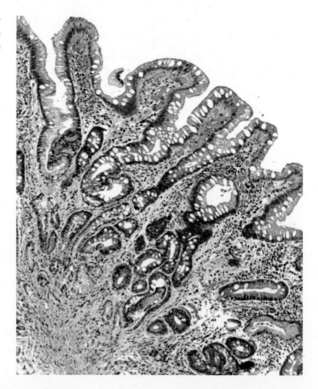

Table 20-3	Phenotypes of intestinal metaplasia		
Intestinal Metaplasia	**Hematoxylin-Eosin**	**PAS and HID**
Type I (complete, mature, small bowel type)	Columnar cells (nonsecreting, mature, absorptive)	Neutral mucins (PAS+)
	Goblet cells	Sialomucins
Type II (incomplete, immature, large bowel type)	Columnar cells (secreting, immature, nonabsorptive)	Neutral mucins (PAS+), Sialomucins
	Goblet cells	Sialomucins and Sulfomucins
Type III (incomplete, immature, large bowel type)	Columnar cells (secreting, immature, nonabsorptive)	Sulfomucins
	Goblet cells	Sialomucins and Sulfomucins

have been distinguished, based on whether the metaplastic epithelium phenotype more closely resembles large bowel epithelia (colonic-type IM) or small intestinal mucosa (small intestinal–type metaplasia). These two main variants of intestinalization can be further classified according to the histochemical type of the mucins (sialomucins or sulfomucins), established using high iron diamine (HID) histochemistry, and according to the cellular location of the mucins (in goblet and/or columnar cells). Cancer risk is thought likely to increase from Type I to Type III IM[36,37] (Table 20-3). IM subtyping is not recommended in routine practice, because there are consistent data demonstrating that the extent of gastric mucosal intestinalization parallels the occurrence of type II–III IM (colonic-type metaplasia); that is, the greater the extent of mucosal intestinalization, the greater the proportion of Type III IM. However, there is a body of evidence supporting the correlation between the extent of Type III IM and the risk of intestinal-type gastric cancer.

Yet, the clinical implications of a diagnosis of gastric IM remain debated. While in countries with high risk for gastric cancer, evaluation of serum levels of pepsinogens and endoscopic follow-up with biopsy may be encouraged, in others such as the United States, surveillance is not indicated in average-risk patients.[38] However, we and others favor an individualized management taking account not only the family history but also the patient's ethnicity and, if relevant, origin of immigration since all these are important risk factors for gastric cancer.[39]

Endocrine cell hyperplasia may be seen in gastric atrophy, and it is secondary to gastric hypochlorhydria/achlorhydria resulting from oxyntic gland loss. Hyperplasia of the antral enterochromaffin-like (ECL) cells is associated with immunomediated atrophy of the corpus mucosa (pernicious anemia) or the oxyntic diffusion of atrophy triggered by long-standing *H. pylori* infection. Neuroendocrine (nodular) tumors (well-differentiated neuroendocrine tumors; i.e., Type I carcinoids) are more common in autoimmune gastritis. It is important to mention that such tumors often regress after the source of gastrin has been removed (i.e., after antral resection), and they almost never metastasize.[40]

As in the antrum, severe inflammation sometimes (and particularly in *H. pylori*–associated gastritis) makes it impossible to determine whether glands that appear to be "lost" are merely obscured by the inflammatory infiltrate or have genuinely disappeared. In such cases, definitive assessment of atrophy should be deferred (until after the *H. pylori* infection has been eradicated, for instance). The cases can be categorized temporarily as "inflammation precluding atrophy assessment"; this category is not meant to represent a biological entity.[12]

In accord with the above criteria, an international group of gastrointestinal pathologists (the Atrophy Club) arranged the histological spectrum of atrophic changes into a formal classification

Table 20-4	Atrophy in the gastric mucosa: histological classification and grading			
		Atrophy		
0 Absent (= score 0)				
1 Indefinite (no score is applicable)				
2 Present	Histological type	Topography and key lesions		Grading
		Antrum	Corpus	
	2.1 Nonmetaplastic	Gland disappearance (shrinking) Fibrosis of the lamina propria		2.1.1 Mild = G1 (1%–30%) 2.1.2 Moderate = G2 (31%–60%) 2.1.3 Severe = G3 (>60%)
	2.2 Metaplastic	Metaplasia Intestinal	Metaplasia Pseudopyloric Intestinal	2.2.1 Mild = G1 (1%–30%) 2.2.2 Moderate = G2 (31%–60%) 2.2.3 Severe = G3 (>60%)

(Table 20-4). After testing it on actual cases, they judged its interobserver consistency in recognizing and scoring atrophic lesions to be more than adequate.[12]

The Histology Report: The OLGA-Staging System

Gastritis can be assessed on two different levels. The basic level consists in recognizing and semi-quantitatively scoring the elementary lesions at each single biopsy level (mononuclear infiltrate, activity, glandular atrophy, and so on). The hierarchically higher level involves comprehensively scoring the lesions featured by all the specimens obtained from the same anatomical compartment (antrum vs. corpus). A combined assessment should give a good global picture of the disease and of atrophy in particular.[33,41,42]

Recently, an international group of gastroenterologists and pathologists (the Operative Link on Gastritis Assessment [OLGA]) proposed a new format for reporting gastritis histology.[40] The OLGA system categorizes gastritis in five stages (from Stage 0 to Stage IV), according to the increasing extent of atrophy as histologically scored in both antral and oxyntic compartments. Consistent with the Houston-updated biopsy protocol, the OLGA proposal suggests taking five biopsies for staging purposes: one each from the greater and lesser curvatures of the distal antrum (A1 and A2, mucus-secreting mucosa), one from the lesser curvature at the *incisura angularis* (A3, where the earliest atrophic-metaplastic changes occur), and one each from the anterior and posterior walls of the proximal corpus (C1 and C2, oxyntic mucosa) (Fig. 20-2).

For each of the two mucosal compartments (mucos secreting and oxyntic), an overall atrophy score expresses the percentage of compartmental atrophic changes: the OLGA stage results from combining the overall antrum score with the overall corpus score. VASs are used to facilitate a consistent assessment for OLGA-staging purposes.[33] The OLGA report also includes etiological information, based on the recognition of specific infectious agents (*H. pylori*) or suggested by the topography/morphology of organic lesions (e.g., the corpus-prevalent location of atrophy in autoimmune gastritis). Gastritis staging helps to identify a patient's approximate position along the path to cancer, based on the notion that chronic gastritis advances from reversible inflammatory lesions (mostly limited to the antrum) at one end to atrophic changes at the other that

Atrophy Score		Corpus			
		No Atrophy (score 0)	Mild Atrophy (score 1)	Moderate Atrophy (score 2)	Severe Atrophy (score 3)
A n t r u m	No Atrophy (score 0) (including *incisura angularis*)	STAGE 0	STAGE I	STAGE II	STAGE II
	Mild Atrophy (score 1) (including *incisura angularis*)	STAGE I	STAGE I	STAGE II	STAGE III
	Moderate Atrophy (score 2) (including *incisura angularis*)	STAGE II	STAGE II	STAGE III	STAGE IV
	Severe Atrophy (score 3) (including *incisura angularis*)	STAGE III	STAGE III	STAGE IV	STAGE IV

FIGURE 20-7 The OLGA-staging system: the stage of gastritis results from combining the atrophy scores of the antral and oxyntic biopsy samples.

extensively involve both functional compartments (antrum and corpus), and is associated with the highest risk of gastric cancer.[43,44]

Ideally, atrophy is assessed on perpendicular (full-thickness) mucosal sections. At each biopsy level, atrophy is easily scored as a percentage of atrophic changes. Nonmetaplastic and metaplastic subtypes are considered together. In each biopsy sample, whatever area it comes from, atrophy is scored on a four-tiered scale (no atrophy – 0%, score 0; mild atrophy = 1%–30%, score 1; moderate atrophy = 31%–60%, score 2; severe atrophy ≥60%, score 3). It is important to note that the atrophic transformation in samples of incisura angularis mucosa is assessed only in terms of glandular shrinkage (with fibrosis of the lamina propria) or IM (replacement of the original mucos-secreting and/or oxyntic glands).

In each of the two mucosal compartments (mucos secreting and oxyntic), an overall atrophy score expresses the percentage of compartmental atrophic changes (pooling all biopsies obtained from the same functional compartment).

The scores obtained (i.e., 0, 1, 2, 3) are used for OLGA staging. The OLGA stage results from the combination of the overall antrum atrophy score with the overall corpus atrophy score (Fig. 20-7).

OTHER GASTRIC PRECANCEROUS CONDITIONS: PEPTIC ULCER AND MUCOSAL HYPERPLASIA

Gastric Ulcer Disease

Chronic gastric ulcer is a focal marker of a disease affecting the whole stomach. It is typically located at or near the atrophic border, so the presence of ulcer in the gastric corpus reflects the level of atrophic (cancer-prone) gastritis.[45–48] Epithelial dysplasia at the margins of chronic gastric ulcers can be considered the most reliable indicator of a higher ulcer-specific risk of cancer, but it must be distinguished from the hyperplastic (repair) changes frequently seen at the edge of ulcers. Such a distinction is sometimes impossible, however, in which case the histological category of "indefinite for noninvasive neoplasia" can be used.

The definition of "ulcer-related cancer" (i.e., adenocarcinoma developing in a preexisting peptic ulcer) requires evidence of a chronic ulcer existing before the malignancy and a definite demonstration of neoplastic changes (invasive or noninvasive) at the edge of the ulcer.[49]

Prudently, when a chronic gastric ulcer is first detected at endoscopy, it should be suspected of being neoplastic until histology has proven otherwise. The edge of the ulcer should be extensively "drilled" to obtain multiple biopsy samples. Because chronic ulcer is part of a whole-stomach disease, the biopsy protocol should always include sampling the oxyntic, *angularis,* and antral mucosa (as recommended for assessing gastritis).

Gastric Mucosa Hyperplasia (Diffuse or Focal/Polypoid)

A comprehensive list of polypoid lesions within gastric mucosa is given in Table 20-5 and those are discussed in Chapter 21 by Lash et al.

Gastric mucosa hyperplasia may be focal (e.g., a hyperplastic polyp) or diffuse (e.g., Ménétrier disease, also known as hyperplastic hypersecretory gastropathy). Noninvasive neoplastic foci may occur in both conditions and are thought to be the main determinant in establishing their cancer risk. The magnitude of the risk parallels the prevalence of noninvasive neoplasia.

Current information on the incidence of diffuse gastric mucosal hyperplasia is inconsistent. Generally speaking, this includes Ménétrier disease and hypertrophic gastropathy (with or without protein loss). Reports of gastric cancers associated with such diseases are largely anecdotal. Focal/polypoid hyperplasia also rarely, if ever, arises in a healthy stomach.[50,51]

In a recent retrospective study, Dirschmid et al.[50] demonstrated that hyperplastic polyps of the stomach can be considered a precancerous condition due to the different diseases coexisting with polypoid lesions (i.e., autoimmune gastritis and *H. pylori*–related gastritis). Hyperplastic polyps are common in areas where *H. pylori* infections and gastric cancers are common. Alone, their malignant potential is very low (<2%). Dysplasia reportedly occurs in 1% to 20% of cases and more frequently in larger polyps.[52] Genetic analyses suggest that simultaneous large gastric hyperplastic polyps have a clonal origin and, therefore, may be considered neoplastic. Hyperplastic polyps also may have a replication error phenotype that has been linked to cancer.[53] The discovery of hyperplastic polyps is strongly suggestive of underlying chronic gastritis and active *H. pylori* infection, so both the antral and the corpus mucosa should be sampled. Any large polyps should be removed, and any *H. pylori* infection should be treated, because the polyp often regresses following *H. pylori* eradication.

Gastritis cystica profunda is a particular hyperplastic lesion (mostly focal/polypoid) seen close to the anastomosis in patients who have undergone partial gastrectomy (Billroth II) for benign diseases. The foveolar epithelium is hyperplastic, and dilated mucos-secreting glands

Table 20-5	Epithelial gastric polyps

Neoplastic
- Adenoma (sporadic or syndromic)
- Carcinoma (primary or metastatic)
- Carcinoid (different histotypes and different clinical behaviors)

Hyperplastic/Inflammatory
- Gastritis related (infectious or chemical [reflux or NSAIDs])
- Polypoid hyperplasia near stomas, ulcers (including gastritis cystica profunda)
- Inflammatory fibroid polyp
- Xanthelasma
- Fundic gland polyp

Hamartomatous/Syndromic
- Peutz-Jeghers
- Juvenile
- Cowden disease
- Pancreatic heterotopia
- Brunner glands

are displaced in the submucosa.[54] The coexisting hyperplasia of the muscularis mucosa may contribute to the disruption of the normal mucosal architecture. Noninvasive neoplastic changes can sometimes be detected in both foveolar and metaplastic (intestinalized) epithelia, usually >10 years after the partial gastrectomy. Noninvasive neoplasia may lie behind the increased carcinoma risk, the incidence of which is three times higher in gastric remnants than in intact stomachs.[55]

In conclusion, despite much needed additional research in this field, there is a growing understanding of the preneoplastic events of the gastric carcinogenesis. Given the clear association among chronic inflammation (gastritis), gastric atrophy (both with and without IM), and increased risk of cancer, proper detection, recognition and reporting of these changes are cardinal. Consequently, appropriate patient's management taking into account individual risk for progression and meaningful surveillance guidelines will be able to be developed.

References

1. Correa P. The biological model of gastric carcinogenesis. *IARC Sci Publ.* 2004;157:301–310.
2. Uemura N, Okamoto S, Yamamoto S, et al. *Helicobacter pylori* infection and the development of gastric cancer. *N Engl J Med.* 2001;345:784–789.
3. McDonald SA, Greaves LC, Gutierrez-Gonzalez L, et al. Mechanisms of field cancerization in the human stomach: the expansion and spread of mutated gastric stem cells. *Gastroenterology.* 2008;134:500–510.
4. Karam SM. Cellular origin of gastric cancer. *Ann N Y Acad Sci.* 2008;1138:162–168.
5. Garcia S, Park HS, Novelli M, et al. Field cancerization, clonality, and epithelial stem cells: the spread of mutated clones in epithelial sheets. *J Pathol.* 1999;187:61–81.
6. Fenoglio-Preiser CM, Isaacson PG, Lantz PE, et al. *Gastrointestinal pathology: an atlas and text.* New York, NY: Lippincott Williams & Wilkins Publishers, 2007.
7. Huntsman DG, Carneiro F, Lewis FR, et al. Early gastric cancer in young, asymptomatic carriers of germ-line E-cadherin mutations. *N Engl J Med.* 2001;344:1904–1909.
8. Guilford P, Humar B, Blair V. Hereditary diffuse gastric cancer: translation of CDH1 germline mutations into clinical practice. *Gastric Cancer.* 2010;13:1–10.
9. Morson BC, Sobin LH, Grundmann E, et al. Precancerous conditions and epithelial dysplasia in the stomach. *J Clin Pathol.* 1980;33:711–721.
10. Amieva MR, El-Omar EM. Host-bacterial interactions in *Helicobacter pylori* infection. *Gastroenterology.* 2008;134:306–323.
11. Malaty HM, Graham DY. Importance of childhood socioeconomic status on the current prevalence of *Helicobacter pylori* infection. *Gut.* 1994;35:742–745.
12. Rugge M, Correa P, Dixon MF, et al. Gastric mucosal atrophy: interobserver consistency using new criteria for classification and grading. *Aliment Pharmacol Ther.* 2002;16:1249–1259.
13. Ruiz B, Garay J, Correa P, et al. Morphometric evaluation of gastric antral atrophy: improvement after cure of *Helicobacter pylori* infection. *Am J Gastroenterol.* 2001;96:3281–3287.
14. Dixon MF, Genta RM, Yardley JH, et al. Classification and grading of gastritis. The updated Sydney System. International Workshop on the Histopathology of Gastritis, Houston 1994. *Am J Surg Pathol.* 1996;20:1161–1181.
15. Alsaigh N, Odze R, Goldman H, et al. Gastric and esophageal intraepithelial lymphocytes in pediatric celiac disease. *Am J Surg Pathol.* 1996;20:865–870.
16. Yantiss RK, Odze RD. Optimal approach to obtaining mucosal biopsies for assessment of inflammatory disorders of the gastrointestinal tract. *Am J Gastroenterol.* 2009;104:774–783.
17. Owen DA. Gastritis and carditis. *Mod Pathol.* 2003;16:325–341.
18. Lynch DA, Dixon MF, Axon AT. Diagnostic criteria in lymphocytic gastritis. *Gastroenterology.* 1997;112:1426–1427.
19. Srivastava A, Lauwers GY. Pathology of non-infective gastritis. *Histopathology.* 2007;50:15–29.
20. Sepulveda AR, Patil M. Practical approach to the pathologic diagnosis of gastritis. *Arch Pathol Lab Med.* 2008;132:1586–1593.

21. Graham DY, Genta RM. Long-term proton pump inhibitor use and gastrointestinal cancer. *Curr Gastroenterol Rep.* 2008;10:543–547.

22. Rugge M, Correa P, Dixon MF, et al. Gastric dysplasia: the Padova international classification. *Am J Surg Pathol.* 2000;24:167–176.

23. Lauwers GY, Riddell RH. Gastric epithelial dysplasia. *Gut.* 1999;45:784–790.

24. Graham DY, Nurgalieva ZZ, El-Zimaity HM, et al. Noninvasive versus histologic detection of gastric atrophy in a Hispanic population in North America. *Clin Gastroenterol Hepatol.* 2006;4:306–314.

25. Graham DY, Kato M, Asaka M. Gastric endoscopy in the 21st century: appropriate use of an invasive procedure in the era of non-invasive testing. *Dig Liver Dis.* 2008;40:497–503.

26. Sipponen P, Graham DY. Importance of atrophic gastritis in diagnostics and prevention of gastric cancer: application of plasma biomarkers. *Scand J Gastroenterol.* 2007;42:2–10.

27. Dinis-Ribeiro M, da Costa-Pereira A, Lopes C, et al. Validity of serum pepsinogen I/II ratio for the diagnosis of gastric epithelial dysplasia and intestinal metaplasia during the follow-up of patients at risk for intestinal-type gastric adenocarcinoma. *Neoplasia.* 2004;6:449–456.

28. Miki K, Morita M, Sasajima M, et al. Usefulness of gastric cancer screening using the serum pepsinogen test method. *Am J Gastroenterol.* 2003;98:735–739.

29. Ren JS, Kamangar F, Qiao YL, et al. Serum pepsinogens and risk of gastric and esophageal cancers in the General Population Nutrition Intervention Trial cohort. *Gut.* 2009;58:636–642.

30. Graham DY, Rugge M. Clinical practice: diagnosis and evaluation of dyspepsia. *J Clin Gastroenterol.* 2010;44:167–172.

31. Graham DY, Asaka M. Eradication of gastric cancer and more efficient gastric cancer surveillance in Japan: two peas in a pod. *J Gastroenterol.* 2010;45:1–8.

32. Mastracci L, Bruno S, Spaggiari P, et al. The impact of biopsy number and site on the accuracy of intestinal metaplasia detection in the stomach A morphometric study based on virtual biopsies. *Dig Liver Dis.* 2008;40:632–640.

33. Rugge M, Correa P, Di Mario F, et al. OLGA staging for gastritis: a tutorial. *Dig Liver Dis.* 2008; 40:650–658.

34. Filipe MI. Mucins in the human gastrointestinal epithelium: a review. *Invest Cell Pathol.* 1979;2: 195–216.

35. Jass JR. Role of intestinal metaplasia in the histogenesis of gastric carcinoma. *J Clin Pathol.* 1980;33: 801–810.

36. Jass JR, Filipe MI. The mucin profiles of normal gastric mucosa, intestinal metaplasia and its variants and gastric carcinoma. *Histochem J.* 1981;13:931–939.

37. Pagnini CA, Bozzola L. Precancerous significance of colonic type intestinal metaplasia. *Tumori.* 1981;67:113–116.

38. Fennerty MB. Gastric intestinal metaplasia on routine endoscopic biopsy. *Gastroenterology.* 2003;125: 586–590.

39. Hirota WK, Zuckerman MJ, Adler DG, et al. ASGE guideline: the role of endoscopy in the surveillance of premalignant conditions of the upper GI tract. *Gastrointest Endosc.* 2006;63:570–580.

40. Rindi G, Kloppel G. Endocrine tumors of the gut and pancreas tumor biology and classification. *Neuroendocrinology.* 2004;80(Suppl 1):12–15.

41. Sipponen P, Stolte M. Clinical impact of routine biopsies of the gastric antrum and body. *Endoscopy.* 1997;29:671–678.

42. Rugge M, Genta RM. Staging gastritis: an international proposal. *Gastroenterology.* 2005;129: 1807–1808.

43. Rugge M, Meggio A, Pennelli G, et al. Gastritis staging in clinical practice: the OLGA staging system. *Gut.* 2007;56:631–636.

44. Rugge M, de Boni M, Pennelli G, et al. Gastritis OLGA-staging and gastric cancer risk: a twelve year clinico-pathological follow-up study. *Aliment Pharmacol Ther.* 2010;31:1104–1111.

45. Correa P. The epidemiology and pathogenesis of chronic gastritis: three etiologic entites. *Front Gastrointest Res.* 1980;6:98–108.

46. Dore MP, Graham DY. Ulcers and gastritis. *Endoscopy.* 2010;42:38–41.

47. Pang SH, Leung WK, Graham DY. Ulcers and gastritis. *Endoscopy.* 2008;40:136–139.

48. Sung JJ, Kuipers EJ, El-Serag HB. Systematic review: update on the global incidence and prevalence of peptic ulcer disease. *Aliment Pharmacol Ther.* 2009;29:938–946.

49. MacDonald WC, Owen DA. Gastric carcinoma after surgical treatment of peptic ulcer: an analysis of morphologic features and a comparison with cancer in the nonoperated stomach. *Cancer*. 2001;91: 1732–1738.
50. Dirschmid K, Platz-Baudin C, Stolte M. Why is the hyperplastic polyp a marker for the precancerous condition of the gastric mucosa? *Virchows Arch*. 2006;448:80–84.
51. Oberhuber G, Stolte M. Gastric polyps: an update of their pathology and biological significance. *Virchows Arch*. 2000;437:581–590.
52. Carmack SW, Genta RM, Graham DY, et al. Management of gastric polyps: a pathology-based guide for gastroenterologists. *Nat Rev Gastroenterol Hepatol*. 2009;6:331–341.
53. Abraham SC, Park SJ, Lee JH, et al. Genetic alterations in gastric adenomas of intestinal and foveolar phenotypes. *Mod Pathol*. 2003;16:786–795.
54. Franzin G, Novelli P. Gastritis cystica profunda. *Histopathology*. 1981;5:535–547.
55. Lim JK, Jang YJ, Jung MK, et al. Menetrier disease manifested by polyposis in the gastric antrum and coexisting with gastritis cystica profunda. *Gastrointest Endosc*. 2010; In Press.

21

Gastric Polyps

▶ Richard H. Lash
▶ Shawn Kinsey
▶ Robert M. Genta
▶ Gregory Y. Lauwers

INTRODUCTION

Gastric polyps are typically found incidentally during upper endoscopy performed for unrelated reasons, as most do not cause clinical symptoms or signs. They are found in about 4% of upper endoscopic procedures, and the relative frequency of each type depends on several factors, including the prevalence of *Helicobacter pylori* infection. Gastric polyps, once detected, may have significant clinical implications, and accurate histopathologic diagnosis is of paramount importance to ensure proper management. This chapter reviews the clinical and pathologic characteristics of both common and uncommon gastric polyps. In addition to the pathologic features of gastric polyps themselves, substantial information about their etiology can be gleaned from the evaluation of the unaffected gastric mucosa and is briefly discussed. Although most gastroenterologists are aware of this fact, in our experience proper sampling of adjacent mucosa is uncommonly performed at the time of polypectomy.

EPIDEMIOLOGY

Published data on the epidemiology of gastric polyps diverge substantially with regard to both absolute and relative prevalence, largely due to variations in the population studied, including age, gender, the prevalence of underlying gastric conditions, the detection methodology used, and the accuracy of the pathologic diagnosis. In general, pathology-based series, in which the denominator is the total of gastric biopsies sampled, are useful to determine the relative frequency of the various types of polyps.[1–10] Regarding prevalence, retrospective reviews of endoscopic reports are likely to underestimate the true rates, because all polyps are typically not excised and characterized,[11,12] while prospective evaluations are necessarily limited to relatively small numbers of patients in single institutions, with resulting population and expertise biases. These pitfalls must be kept in mind when interpreting the prevalence data in Table 21-1.

A diverse array of polyps and polypoid lesions may be found in the stomach. Polyps may be epithelial (e.g., fundic gland, adenomatous), neuroendocrine (e.g., carcinoid), lymphohistiocytic (e.g., xanthelasma, lymphoid hyperplasia), mesenchymal (e.g., gastrointestinal [GI] stromal, neural, vascular), or mixed. Some are sporadic and some syndromic. This review excludes carcinomas, lymphomas, carcinoids, mesenchymal tumors, and all other malignancies, which are discussed in other chapters.

Table 21-1	Gastric polyp prevalence studies, including year published and number of years during which polyps were collected							
Authors	Country	Pub. Year	Years	No. Polyps	Hyperplastic	Fundic Gland	Adenoma	Carcinoma
Carmack et al.[1]	United States	2009	1	7,878	14.3%	77.0%	0.7%	1.35%
Morais et al.[12]	Brazil	2007	5	153	71.30%	16.30%	12.40%	2%
Gencosmanoglu et al.[4]	Turkey	2003	5	150	64%**	14%	3%	NR
Ljubicic et al.[10]	Croatia	2002	1	42	50%	7%	17%	NR
Sivelli et al.[9]	Italy	2002	6	164	44.50%	NR	16.40%	0.60%
Attard et al.[23]	United States–pediatric*	2002	18	41	42%	40%	5%	NR
Papa et al.[6]	Italy	1998	7	121	55.4%	3.3%	9.90%	0.8%
Archimandritis et al.[11]	Greece	1996	4	258	75.6%	NR	6.60%	NR
Stolte et al.[2]	Germany	1994	20	5515	28.3%	47%	9%	7.20%
Rattan et al.[7]	Israel	1993	8	188	45.2%	NR	3.2%	5.3%
Roseau et al.[8]	France	1990	4	191	25.1%	9.9%	3.1%	NR
Deppish et al.[3]	United States	1989	10	121	75%	17%	8.60%	NR
Niv et al.[5]	Israel	1985	8	99	23.2%	17.2%	10.1%	NR
Laxen et al.[67]	Finland	1982	10	357	55%**	NR	8%	NR

*10% reported as hamartomatous.
**Includes polypoid foveolar hyperplasia.
NR, not reported.

Source: Modified from Carmack SW, Genta RM, Schuler CM, et al. The current spectrum of gastric polyps: a 1-year national study of over 120,000 patients. *Am J Gastroenterol.* 2009;104:1524–1532.

FUNDIC GLAND POLYPS

Fundic gland polyps (FGPs) are the most common type of polyps detected at Esophago-gastro-dvodenoscopy (EGD) in Western countries (up to 50%),[13] apparently due to the relatively low incidence of *H. pylori* infection and relatively high level of proton pump inhibitor (PPI) use.[1] In fact, FGPs are negatively associated with *H. pylori* infection.[13–16] This negative association is further, if indirectly, supported by reports of the disappearance of FGPs upon *H. pylori* infection and their subsequent recurrence after eradication.[17]

The reported prevalence of FGPs ranges from 3.2% to 11%.[18–20] While most FGPs are sporadic, they were originally described in patients with familial adenomatous polyposis (FAP) syndrome.[21–23] Sporadic FGPs are most prevalent among middle-aged women,[13,15,19] although this gender difference is not observed in all studies. Among FAP patients, the prevalence of FGPs is much higher than in the general population, occurs at a younger age, and is equally likely to develop in both genders.[13,22]

Endoscopically, FGPs appear as smooth, glassy, sessile, circumscribed elevations in the oxyntic mucosa, usually measuring <0.5 cm. Sporadic polyps are typically single or few; however, in PPI users, there may be large numbers of polyps, although these may regress with cessation of therapy.[24] In contrast, syndromic patients may have 50 polyps or more, sometimes becoming confluent and measuring as large as 5 to 8 cm ("giant FGPs").[25]

Histologically, FGPs comprise cystically dilated oxyntic glands, with the lining cells appearing variably flattened or hobnail-like (Fig. 21-1A and B). These lining cells may become difficult to recognize as oxyntic when markedly dilated (Fig. 21-2). While dysplasia is frequent in FAP patients with FGPs (up to half), almost all are low-grade.[21,22] In sporadic cases, true dysplasia is very unusual, and high-grade dysplasia is distinctly rare.[26] Given the extreme rarity of advanced gastric neoplasia in patients with FGPs, we recommend being very conservative in the interpretation of focal nuclear enlargement of the pit epithelium that occasionally occurs in FGPs and is likely not biologically true dysplasia. Nevertheless, when multiple FGPs are diagnosed in a young patient and when true dysplasia is encountered, FAP should be considered, and it is incumbent upon the pathologist to alert the clinician about this possibility.

Little is known about the etiology of FGPs. In the past, these polyps were considered to be hamartomatous; however, the recently recognized association of FGPs with long-term use of PPIs suggests that mechanisms related to the suppression of acid secretion may be involved in their pathogenesis.[27] In recent years, there has been somewhat conflicting evidence of genetic alterations in sporadic and syndromic FGPs that are intriguing but do little to further our understanding of pathogenesis or enhance our ability to discern these two pathogenic types. For example, the Wnt signaling pathway is implicated in both syndromic and sporadic FGPs. Also, up to 75% of patients with FAP-associated polyps demonstrate a somatic second-hit mutation of the *APC* gene that leads to the inactivation of both copies of this tumor suppressor gene and occurs independently of the presence of histologic dysplasia.[28–30] While most sporadic FGPs are devoid of APC mutations and 65% to 90% harbor somatic mutations in the β-catenin gene,[28–30] rare cases of sporadic dysplastic FGP have been shown to demonstrate APC mutations without β-catenin mutations.[28,31] In addition, methylation of promoters of genes associated with gastric cancer has been observed in a small proportion of FGPs and mainly affects the promoters of the p16 and p14 genes.[32] Finally, tuberin has been hypothesized to play a role in the pathogenesis of sporadic FGPs with loss of tuberin nuclear expression and its cytoplasmic accumulation associated with loss of negative regulation of nuclear glucocorticoid receptors.[33]

For the typical patient on PPI therapy with multiple small (<0.5 cm) FGPs, a biopsy of one polyp should suffice to confirm the diagnosis. Biopsy specimens should be taken from all polyps ranging from 0.5 to 1 cm. It is not recommended to discontinue PPI therapy for these patients with smaller polyps. Larger polyps (>1 cm) should also be removed, and PPI therapy discontinued in these patients, if clinically appropriate.

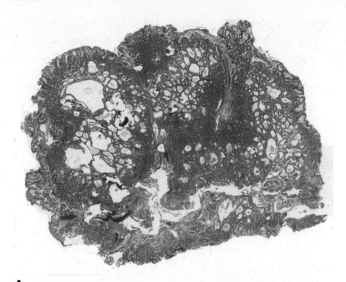

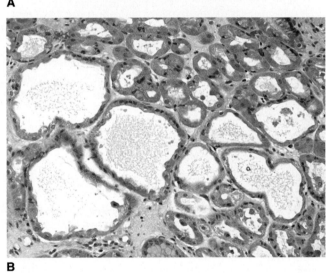

FIGURE 21-1 Fundic gland polyps at low magnification with a smooth surface (**A**) and dilated oxyntic glands (**B**).

A

B

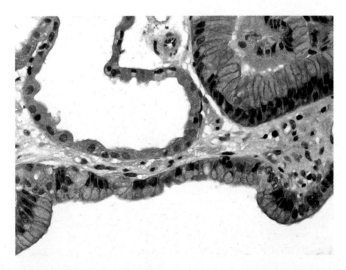

FIGURE 21-2 Fundic gland polyps at high magnification showing the lining of the dilated glands, which include a mixture of oxyntic and mucinous cells.

Since some studies have suggested that FGPs are associated with a higher frequency of colonic adenoma, some authors have recommended that a colonoscopy be performed when FGPs are diagnosed.[19,34–36] However, a recent study by Genta et al. of over 100,000 patients with simultaneous EGD and colonoscopy, >6,000 of whom had FGPs, found that there was no relationship between the presence of sporadic FGPs and neoplasia elsewhere in the GI tract. They concluded that the detection of sporadic FGPs does not warrant the performance of a colonoscopy.[13]

HYPERPLASTIC POLYPS

Hyperplastic polyps are traditionally believed to arise most frequently in patients with an inflamed or atrophic gastric mucosa.[37] In the industrialized world, both their absolute and relative prevalence has been decreasing along with the declining prevalence of *H. pylori* infection.[38,39] In a review of almost 8,000 gastric polyps examined over a 1-year period, only 14.3% were hyperplastic.[1] Solid organ transplantation has also been reported as a risk factor, with as many as 15% of hyperplastic polyps arising in transplant patients.[40,41] Hyperplastic polyps usually arise in adults (mean age: 60 years), and in most studies, a female predominance is reported, although others report an equal sex ratio or even a male predominance.[12,42,43]

Hyperplastic polyps are multiple in about 20% of the patients and are more frequently observed in the antrum. They are usually small (0.5–1.5 cm) with a smooth, dome shape, but they may grow much larger, becoming lobulated and pedunculated, some with surface erosions (Fig. 21-3).[42,44] Protracted erosion may result in chronic blood loss and iron-deficiency anemia, one of the most common clinical manifestations of these polyps. Gastric outlet obstruction has also been described for large antral polyps that protrude into the duodenal lumen.[45,46] Nevertheless, most hyperplastic polyps remain asymptomatic.

Hyperplastic gastric polyps comprise both epithelial and stromal components in varying proportions. There are elongated, grossly distorted, branching and dilated foveolae lying in an edematous stroma rich in vasculature and sparse, haphazardly distributed smooth muscle bundles along with a variable degree of chronic and active inflammatory cells (Fig. 21-4). The epithelial lining consists of a single layer of regularly arranged hypertrophic foveolar epithelium containing abundant neutral mucin. In some regions, the cells may be cuboidal with a granular eosinophilic cytoplasm.[47,48] Parietal and chief cells are uncommon, even in polyps from the corpus. Intestinal metaplasia may be seen but is rarely a conspicuous feature. At the smaller end of the spectrum, it may be difficult to distinguish exuberant reactive gastropathy (i.e., "polypoid foveolar hyperplasia") from a small hyperplastic gastric polyp; the latter term may be best used

FIGURE 21-3 Hyperplastic polyp at low magnification, highlighting the dominant stromal component that characterizes these polyps.

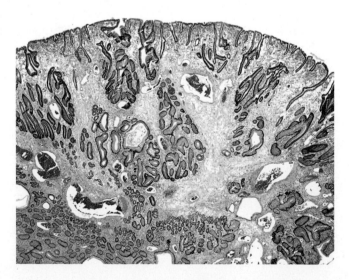

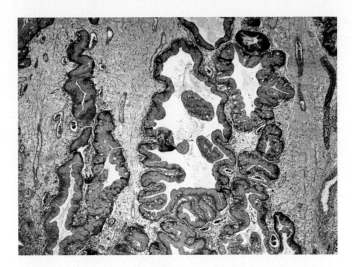

FIGURE 21-4 Hyperplastic polyp at high magnification showing elongated and dilated foveolae.

when the endoscopist identifies a discrete polypoid lesion. Finally, other hamartomatous polyps (see below) can be histologically indistinguishable from hyperplastic gastric polyps and can be discerned only in the proper clinical context.

It is believed that hyperplastic gastric polyps arise as a hyperproliferative foveolar response to tissue injury (erosions or ulcers) (Fig. 21-5). Foveolar hyperplasia has long been recognized as a fundamental feature of chemical gastropathy[49] (caused by bile reflux or NSAIDs) and, to a lesser extent, of *H. pylori* gastritis.[50] Polypoid foveolar hyperplasia, gastric foveolar polyps, gastritis cystica polyposa (characteristic of post Billroth I and II gastric stumps), and gastric hyperplastic polyps are considered variants of the same basic hyperproliferative disturbance. Removal of the underlying injury (e.g., eradication of *H. pylori* infection) resulted in regression of hyperplastic polyps in 70% of patients in one study.[51,52] Both isolated hyperplastic polyps and the polypoid lesions found at gastrectomy sites have a low but definite potential for the development of carcinoma. Between 1% and 20% of hyperplastic polyps have been reported to harbor foci of dysplasia; furthermore, mutations of the p53 gene, chromosomal aberrations, and microsatellite instability have been detected in these polyps.[43,53–55] (Fig. 21-6). The overall prevalence of dysplasia in hyperplastic polyps is most frequently reported at <2%, but higher frequencies have been noted in large polyps (>2 cm).[48,56] These data from academic centers are likely overestimating the actual rate of dysplasia found in routine practice; nevertheless, large hyperplastic polyps should be completely excised for thorough histologic evaluation. If dysplasia or intramucosal carcinoma is present,

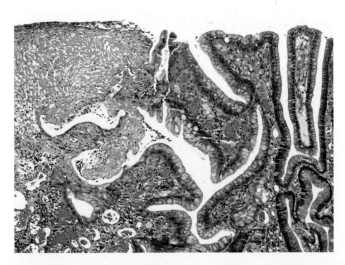

FIGURE 21-5 Hyperplastic polyp with erosion, a common feature of these polyps.

FIGURE 21-6 Low-grade dysplasia in a hyperplastic polyp.

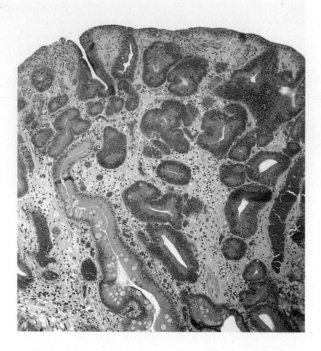

complete removal would be expected to result in a cure. When present, most adenocarcinomas are well-differentiated, but rare cases of signet-ring cell carcinoma have been reported.[57] The risk of malignant transformation correlates with size,[43] and the two most common underlying etiologies of carcinoma arising in hyperplastic polyps are autoimmune gastritis and *H. pylori*[37,58] with the risk correlating with the severity of gastric mucosal atrophy, especially in the gastric corpus.[59] Because of this association with gastric atrophy and intestinal metaplasia, two well-known risk factors of gastric cancer,[37] hyperplastic polyps can be seen as surrogate markers for cancer risk, and synchronous or metachronous gastric cancer has been reported in 4% to 6% of cases. Therefore, when a hyperplastic polyp (with or without dysplasia) is diagnosed, a set of topographically defined biopsy specimens (following the guidelines of the Updated Sydney System[60]) should be obtained. If *H. pylori* gastritis is present, eradication is warranted with a follow-up endoscopy after several months to monitor not only cure of the infection but also the presence or regression of polyps.[51,52] If extensive metaplastic atrophy is found, the patient should be considered at risk for gastric cancer, and an individualized surveillance plan (for which guidelines do not yet exist) should be implemented.[37] If a hyperplastic polyp without dysplasia is obtained from a gastrectomy site, the optimal management remains uncertain.

Gastric hyperplastic polyposis (characterized by the presence of 50 or more hyperplastic polyps) has been described but remains very rare.[61] Finally, another rare variant, the so-called inverted hyperplastic polyp, is caused by a dense submucosal glandular proliferation with cystic dilatation leading to a polyp covered by normal-appearing mucosa. These may be related to *gastritis cystica profunda*,[62] and one case of malignant transformation has been reported.[63]

INTESTINAL-TYPE ADENOMATOUS POLYPS

Gastric intestinal-type adenomas may occur either sporadically or in association with FAP. They are most common in patients over 50 years of age and three times more frequent in men. Their prevalence varies widely, estimated at 0.5% to 3.75% in Western countries and 9% to 27% in areas with higher rates of gastric carcinoma, such as China and Japan.[2,64,65] In a 2008 Caris series, they represented <0.7% of approximately 8,000 gastric polyps detected in a cohort of over 121,000 U.S. patients (as compared to FGPs comprising 77%).[1]

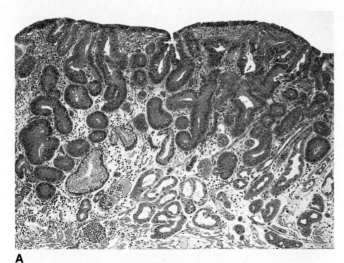

A

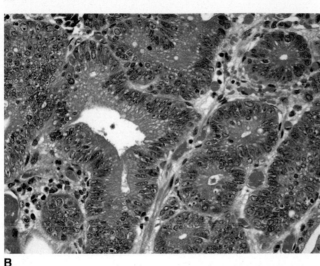

B

FIGURE 21-7 **A,B:** Intestinal-type adenomatous polyp, at low (**A**) and high magnification (**B**), with characteristic epithelial dysplasia.

Endoscopically, intestinal-type adenomas are usually solitary (82%), circumscribed, and pedunculated or sessile. Most are found in the lesser curve of the antrum or angulus, typically <2 cm in diameter, with a velvety, lobulated surface.[66] Histologically, epithelial dysplasia is the hallmark, with surface proliferation, loss of mucin, and pencillate, pseudostratified, and hyperchromatic nuclei, analogous to those found in colonic adenomas (Fig. 21-7A and B). The criteria for high-grade dysplasia are also the same as for colonic adenomas (architectural complexity including cribriform growth along with the nuclear changes of further enlargement and rounding, loss of polarity, and cleared irregular chromatin with large nucleoli). Unlike in the colon, however, where the virtual absence of lymphatics in the *lamina propria* results in minimal risk of metastasis and allows for intramucosal carcinoma to be combined under the terminological umbrella of "high-grade dysplasia," the lamina propria of the stomach is rich in lymphatics, and intramucosal carcinoma (defined as infiltrating glands in the *lamina propria*) is important to distinguish.

Sporadic adenomatous polyps (i.e., polypoid dysplasia) are precursors of intestinal-type gastric adenocarcinoma. Both conditions arise most often in patients with chronic atrophic gastritis with intestinal metaplasia, and they share a common epidemiology. The larger the adenoma, the greater is the probability that it contains foci of high-grade dysplasia and adenocarcinoma, as up to 50% of adenomatous polyps larger than 2 cm harbor a focus of adenocarcinoma.[67] Additionally, a synchronous adenocarcinoma in another area of the stomach has been found in up to 30% of patients with an adenomatous polyp.[67,68] COX-2 has been reported to be overexpressed in 79% of cases, showing a correlation with high-grade dysplasia, size >1 cm, and presence of a synchronous carcinoma.[69]

The management approach to gastric intestinal-type adenomas has not changed significantly, Gastric mapping is useful to determine the phenotype of gastritis in which the adenoma arises; metaplastic atrophic gastritis with an adenoma is an indication for a surveillance program.[70] In addition, synchronous adenocarcinoma should be excluded, and complete excision of the adenoma should be confirmed with a follow-up endoscopy. The guidelines of the American Society of Gastrointestinal Endoscopy recommend endoscopic surveillance at 1-year follow-up for patients with gastric adenoma and recommend that specific biopsy techniques be implemented when large or multiple polyps exist.[70]

NONINTESTINAL-TYPE GASTRIC ADENOMAS

Unlike the classic intestinal-type gastric adenoma described above, the more recently recognized nonintestinal types of adenomas are much less common, are characterized by gastric rather than intestinal differentiation, and are more difficult to diagnose. Their biologic behavior is not as well characterized as intestinal-type gastric adenomas.

Pyloric Gland Adenoma

The characteristics of pyloric gland adenomas were described in 1990 by Borchard et al.[71] and Jass et al.[72] Like intestinal-type adenomas, these polyps often occur in a background of autoimmune gastritis or *H. pylori* infection. The mean age of these patients is 70 years, with a threefold predominance in women, corresponding to the high prevalence autoimmune gastritis in that population. Although 85% of pyloric gland adenomas occur in the stomach, they also can be found in the duodenum, gall bladder, bile duct, pancreatic duct, and the uterine cervix.[73]

Histologically, pyloric gland adenomas are composed of closely packed pyloric-type glands, lined by cuboidal or columnar mucus-secreting cells, forming a nodule that, although discrete, is less easy to discern from adjacent normal tissue than an intestinal-type adenoma. (Fig. 21-8) Notably, the apical mucin caps that characterize foveolar cells are lacking, as are prominent nucleoli.[74] The mucin is immunoreactive to antibodies directed at MUC 6 (Table 21-2). In contrast to the dysplasia found in classic intestinal-type adenomas, "dysplasia" in pyloric gland adenomas ranges from very subtle (*sc.* undetectable) to appreciable (Fig. 21-9), and some authors have used a three-tier system: none, low-grade, and high-grade.[74] In one study, 30% contained an invasive adenocarcinoma.[73] While this study may overestimate the risk at large, the reported risk of progression suggests that complete removal of these polyps is advised.

FIGURE 21-8 Pyloric gland adenoma. The atypical glands are characterized by low columnar to cuboidal cells with eosinophilic cytoplasm and round nuclei.

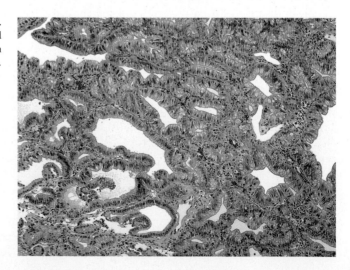

Table 21-2	Immunophenotypic expression of gastric adenomas			
	CD10	MUC2	MUC5AC	MUC6
Intestinal type	Expressed on the luminal surface along the apical membrane	Positive goblet cells are distributed in the upper portion of adenoma glands	Adenoma cells are negative. Residual nondysplastic glands are positive	Negative
Foveolar adenoma	Generally negative	Positive cells in intestinal metaplasia and few scattered in adenoma	Positive	Positive in adenoma cells deep in the mucosa
Mixed gastric and intestinal type (incomplete intestinal type)	Negative in adenoma tissue	Positive adenoma cells are in the mid to superficial layer	Most adenoma positive cells distributed superficially	Positive adenoma cells distributed basally
Pyloric gland adenoma	Generally negative	Generally negative	Positive in the foveolae on the surface and in some pyloric type glands	Strongly positive in pyloric type glands. Foveolar-like structures are negative

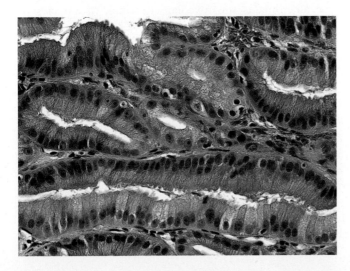

FIGURE 21-9 Pyloric gland adenoma. The dysplasia is more subtle and does not resemble that of intestinal-type adenomas.

FIGURE 21-10 A,B: Foveolar adenoma (low and high magnification). Note the sharp demarcation between the normal (right) and atypical (left) foveolar cells.

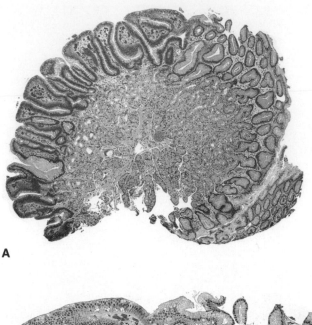

A

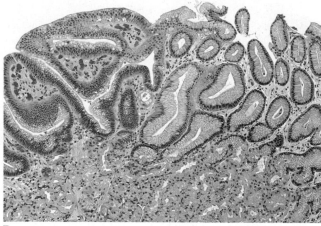

B

Foveolar Adenoma

The other nonintestinal, gastric-type adenoma is the foveolar adenoma. In a series of 69 cases of gastric dysplasia removed endoscopically, foveolar dysplasia represented 21.7% of the cases and intestinal/adenomatous dysplasia 45% of the cases, with hybrid cases representing the difference.[75,76] There is a report of increased incidence of foveolar adenomas in patients with FAP with only rare sporadic examples, but in our practice, we find the opposite to be true.

Foveolar adenomas, like pyloric gland adenomas, can be deceptively bland (Fig. 21-10A and B). They are formed by a superficial epithelial proliferation that may impart a villous or papillary configuration. The superficial location of the proliferation is in contradistinction to pyloric gland adenomas. The lining cells are tall columnar with a low nuclear-cytoplasmic ratio and an apical neutral mucin cap, resembling normal (albeit larger) foveolar cells. Nuclei may also be more elongated and stratified than normal.[74] Intestinal metaplasia is not a feature of these polyps or the uninvolved gastric mucosa. The biologic nature of these polyps is still unknown, although in one series the dysplasia was reported to be more commonly high-grade than in intestinal-type adenomas (Fig. 21-11).[75,76] Rarely, they may develop into adenocarcinomas (Fig. 21-12A and B).

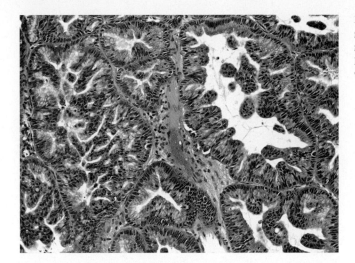

FIGURE 21-11 Foveolar adenoma high-grade dysplasia characterized by complex glands of variable size and shape with papillary infoldings, serration, and cystic dilatation.

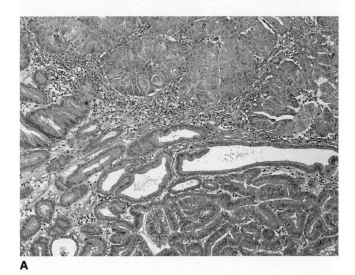

A

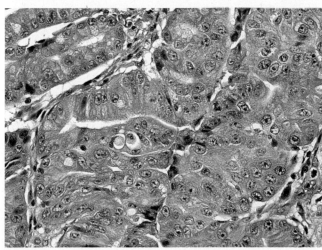

B

FIGURE 21-12 **A,B:** Foveolar adenoma with progression into a moderately differentiated adenocarcinoma (**A**); higher magnification of the adenocarcinoma component (**B**).

FIGURE 21-13 **A:** Chief cell adenoma. There is absence of parietal cells within the polyp, and some of the nuclei are large. The lesion contained only rare mitoses. **B:** Chief cell adenoma at higher magnification. Considerable nuclear polymorphism is noted.

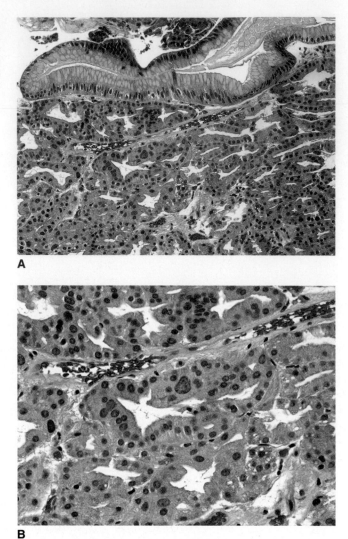

A

B

Chief Cell "Adenoma"

There are very few reports in the literature of lesions that are composed entirely of chief cells and these have been referred to as chief cell proliferation, hyperplasia, and adenoma. They have been described as irregular tubules composed of chief cells with nuclear atypia but without mitotic activity[77,78] (Fig. 21-13A and B). In addition, there are also reports of polyps similar to these but composed entirely of oxyntic mucosa. It remains to be determined if these lesions truly represent a neoplasm and if so, what their biological behavior is.[79]

POLYPOSIS SYNDROMES

Polyposis syndromes affecting the stomach are rare, and patients with these syndromes often present with clinical manifestations unrelated to gastric polyps. However, some cases of juvenile polyposis may affect the stomach alone.[80,81] The histologic features of the hamartomatous polyps found in juvenile polyposis, Cronkite-Canada syndrome, and Cowden disease essentially overlap those of hyperplastic gastric polyps, and therefore the diagnosis of a syndromic polyp must rest upon a high index of suspicion, as when polyps are multiple and/or there is suggestive clinical

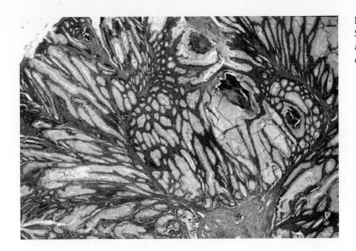

FIGURE 21-14 Peutz-Jeghers polyp. Smooth muscles are present, but not as arborizing as seen in small intestinal examples.

context.[82,83] By contrast, hamartomatous polyps in patients with the Peutz-Jeghers (PJ) syndrome (PJS) are more readily recognized histologically (see below).

Peutz-Jeghers Polyps

Although solitary PJ gastric polyps have been described, they are very rare and most cases are seen in the context of PJS.[84,85] This autosomal dominant syndrome is rare, with a prevalence estimated to be about 1/200,000. The clinical criteria required to make this diagnosis are (a) the presence of at least two PJ polyps or (b) the presence of one PJ polyp and either characteristic mucosal pigmentation or a family history of PJ polyps.[86] These hamartomatous polyps develop all along the GI tract but are more frequent in the small intestine (90%) than in the colon (78%) or stomach (74%). While classically described as pedunculated, PJ polyps tend to be sessile when located in the stomach.[87] The core of the polyps is composed of branching bundles of smooth muscles emerging from the *muscularis mucosae*, extending well into the peripheral portions of the polyp, along with a paucity of stromal edema and inflammation in the *lamina propria*. The epithelium is frequently hyperplastic but follows closely the underlying stroma. Note that the characteristic features of PJ polyps in the stomach are typically more subtle than the classic examples in the small bowel, with thinner and less arborizing smooth muscle bundles, and as a result are often mistaken for hyperplastic gastric polyps (Fig. 21-14).[81]

Individuals with PJS are at risk for cancer at a young age in a wide variety of organs, including breast, colon, pancreas, stomach, small intestine, ovaries, uterus, and testes. The lifetime risk for gastric cancer has been estimated to be around 30% in patients with PJS[88]; therefore, most authorities suggest surveillance of the stomach and small intestine with upper endoscopy and small bowel series, starting at 18 years of age.[89] Surveillance should continue every 2 to 3 years if polyps are noted at baseline evaluation.[80,90] However, the origin of GI adenocarcinomas that arise in patients with PJS is still a subject of debate. Some studies have confirmed the hamartomatous nature of the polyp by proving they are polyclonal.[91,92] However, other studies have described dysplasia in PJ polyps, supporting a neoplastic and premalignant condition.[93,94]

Molecular analysis of PJ polyps has yielded some insight into pathogenesis and biology. In up to 80% of patients, there is a germline mutation of the STK11/LKB1 gene that encodes the enzyme serine/threonine kinase, which is responsible for cell division, differentiation, and signal transduction.[87] Notably, truncation mutations, which are observed in about 75% of patients, tend to be associated with a higher frequency of gastric involvement and a higher risk of developing carcinoma than nonsense mutations.[94] As COX-2 has been reported to be upregulated in such lesions, the use of COX-2 inhibitors has been recommended in patients with severe gastric involvement, and their use has been proven to actually decrease the number of gastric polyps.[95]

Juvenile Polyposis

Juvenile Polyposis (JP) is a rare autosomal dominant disease with variable penetrance that is characterized by the presence of multiple juvenile polyps throughout the GI tract and is associated with an increased risk of cancer.[96] The clinical criteria for the diagnosis of JP include (a) the presence of at least five juvenile polyps in the colon, (b) the presence of juvenile polyps throughout the GI tract, or (c) the presence of single or multiple juvenile polyps in a patient with an established family history of JP.[97] While reported to be more common in the antrum,[98] gastric juvenile polyps have also been described in the body and fundus.[98–100] As described above, these polyps are histologically indistinguishable from hyperplastic gastric polyps and are only suspected when they are multiple or associated with juvenile polyps elsewhere in the GI tract.

Data regarding gastric malignancy in the setting of JP are limited, but the risk in patients with this condition is estimated to be 15% to 20%. Although the underlying mechanisms that predispose these patients to cancer remain unknown, the development of cancer seems to follow a dysplasia-carcinoma sequence, with the risk increasing with the size of the polyps.[101] Germline mutations of SMAD4 or BMPR1A, two genes that are implicated in the TGFβ-signaling pathway, are the most common encountered genetic abnormalities in JP, each representing 20% of the genetic alterations,[96,99,102] but this genotypic-phenotypic association remains controversial.[100] Given the present data it seems reasonable to offer gastric endoscopic surveillance at intervals of 1 to 2 years, simultaneously with colonoscopy.[80,103]

Cronkhite-Canada Syndrome

Cronkhite-Canada syndrome (CCS) is a rare noninherited GI polyposis of unknown pathogenesis, although some authors suspect an autoimmune mechanism.[104] This syndrome typically affects men and women in the sixth to seventh decades of life and occurs worldwide, though most cases are described in Japan. The polyposis causes malabsorption, diarrhea, hypoproteinemia, and weight loss, and there are associated ectodermal signs, primarily changes in skin pigmentation, alopecia, and onychodystrophy. In the stomach, the polyps are usually sessile reddish lesions that sometimes appear cystic. As with juvenile polyps, these polyps are essentially histologically indistinguishable to hyperplastic gastric polyps, with foveolar hyperplasia, cystic dilated glands, and stromal inflammation and edema (Fig. 21-15)[104,105]; however, the intervening mucosa in CCS patients does tend to be

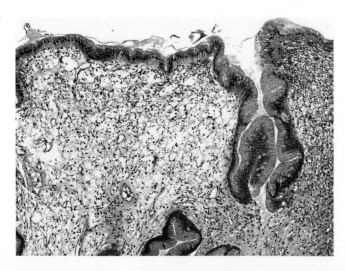

FIGURE 21-15 Gastric polyp of Cronkhite-Canada syndrome. Although not pathognomonic, this hyperplastic-like polyp had a markedly edematous stroma. The patient, a 55-year-old man, presented with polyps carpeting the stomach and duodenum and had a rectal adenocarcinoma.

more inflamed than in juvenile polyps.[106] The risk of associated cancers in CCS remains controversial, even though colorectal and gastric carcinomas seem to be more frequent,[104,105,107] with a 5% incidence in these patients.[108] Recommendations for the management have focused on pharmacologic therapy and surgical resection.[109]

Cowden Disease

Cowden disease is a rare autosomal dominant disorder that is a component of PTEN (phosphatase and tensin homolog) hamartoma syndrome. This syndrome includes Cowden disease, Bannayan-Riley-Ruvalcaba syndrome, Proteus syndrome, and other syndromes caused by germline mutations of the tumor suppressor gene PTEN that is deleted in chromosome 10. In Cowden disease, the mutation is responsible for a combination of endodermal, mesodermal, and ectodermal alterations, and results in the development of multiple hamartomas involving various organs. GI polyps are observed in 35% to 65% of cases.[83,110] In the stomach, these polyps (as with the other non-PJ hamartomatous polyps) resemble hyperplasic polyps but are described as having more basal, cystically dilated glands containing papillary infolding.[111] Some smooth muscle fibers may be interspersed among the glands, but the organized bundles of PJ polyps are not present. Also, the glandular cysts sometimes extend into the submucosa.[112] Occasionally, adenomatous polyps have also been reported to occur in Cowden disease.[83]

Cowden disease is associated with an increased risk of cancer, most frequently of breast, but urogenital, thyroid, and GI cancers (albeit rarely gastric) have also been reported.[113] There are no clear guidelines concerning the follow-up of such patients, but screening is aimed primarily at detecting breast and thyroid cancers.[114]

INFLAMMATORY FIBROID POLYPS

Inflammatory fibroid polyps (IFPs) are rare lesions. In the 2008 Caris series of over 6,600 polyps in 120,000 patients, there were only 6 IFPs, representing <0.1% of all gastric polyps.[1] Occurring slightly more commonly in women, the average age of affected patients is in the mid-sixties. These polyps can occur throughout the GI tract, and over 80% of those in the stomach arise in the antrum and angulus.[115] Known associations include hypochlorydia or achlorhydria, as well as gastric adenomas.[115] Although they are usually found incidentally, symptoms of bleeding and gastric outlet obstruction have been reported.[116] IFPs are firm, solitary, sessile or pedunculated polyps that are often ulcerated.

Histologically, they consist of a submucosal proliferation of spindle cells, small vessels, and a mixed inflammatory infiltrate with mast cells and prominent eosinophils (Fig. 21-16A and B). Perivascular "onion-skin" reticular fibers are characteristic. Because of their conspicuous eosinophilic infiltrates, these polyps have been referred to as eosinophilic granulomas; however, this term is best avoided since it more specifically refers to Langerhan cell histiocytosis. The mucosa adjacent to these polyps is usually unremarkable, but associated chronic atrophic gastritis has been reported. Immunoreactivity with CD34 suggests that these polyps have dendritic cell differentiation.[117] The differential diagnoses of IFPs include eosinophilic gastroenteritis, inflammatory pseudotumor, hemangioendothelioma, and hemangiopericytoma.[118] IFPs may also be mistaken for sarcoma (particularly GIST) on small endoscopic biopsies of more cellular areas.[119]

The etiology of inflammatory fibroid polyps is unknown. A familial tendency has been suggested by the finding of a family in Devon, UK, whose female members had a high rate of these polyps.[120] Given the prominent eosinophilic component, one might suspect an allergic etiology; however, no supportive evidence currently exists. A recent study found that 70% of IFPs contain gain-of-function mutations in the platelet-derived growth factor receptor-alpha polypeptide gene, similar to those found in KIT-negative GI stromal tumors, suggesting that these lesions may be neoplastic rather than purely inflammatory.[121] Most inflammatory fibroid polyps are found

FIGURE 21-16 A,B: Inflammatory fibroid polyp. The polyp results in the expansion of the submucosa (**A**). Higher magnification shows the spindle cell proliferation with numerous small vessels and mixed inflammatory infiltrate (**B**).

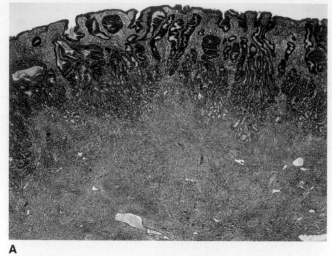

A

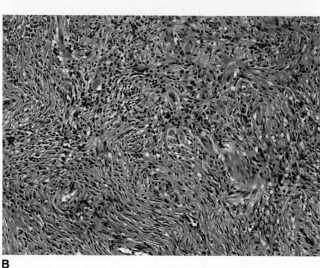

B

incidentally and do not recur after excision; therefore, neither further treatment beyond local excision nor surveillance is recommended.[118]

XANTHOMAS

Xanthomas (also known as xanthelasmas) are small (usually <3 mm) yellowish nodules or plaques that barely protrude from the surrounding pink gastric mucosa. Their reported prevalence ranges from <1% to as many as 7% (in Asia) of patients undergoing gastric biopsy.[122,123]

These sessile lesions are usually associated with chronic gastritis and are often found near sites of mucosal repair, such as gastrectomy stomas, ulcers, or, less commonly, the mucosa adjacent to an adenocarcinoma. They may be found in small clusters along the lesser curvature, antrum, and prepyloric areas of the stomach. Importantly, xanthomas represent a local reparative response and are not associated with hypercholesterolemia.[123] Histologically, they consist of aggregates of lipid-laden macrophages containing cholesterol and neutral fat, loosely embedded in the lamina propria (Fig. 21-17). The ill-defined, pale round cells may initially suggest signet-ring cell carcinoma or Whipple disease to those less familiar with xanthomas; however, the vacuoles in these foamy macrophages are characteristic, and special stains for mucins and bacteria are negative, as are immunohistochemical stains for epithelial cells.

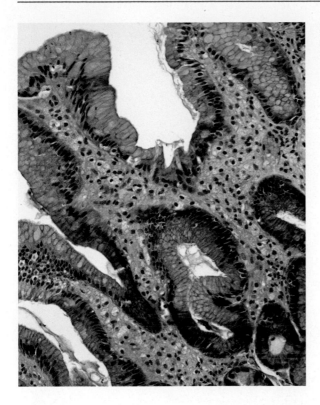

FIGURE 21-17 Xanthoma at high magnification showing aggregates of lipid-laden macrophages in the lamina propria. Reactive elongated foveolae are common.

LIPOMA

Lipomas are rare in the stomach, accounting for 2% to 3% of all benign gastric tumors. They are frequently observed in adults, although some pediatric cases have been reported.[124] Most are found in the antrum, and symptoms when present include abdominal pain and bleeding[125] or even GI intussusception and gastric outlet obstruction.[126–128] Endoscopically, lipomas present as smooth, submucosal lesions that protrude into the gastric lumen, and mucosal ulcerations or central depressions are sometimes reported. Gastric lipomas vary in size, reaching up to 10 cm ("giant gastric lipomas").[125,128,129]

These circumscribed masses of adipose tissue are composed of mature, well-differentiated adipocytes devoid of atypia. Typically, endoscopic biopsies contain little or no submucosa, and the diagnosis can only be surmised based upon the endoscopy and the lack of a mucosal polyp. Even when some superficial submucosa is present, it can be difficult to discern normal submucosal fat from a lipoma. Larger specimens will reveal the homogeneous nature and circumscription of a true lipoma.

PANCREATIC HETEROTOPIA

The term "pancreatic heterotopia" encompasses two clinical and pathologic entities. One presentation, only rarely seen endoscopically but found frequently on microscopic examination, consists of small, mucosal or submucosal foci of pancreatic acinar tissue at the gastroesophageal junction; this finding is more often named "pancreatic metaplasia," although it is unclear whether it actually represents metaplasia or heterotopia. In 5% to 15% of junctional biopsies for Gastroesophageal Reflux Disease (GERD), such foci of benign pancreatic acinar tissue will be found and may be related to inflammation and repair. The significance of this condition is unclear, but there is no indication that these small foci of pancreatic tissue have any neoplastic potential.[130,131]

The other presentation, "true" pancreatic heterotopia, is uncommon and is usually discovered endoscopically as a submucosal nodule in the antrum and prepyloric region,

FIGURE 21-18 A,B: Pancreatic heterotopia presenting as a large submucosal
nodule (A). Higher magnification shows
benign ducts and acinar tissue.

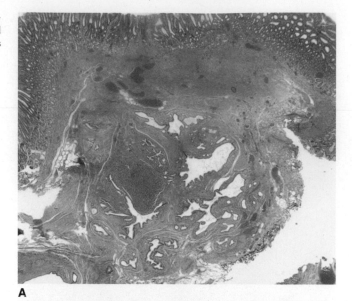

A

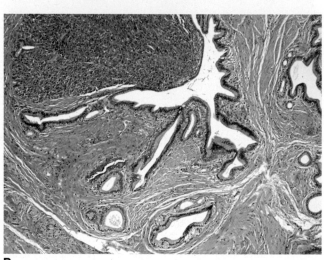

B

sometimes with a central dimple if a duct is present.[132] These nodules are typically solitary, representing <1% of all gastric polyps. Unlike metaplasia, there are often ducts along with the pancreatic acinar tissue, and even islets may rarely be seen, creating a lobular configuration resembling normal pancreas. As is the case with all submucosal lesions, they can be missed in superficial biopsies (Fig. 21-18A and B). The gastric mucosa surrounding these lesions is usually unremarkable.

Pancreatic heterotopia is a benign and usually asymptomatic lesion; thus, no therapy is warranted.[132] Symptomatic lesions (large enough to cause gastric outlet obstruction) are rare and can be treated by excision.[133] Ductal adenocarcinomas, islet cell tumors, and pancreatitis arising in heterotopic pancreatic tissue have been reported, but the rarity of such occurrences suggests that neither surgical excision nor endoscopic surveillance is warranted.[134,135]

WHEN A POLYP IS NOT A POLYP

In the Caris 2008 series,[1] 16.1% of all gastric biopsy specimens described endoscopically as polyp or nodule revealed no evidence of any recognized gastric polyp microscopically. The overwhelming majority of these specimens consisted of normal or inflamed gastric mucosa. Mucosal folds, edema of the lamina propria, foveolar hyperplasia, and prominent lymphoid follicles may cause the endoscopic appearance of a small polyp. Having reliable clinical and endoscopic information can be crucial to the formulation of an informed report. For example, if endoscopy shows a smooth round antral nodule and the biopsy specimen reveals a perfectly normal mucosa, an appropriate comment should be added to the report suggesting that the biopsy specimen may not be representative of the endoscopically identified lesion and that a submucosal lesion may not have been sampled.

In cases where no polyp is found, one should avoid nonspecific diagnoses, such as "polypoid mucosa," "mild hyperplastic features," or similar vacuous expressions, as gastroenterologists could suspect that their pathologist is merely trying to appease them with a diagnosis that fits their expectations, undermining their confidence. A frank conversation between the pathologist and the clinician, ideally accompanied by a few sessions at the microscope, can go a long way toward improving the specificity of the diagnoses and, ultimately, patient care.

References

1. Carmack SW, Genta RM, Schuler CM, et al. The current spectrum of gastric polyps: a 1-year national study of over 120,000 patients. *Am J Gastroenterol.* 2009;104:1524–1532.
2. Stolte M, Sticht T, Eidt S, et al. Frequency, location, and age and sex distribution of various types of gastric polyp. *Endoscopy.* 1994;26:659–665.
3. Deppisch LM, Rona VT. Gastric epithelial polyps. A 10-year study. *J Clin Gastroenterol.* 1989;11:110–115.
4. Gencosmanoglu R, Sen-Oran E, Kurtkaya-Yapicier O, et al. Gastric polypoid lesions: analysis of 150 endoscopic polypectomy specimens from 91 patients. *World J Gastroenterol.* 2003;9:2236–2239.
5. Niv Y, Bat L. Gastric polyps—a clinical study. *Isr J Med Sci.* 1985;21:841–844.
6. Papa A, Cammarota G, Tursi A, et al. Histologic types and surveillance of gastric polyps: a seven year clinico-pathological study. *Hepatogastroenterology.* 1998;45:579–582.
7. Rattan J, Arber N, Tiomny E, et al. Gastric polypoid lesions—an eight-year study. *Hepatogastroenterology.* 1993;40:107–109.
8. Roseau G, Ducreux M, Molas G, et al. Epithelial gastric polyps in a series of 13000 gastroscopies. *Presse Med.* 1990;19:650–654.
9. Sivelli R, Del RP, Bonati L, et al. Gastric polyps: a clinical contribution. *Chir Ital.* 2002;54:37–40.
10. Ljubicic N, Kujundzic M, Roic G, et al. Benign epithelial gastric polyps—frequency, location, and age and sex distribution. *Coll Antropol.* 2002;26.55–60.
11. Archimandritis A, Spiliadis C, Tzivras M, et al. Gastric epithelial polyps: a retrospective endoscopic study of 12974 symptomatic patients. *Ital J Gastroenterol.* 1996;28:387–390.
12. Morais DJ, Yamanaka A, Zeitune JM, et al. Gastric polyps: a retrospective analysis of 26,000 digestive endoscopies. *Arq Gastroenterol.* 2007;44:14–17.
13. Genta RM, Schuler CM, Robiou CI, et al. No association between gastric fundic gland polyps and gastrointestinal neoplasia in a study of over 100,000 patients. *Clin Gastroenterol Hepatol.* 2009;7: 849–854.
14. Fossmark R, Jianu CS, Martinsen TC, et al. Serum gastrin and chromogranin A levels in patients with fundic gland polyps caused by long-term proton-pump inhibition. *Scand J Gastroenterol.* 2007;43:1–5.
15. Jalving M, Koornstra JJ, Wesseling J, et al. Increased risk of fundic gland polyps during long-term proton pump inhibitor therapy. *Aliment Pharmacol Ther.* 2006;24:1341–1348.
16. Shand AG, Taylor AC, Banerjee M, et al. Gastric fundic gland polyps in south-east Scotland: absence of adenomatous polyposis coli gene mutations and a strikingly low prevalence of *Helicobacter pylori* infection. *J Gastroenterol Hepatol.* 2002;17:1161–1164.
17. Watanabe N, Seno H, Nakajima T, et al. Regression of fundic gland polyps following acquisition of *Helicobacter pylori.* Gut. 2002;51:742–745.
18. Ally MR, Veerappan GR, Maydonovitch CL, et al. Chronic proton pump inhibitor therapy associated with increased development of fundic gland polyps. *Dig Dis Sci.* 2009;54:2617–2622.

19. Samarasam I, Roberts-Thomson J, Brockwell D. Gastric fundic gland polyps: a clinico-pathological study from North West Tasmania. *ANZ J Surg*. 2009;79:467–470.

20. Vieth M, Stolte M. Fundic gland polyps are not induced by proton pump inhibitor therapy. *Am J Clin Pathol*. 2001;116:716–720.

21. Bertoni G, Sassatelli R, Nigrisoli E, et al. Dysplastic changes in gastric fundic gland polyps of patients with familial adenomatous polyposis. *Ital J Gastroenterol Hepatol*. 1999;31:192–197.

22. Bianchi LK, Burke CA, Bennett AE, et al. Fundic gland polyp dysplasia is common in familial adenomatous polyposis. *Clin Gastroenterol Hepatol*. 2008;6:180–185.

23. Attard TM, Cuffari C, Tajouri T, et al. Multicenter experience with upper gastrointestinal polyps in pediatric patients with familial adenomatous polyposis. *Am J Gastroenterol*. 2004;99:681–686.

24. Kim JS, Chae HS, Kim HK, et al. Spontaneous resolution of multiple fundic gland polyps after cessation of treatment with omeprazole. *Korean J Gastroenterol*. 2008;51:305–308.

25. Winkler A, Hinterleitner TA, Langner C. Giant fundic gland polyp mimicking a gastric malignancy. *Endoscopy*. 2007;39(Suppl 1):E34. Epub;%2007 Feb 7.:E34.

26. Stolte M, Vieth M, Ebert MP. High-grade dysplasia in sporadic fundic gland polyps: clinically relevant or not? *Eur J Gastroenterol Hepatol*. 2003;15:1153–1156.

27. Raghunath AS, O'Morain C, McLoughlin RC. Review article: the long-term use of proton-pump inhibitors. *Aliment Pharmacol Ther*. 2005;22(Suppl 1):55–63.

28. Abraham SC, Park SJ, Mugartegui L, et al. Sporadic fundic gland polyps with epithelial dysplasia: evidence for preferential targeting for mutations in the adenomatous polyposis coli gene. *Am J Pathol*. 2002;161:1735–1742.

29. Abraham SC, Nobukawa B, Giardiello FM, et al. Sporadic fundic gland polyps: common gastric polyps arising through activating mutations in the beta-catenin gene. *Am J Pathol*. 2001;158:1005–1010.

30. Sekine S, Shimoda T, Nimura S, et al. High-grade dysplasia associated with fundic gland polyposis in a familial adenomatous polyposis patient, with special reference to APC mutation profiles. *Mod Pathol*. 2004;17:1421–1426.

31. Jalving M, Koornstra JJ, Boersma-van EW, et al. Dysplasia in fundic gland polyps is associated with nuclear beta-catenin expression and relatively high cell turnover rates. *Scand J Gastroenterol*. 2003;38: 916–922.

32. Abraham SC, Park SJ, Cruz-Correa M, et al. Frequent CpG island methylation in sporadic and syndromic gastric fundic gland polyps. *Am J Clin Pathol*. 2004;122:740–746.

33. Wei J, Chiriboga L, Yee H, et al. Altered cellular distribution of tuberin and glucocorticoid receptor in sporadic fundic gland polyps. *Mod Pathol*. 2002;15:862–869.

34. Declich P, Ambrosiani L, Bellone S, et al. Do fundic gland polyps enter the mainstream of gastric carcinogenesis? *Am J Gastroenterol*. 1998;93:2636.

35. Declich P, Tavani E, Ferrara A, et al. Sporadic fundic gland polyps: clinico-pathologic features and associated diseases. *Pol J Pathol*. 2005;56:131–137.

36. Eidt S, Stolte M. Gastric glandular cysts—investigations into their genesis and relationship to colorectal epithelial tumors. *Z Gastroenterol*. 1989;27:212–217.

37. Dirschmid K, Platz-Baudin C, Stolte M. Why is the hyperplastic polyp a marker for the precancerous condition of the gastric mucosa? *Virchows Arch*. 2006;448:80–84.

38. Malaty HM. Epidemiology of *Helicobacter pylori* infection. *Best Pract Res Clin Gastroenterol*. 2007;21:205–214.

39. Carmack SW, Genta RM. *Helicobacter pylori* seroprevalence in symptomatic veterans: a study of 7310 patients over 11 years. *Helicobacter*. 2009;14:298–302.

40. Amaro R, Neff GW, Karnam US, et al. Acquired hyperplastic gastric polyps in solid organ transplant patients. *Am J Gastroenterol*. 2002;97:2220–2224.

41. Jewell KD, Toweill DL, Swanson PE, et al. Gastric hyperplastic polyps in post transplant patients: a clinicopathologic study. *Mod Pathol*. 2008;21:1108–1112.

42. Abraham SC, Singh VK, Yardley JH, et al. Hyperplastic polyps of the stomach: associations with histologic patterns of gastritis and gastric atrophy. *Am J Surg Pathol*. 2001;25:500–507.

43. Murakami K, Mitomi H, Yamashita K, et al. p53, but not c-Ki-ras, mutation and down-regulation of p21WAF1/CIP1 and cyclin D1 are associated with malignant transformation in gastric hyperplastic polyps. *Am J Clin Pathol*. 2001;115:224–234.

44. Abraham SC, Singh VK, Yardley JH, et al. Hyperplastic polyps of the esophagus and esophagogastric junction: histologic and clinicopathologic findings. *Am J Surg Pathol*. 2001;25:1180–1187.

45. Alper M, Akcan Y, Belenli O. Large pedinculated antral hyperplastic gastric polyp traversed the bulbus causing outlet obstruction and iron deficiency anemia: endoscopic removal. *World J Gastroenterol.* 2003;9:633–634.

46. Gencosmanoglu R, Sen-Oran E, Kurtkaya-Yapicier O, et al. Antral hyperplastic polyp causing intermittent gastric outlet obstruction: case report. *BMC Gastroenterol.* 2003;3:16.

47. Muto T, Ota K. Polypogenesis of gastric mucosa. *Gann.* 1970;61:435–442.

48. Hattori T. Morphological range of hyperplastic polyps and carcinomas arising in hyperplastic polyps of the stomach. *J Clin Pathol.* 1985;38:622–630.

49. Dixon MF, O'Connor HJ, Axon AT, et al. Reflux gastritis: distinct histopathological entity? *J Clin Pathol.* 1986;39:524–530.

50. Genta RM. Differential diagnosis of reactive gastropathy. *Semin Diagn Pathol.* 2005;22:273–283.

51. Ljubicic N, Banic M, Kujundzic M, et al. The effect of eradicating *Helicobacter pylori* infection on the course of adenomatous and hyperplastic gastric polyps. *Eur J Gastroenterol Hepatol.* 1999;11: 727–730.

52. Ohkusa T, Takashimizu I, Fujiki K, et al. Disappearance of hyperplastic polyps in the stomach after eradication of *Helicobacter pylori*. A randomized, clinical trial. *Ann Intern Med.* 1998;129:712–715.

53. Lauwers GY, Wahl SJ, Melamed J, et al. p53 expression in precancerous gastric lesions: an immunohistochemical study of PAb 1801 monoclonal antibody on adenomatous and hyperplastic gastric polyps. *Am J Gastroenterol.* 1993;88:1916–1919.

54. Nogueira AM, Carneiro F, Seruca R, et al. Microsatellite instability in hyperplastic and adenomatous polyps of the stomach. *Cancer.* 1999;86:1649–1656.

55. Yao T, Kajiwara M, Kuroiwa S, et al. Malignant transformation of gastric hyperplastic polyps: alteration of phenotypes, proliferative activity, and p53 expression. *Hum Pathol.* 2002;33:1016–1022.

56. Zea-Iriarte WL, Sekine I, Itsuno M, et al. Carcinoma in gastric hyperplastic polyps. A phenotypic study. *Dig Dis Sci.* 1996;41:377–386.

57. Hirasaki S, Suzuki S, Kanzaki H, et al. Minute signet ring cell carcinoma occurring in gastric hyperplastic polyp. *World J Gastroenterol.* 2007;13:5779–5780.

58. Di GE, Lahner E, Micheletti A, et al. Occurrence and risk factors for benign epithelial gastric polyps in atrophic body gastritis on diagnosis and follow-up. *Aliment Pharmacol Ther.* 2005;21:567 574.

59. Borch K, Skarsgard J, Franzen L, et al. Benign gastric polyps: morphological and functional origin. *Dig Dis Sci.* 2003;48:1292–1297.

60. Dixon MF, Genta RM, Yardley JH, et al. Classification and grading of gastritis. The updated Sydney System. International Workshop on the Histopathology of Gastritis, Houston 1994. *Am J Surg Pathol.* 1996;20:1161–1181.

61. Hu TL, Hsu JT, Chen HM, et al. Diffuse gastric polyposis: report of a case. *J Formos Med Assoc.* 2002;101:712–714.

62. Yamashita M, Hirokawa M, Nakasono M, et al. Gastric inverted hyperplastic polyp. Report of four cases and relation to gastritis cystica profunda. *APMIS.* 2002;110:717–723.

63. Kono T, Imai Y, Ichihara T, et al. Adenocarcinoma arising in gastric inverted hyperplastic polyp: a case report and review of the literature. *Pathol Res Pract.* 2007;203:53–56.

64. Nakamura T, Nakano G. Histopathological classification and malignant change in gastric polyps. *J Clin Pathol.* 1985;38:754–764.

65. Yoshihara M, Sumii K, Haruma K, et al. Correlation of ratio of serum pepsinogen I and II with prevalence of gastric cancer and adenoma in Japanese subjects. *Am J Gastroenterol.* 1998;93:1090–1096.

66. Park dY, Lauwers GY. Gastric polyps: classification and management. *Arch Pathol Lab Med.* 2008;132:633–640.

67. Laxen F, Sipponen P, Ihamaki T, et al. Gastric polyps; their morphological and endoscopical characteristics and relation to gastric carcinoma. *Acta Pathol Microbiol Immunol Scand A.* 1982;90:221–228.

68. Abraham SC, Park SJ, Lee JH, et al. Genetic alterations in gastric adenomas of intestinal and foveolar phenotypes. *Mod Pathol.* 2003;16:786–795.

69. Rocco A, Caruso R, Toraccio S, et al. Gastric adenomas: relationship between clinicopathological findings, *Helicobacter pylori* infection, APC mutations and COX-2 expression. *Ann Oncol.* 2006;17(Suppl 7):vii103–vii108.

70. Hirota WK, Zuckerman MJ, Adler DG, et al. ASGE guideline: the role of endoscopy in the surveillance of premalignant conditions of the upper GI tract. *Gastrointest Endosc.* 2006;63:570–580.

71. Borchard F, Ghanei A, Koldovsky U. Gastrale Differenzierung in Adenomen der Magenschleimhaut. Immunocytochemische Untersuchungen. *Verh Ges Pathol.* 1990;74:528–541.

72. Jass JR, Sobin LH, Watanabe H. The World Health Organization's histologic classification of gastrointestinal tumors. A commentary on the second edition. *Cancer*. 1990;66:2162–2167.

73. Vieth M, Kushima R, Borchard F, et al. Pyloric gland adenoma: a clinico-pathological analysis of 90 cases. *Virchows Arch*. 2003;442:317–321.

74. Chen ZM, Scudiere JR, Abraham SC, et al. Pyloric gland adenoma: an entity distinct from gastric foveolar type adenoma. *Am J Surg Pathol*. 2009;33:186–193.

75. Park DY, Srivastava A, Kim GH, et al. Adenomatous and foveolar gastric dysplasia: distinct patterns of mucin expression and background intestinal metaplasia. *Am J Surg Pathol*. 2008;32:524–533.

76. Park dY, Srivastava A, Kim GH, et al. CDX2 expression in the intestinal-type gastric epithelial neoplasia: frequency and significance. *Mod Pathol*. 2010;23:54–61.

77. Matsukawa A, Kurano R, Takemoto T, et al. Chief cell hyperplasia with structural and nuclear atypia: a variant of fundic gland polyp. *Pathol Res Pract*. 2005;200:817–821.

78. Muller-Hocker J, Rellecke P. Chief cell proliferation of the gastric mucosa mimicking early gastric cancer: an unusual variant of fundic gland polyp. *Virchows Arch*. 2003;442:496–500.

79. Hemminki A, Markie D, Tomlinson I, et al. A serine/threonine kinase gene defective in Peutz-Jeghers syndrome. *Nature*. 1998;391:184–187.

80. Dunlop MG. Guidance on gastrointestinal surveillance for hereditary non-polyposis colorectal cancer, familial adenomatous polypolis, juvenile polyposis, and Peutz-Jeghers syndrome. *Gut*. 2002;51(Suppl 5):V21–V27.

81. Hizawa K, Iida M, Yao T, et al. Juvenile polyposis of the stomach: clinicopathological features and its malignant potential. *J Clin Pathol*. 1997;50:771–774.

82. Johnson GK, Soergel KH, Hensley GT, et al. Cronkite-Canada syndrome: gastrointestinal pathophysiology and morphology. *Gastroenterology*. 1972;63:140–152.

83. Hizawa K, Iida M, Matsumoto T, et al. Gastrointestinal manifestations of Cowden's disease. Report of four cases. *J Clin Gastroenterol*. 1994;18:13–18.

84. Kantarcioglu M, Kilciler G, Turan I, et al. Solitary Peutz-Jeghers-type hamartomatous polyp as a cause of recurrent acute pancreatitis. *Endoscopy*. 2009;41(Suppl 2):E117–E118.

85. Oncel M, Remzi FH, Church JM, et al. Course and follow-up of solitary Peutz-Jeghers polyps: a case series. *Int J Colorectal Dis*. 2003;18:33–35.

86. Tomlinson IP, Houlston RS. Peutz-Jeghers syndrome. *J Med Genet*. 1997;34:1007–1011.

87. Volikos E, Robinson J, Aittomaki K, et al. LKB1 exonic and whole gene deletions are a common cause of Peutz-Jeghers syndrome. *J Med Genet*. 2006;43:e18.

88. Giardiello FM, Brensinger JD, Tersmette AC, et al. Very high risk of cancer in familial Peutz-Jeghers syndrome. *Gastroenterology*. 2000;119:1447–1453.

89. McGrath DR, Spigelman AD. Preventive measures in Peutz-Jeghers syndrome. *Fam Cancer*. 2001;1:121–125.

90. Giardiello FM, Trimbath JD. Peutz-Jeghers syndrome and management recommendations. *Clin Gastroenterol Hepatol*. 2006;4:408–415.

91. de Leng WW, Jansen M, Keller JJ, et al. Peutz-Jeghers syndrome polyps are polyclonal with expanded progenitor cell compartment. *Gut*. 2007;56:1475–1476.

92. Jansen M, de Leng WW, Baas AF, et al. Mucosal prolapse in the pathogenesis of Peutz-Jeghers polyposis. *Gut*. 2006;55:1–5.

93. Ben BE, Jouini R, Khayat O, et al. Adenomatous transformation in hamartomatous polyps cases of two patients with Peutz-Jeghers syndrome. *Int J Colorectal Dis*. 2009;24:1361–1363.

94. Salloch H, Reinacher-Schick A, Schulmann K, et al. Truncating mutations in Peutz-Jeghers syndrome are associated with more polyps, surgical interventions and cancers. *Int J Colorectal Dis*. 2010;25:97–107.

95. Udd L, Katajisto P, Rossi DJ, et al. Suppression of Peutz-Jeghers polyposis by inhibition of cyclooxygenase-2. *Gastroenterology*. 2004;127:1030–1037.

96. Friedl W, Uhlhaas S, Schulmann K, et al. Juvenile polyposis: massive gastric polyposis is more common in MADH4 mutation carriers than in BMPR1A mutation carriers. *Hum Genet*. 2002;111:108–111.

97. Jass JR, Williams CB, Bussey HJ, et al. Juvenile polyposis—a precancerous condition. *Histopathology*. 1988;13:619–630.

98. Jarvinen HJ, Sipponen P. Gastroduodenal polyps in familial adenomatous and juvenile polyposis. *Endoscopy*. 1986;18:230–234.

99. Shikata K, Kukita Y, Matsumoto T, et al. Gastric juvenile polyposis associated with germline SMAD4 mutation. *Am J Med Genet A*. 2005;134:326–329.

100. Yamashita K, Saito M, Itoh M, et al. Juvenile polyposis complicated with protein losing gastropathy. *Intern Med*. 2009;48:335–338.

101. Coffin CM, Dehner LP. What is a juvenile polyp? An analysis based on 21 patients with solitary and multiple polyps. *Arch Pathol Lab Med*. 1996;120:1032–1038.

102. Pintiliciuc OG, Heresbach D, de-Lajarte-Thirouard AS, et al. Gastric involvement in juvenile polyposis associated with germline SMAD4 mutations: an entity characterized by a mixed hypertrophic and polypoid gastropathy. *Gastroenterol Clin Biol*. 2008;32:445–450.

103. Howe JR, Mitros FA, Summers RW. The risk of gastrointestinal carcinoma in familial juvenile polyposis. *Ann Surg Oncol*. 1998;5:751–756.

104. Takeuchi Y, Yoshikawa M, Tsukamoto N, et al. Cronkhite-Canada syndrome with colon cancer, portal thrombosis, high titer of antinuclear antibodies, and membranous glomerulonephritis. *J Gastroenterol*. 2003;38:791–795.

105. Yamaguchi K, Ogata Y, Akagi Y, et al. Cronkhite-Canada syndrome associated with advanced rectal cancer treated by a subtotal colectomy: report of a case. *Surg Today*. 2001;31:521–526.

106. Samet JD, Horton KM, Fishman EK, et al. Cronkhite-Canada syndrome: gastric involvement diagnosed by MDCT. *Case Report Med*. 2009;2009:148795.

107. Watanabe T, Kudo M, Shirane H, et al. Cronkhite-Canada syndrome associated with triple gastric cancers: a case report. *Gastrointest Endosc*. 1999;50:688–691.

108. Egawa T, Kubota T, Otani Y, et al. Surgically treated Cronkhite-Canada syndrome associated with gastric cancer. *Gastric Cancer*. 2000;3:156–160.

109. Ward EM, Wolfsen HC. Pharmacological management of Cronkhite-Canada syndrome. *Expert Opin Pharmacother*. 2003;4:385–389.

110. Vasovcak P, Krepelova A, Puchmajerova A, et al. A novel mutation of PTEN gene in a patient with Cowden syndrome with excessive papillomatosis of the lips, discrete cutaneous lesions, and gastrointestinal polyposis. *Eur J Gastroenterol Hepatol*. 2007;19:513–517.

111. Campos FG, Habr-Gama A, Kiss DR, et al. Cowden syndrome: report of two cases and review of clinical presentation and management of a rare colorectal polyposis. *Curr Surg*. 2006;63:15–19.

112. Carlson GJ, Nivatvongs S, Snover DC. Colorectal polyps in Cowden's disease (multiple hamartoma syndrome). *Am J Surg Pathol*. 1984;8:763–770.

113. Hamby LS, Lee EY, Schwartz RW. Parathyroid adenoma and gastric carcinoma as manifestations of Cowden's disease. *Surgery*. 1995;118:115–117.

114. Wirtzfeld DA, Petrelli NJ, Rodriguez-Bigas MA. Hamartomatous polyposis syndromes: molecular genetics, neoplastic risk, and surveillance recommendations. *Ann Surg Oncol*. 2001;8:319–327.

115. Hasegawa T, Yang P, Kagawa N, et al. CD34 expression by inflammatory fibroid polyps of the stomach. *Mod Pathol*. 1997;10:451–456.

116. Puri AS, Gupta B, Bhalla S. Giant inflammatory fibroid polyp of stomach causing massive upper gastrointestinal bleeding. *Indian J Gastroenterol*. 1991;10:23–24.

117. Pantanowitz L, Antonioli DA, Pinkus GS, et al. Inflammatory fibroid polyps of the gastrointestinal tract: evidence for a dendritic cell origin. *Am J Surg Pathol*. 2004;28:107–114.

118. Paikos D, Moschos J, Tzilves D, et al. Inflammatory fibroid polyp or Vanek's tumour. *Dig Surg*. 2007;24:231–233.

119. Ozolek JA, Sasatomi E, Swalsky PA, et al. Inflammatory fibroid polyps of the gastrointestinal tract: clinical, pathologic, and molecular characteristics. *Appl Immunohistochem Mol Morphol*. 2004;12:59–66.

120. Allibone RO, Nanson JK, Anthony PP. Multiple and recurrent inflammatory fibroid polyps in a Devon family ('Devon polyposis syndrome'): an update. *Gut*. 1992;33:1004–1005.

121. Schildhaus HU, Cavlar T, Binot E, et al. Inflammatory fibroid polyps harbour mutations in the platelet-derived growth factor receptor alpha (PDGFRA) gene. *J Pathol*. 2008;216:176–182.

122. Gursoy S, Yurci A, Torun E, et al. An uncommon lesion: gastric xanthelasma. *Turk J Gastroenterol*. 2005;16:167–170.

123. Yi SY. Dyslipidemia and *H. pylori* in gastric xanthomatosis. *World J Gastroenterol*. 2007;13:4598–4601.

124. Antoniou D, Soutis M, Stefanaki K, et al. Gastric fibrolipoma causing bleeding in a child. *Eur J Pediatr Surg*. 2007;17:282–284.

125. Thompson WM, Kende AI, Levy AD. Imaging characteristics of gastric lipomas in 16 adult and pediatric patients. *Am J Roentgenol*. 2003;181:981–985.

126. Vinces FY, Ciacci J, Sperling DC, et al. Gastroduodenal intussusception secondary to a gastric lipoma. *Can J Gastroenterol.* 2005;19:107–108.

127. Ha JP, Tang CN, Cheung HY, et al. An unusual cause of gastric outlet obstruction. *Gut.* 2007;56:967, 1018.

128. Moues CM, Steenvoorde P, Viersma JH, et al. Jejunal intussusception of a gastric lipoma: a review of literature. *Dig Surg.* 2002;19:418–420.

129. Zak Y, Biagini B, Moore H, et al. Submucosal resection of giant gastric lipoma. *J Surg Oncol.* 2006;94:63–67.

130. El-Serag HB, Graham DY, Rabeneck L, et al. Prevalence and determinants of histological abnormalities of the gastric cardia in volunteers. *Scand J Gastroenterol.* 2007;42:1158–1166.

131. Polkowski W, van Lanschot JJ, ten Kate FJ, et al. Intestinal and pancreatic metaplasia at the esophago-gastric junction in patients without Barrett's esophagus. *Am J Gastroenterol.* 2000;95:617–625.

132. Christodoulidis G, Zacharoulis D, Barbanis S, et al. Heterotopic pancreas in the stomach: a case report and literature review. *World J Gastroenterol.* 2007;13:6098–6100.

133. Ormarsson OT, Gudmundsdottir I, Marvik R. Diagnosis and treatment of gastric heterotopic pancreas. *World J Surg.* 2006;30:1682–1689.

134. Ayantunde AA, Pinder E, Heath DI. Symptomatic pyloric pancreatic heterotopia: report of three cases and review of the literature. *Med Sci Monit.* 2006;12:CS49–CS52.

135. Chetty R, Weinreb I. Gastric neuroendocrine carcinoma arising from heterotopic pancreatic tissue. *J Clin Pathol.* 2004;57:314–317.

Gastric Dysplasia

▶ Mikhail Lisovsky
▶ Gregory. Y. Lauwers

INTRODUCTION

Gastric epithelial dysplasia (GED), defined as histologically unequivocal neoplastic epithelium devoid of evidence of invasion into the lamina propria or submucosa, encompasses a wide spectrum of cytologic and/or architectural alterations. GED is recognized as precursor of gastric adenocarcinoma and also as a marker of risk for cancer elsewhere in the gastric mucosa.[1] Evidence supporting that GED is a direct precursor of gastric adenocarcinoma stems primarily from observations in surgically resected gastric cancers. In this setting, high-grade dysplasia has been identified in 40% to 100% of early gastric cancers and 5% to 80% of advanced adenocarcinomas.[2] Subsequent prospective and cohort studies have shown an increased risk of progression of dysplastic lesions to adenocarcinoma, which supports initial observations.[3,4] Notably, while the more differentiated tubular (intestinal) type of gastric adenocarcinoma is associated with well characterized dysplastic lesions, a specific precursor lesion for sporadic discohesive (diffuse) cancer is not as well defined (i.e., "neck dysplasia") and its existence is questioned by some authors. As dysplastic lesions show molecular abnormalities similar to those of adenocarcinoma, the etiology of GED is thought to be the same as of gastric adenocarcinoma. Approximately 80% of gastric adenocarcinomas develop in the background of *Helicobacter pylori* atrophic gastritis; 5% are associated with Epstein-Barr virus; 5% arise in the setting of hereditary syndromes, such as Peutz-Jeghers, Cowden, Li-Fraumeni, hereditary nonpolyposis colonic cancer, hereditary diffuse gastric cancer, familial adenomatous polyposis (FAP), and juvenile polyposis.[5–8] Rarer causes of gastric adenocarcinoma are autoimmune gastritis, atrophic gastritis in a gastric remnant, and Ménétrier disease.[9,10] One of the consequences of this etiologic diversity is the heterogeneity of molecular pathways that leads to dysplasia and adenocarcinoma, which will be addressed later.

PREDYSPLASTIC MUCOSAL ABNORMALITIES
(See Chapter By M. Rugge)

A widely accepted model of gastric carcinogenesis, where dysplasia plays an essential role has been described by Correa in the 1980s. Based on epidemiological and morphological studies, Correa postulated a sequence of progressive changes where chronic gastritis, mainly caused by *H. pylori* infection, causes mucosal atrophy, leading to intestinal metaplasia, then dysplasia and intestinal-type adenocarcinoma. Diffuse gastric cancer is thought not to arise through this cascade. The general validity of this pathway has been confirmed using mouse models.[11] Gastric atrophy is defined as the loss of native glandular elements, with their replacement by stromal fibrosis and/or metaplasia of intestinal or pseudopyloric type. Currently, it is thought that metaplasia represents the first permanent alteration of the genetic/epigenetic program of precursor epithelial cells that give rise to metaplastic glands.[12] Pseudopyloric metaplasia seen in the corpus/fundus shows a phenotype similar to antral or pyloric glands. It is characterized by expression of trefoil factor 2/spasmolytic polypeptide and by expression of pepsinogen I, a marker of chief cells. It is also referred to as spasmolytic polypeptide-expressing metaplasia.[13] In a seminal study, showing a role of pseudopyloric metaplasia in gastric carcinogenesis, stomachs with early intestinal-type adenocarcinoma were subjected to sectioning in toto. Atrophy was present as a continuous sheet of pseudopyloric metaplasia with islands of intestinal metaplasia seen only within the atrophic zone. All carcinomas were found within the atrophic zone, suggesting that the extent of mucosal atrophy defined by pseudopyloric metaplasia is more closely related to gastric carcinoma than is the presence or type of intestinal metaplasia.[14] Independently, pseudopyloric metaplasia was found to be associated with >90% of gastric adenocarcinomas in patients from the United States, Japan, and Iceland, implicating it as an important preneoplastic lesion.[15–17] Furthermore, in a mouse model of gastric cancer caused by *H. felis*, pseudopyloric metaplasia appears to be an essential step and the only type of metaplasia observed.[18,19] Finally, in transgenic mouse models expressing transcription factors Cdx1 and Cdx2, pseudopyloric metaplasia and gastric cancer developed consistently in Cdx2 transgenic mice but were not reported in the Cdx1 transgenic mice, although in both models, gastric mucosa converted to intestinal metaplasia.[20,21]

CLINICAL FEATURES

The prevalence of GED is characterized by variation worldwide, from 9% to 20% in high-risk areas such as Colombia and China to 0.5% to 3.75% in Western countries where gastric cancer is less common.[22,23] This difference is likely a result of variations in the genetic makeup of the respective populations, defined by polymorphisms of IL-1B, IL-1RN, and TNF-α and by environmental factors, including the prevalence of *H. pylori* infection. The genotype of *H. pylori* also affects the risk of neoplastic progression. For instance, cagA, vacA, and babA genotypes have been associated with increased cancer risk. Moreover, the frequency of GED varies with the underlying etiology. GED prevalence of up to 40% has been reported in patients with pernicious anemia.[24] However, the disease confers an only moderately increased risk of gastric cancer.[25] Patients with FAP are also at higher risk of developing either flat or, more commonly, polypoid dysplasia (i.e., adenomas). These adenomas typically are located in the antrum, are frequently multiple, and are observed in 2% to 5% of patients.[26–29]

Most patients diagnosed with GED are in the sixth to seventh decade of life,[29,30] with men affected more often than women (male-female ratios range from 2.4 to 3.9:1).[30,31] Although GED may be diagnosed in any segment of the stomach, it most commonly affects the lesser curvature, particularly the antrum or the incisura angularis.[29,32] Although GED is often diagnosed on random biopsies without corresponding endoscopic abnormalities, various abnormal endoscopic patterns may be seen.[30,31] These include mucosal irregularity in a background of atrophic mucosa, erosions, ulcers,[30] mucosal scars,[29] diffuse inflammatory changes,[33] plaques, and polyps.[29]

HISTOLOGIC FEATURES, GRADING, AND CLASSIFICATION

GED is characterized by variable cellular and architectural atypia. In the United States, the term "adenoma" has been used when a discrete grossly appreciable lesion is observed or "dysplasia" when it is flat. However, in Japan, for example, the term "adenoma" encompasses all macroscopic types. GED is divided into several histologic subtypes and is graded according to the prominence of the atypia. The current two-tier scheme of low-grade and high-grade dysplasia has proven to be more reproducible than the obsolete three-tier system of mild, moderate, and severe dysplasia.[34] Determination of the correct grade is critical, because it predicts both the risk of malignant transformation and the risk of developing gastric cancer elsewhere in the stomach. It also provides a clinically meaningful risk stratification method that can be used to guide patient management (see below).[35]

Most cases of GED have an intestinal phenotype resembling colonic adenomas and express intestinal type mucin Muc2 and CDX2.[36,37] This type of dysplasia is referred to as adenomatous dysplasia or type I. When low-grade, it is characterized architecturally by crowded but simple tubular glands with little branching or budding. The glands are lined by atypical columnar cells with increased nuclear-to-cytoplasmic ratio and mucin depletion (Fig. 22-1A and B). The nuclei

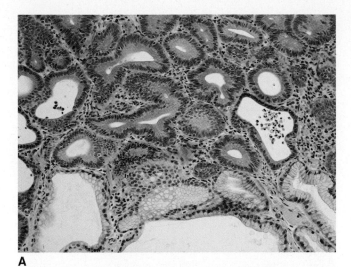

FIGURE 22-1 **A,B:** Low-grade adenomatous dysplasia, characterized by limited gland crowding, pencillate, hyperchromatic nuclei, and pseudostratification.

A

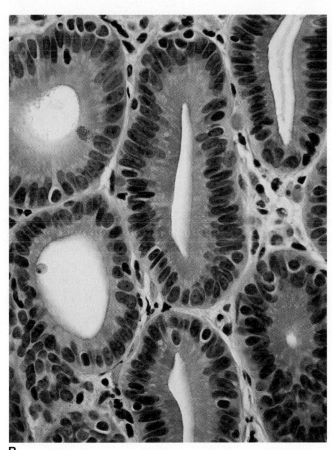

B

are overlapping, pencillate, and hyperchromatic, with pseudostratification and inconspicuous nucleoli.[38] The dysplastic cells extend to the mucosal surface, and this lack of surface maturation is an essential feature of dysplasia.[34,35,39]

High-grade dysplasia is characterized by marked architectural and cytologic abnormalities, and the diagnosis can be made when either abnormality is present unequivocally. Glands show back-to-back crowding and limited branching (Fig. 22-2A and B). Intraluminal necrotic debris is

FIGURE 22-2 A,B: High-grade adenomatous dysplasia, characterized by more
irregular glandular structure, rounded
large nuclei with an open chromatin
pattern, prominent nucleoli, and full
stratification.

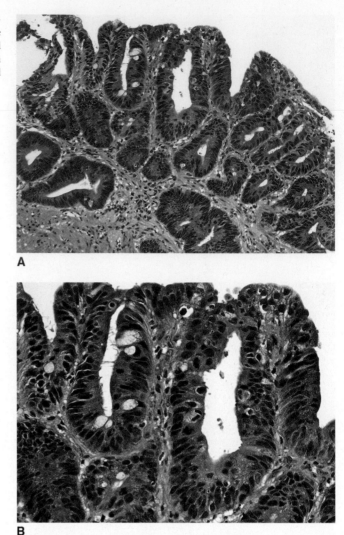

A

B

commonly present. However, cribriforming and budding are not part of high-grade dysplasia and
are consistent with intramucosal carcinoma. In contrast to low-grade dysplasia, dysplastic cells
are usually cuboidal rather than columnar, with a high nuclear-cytoplasmic ratio. The nuclei vary
in size, are round to oval, and are vesicular with prominent nucleoli and a thickened and irregular
nuclear membrane. Cells show distinct loss of cell polarity, defined either as marked pseudostratification of the nuclei (to the level of the luminal surface) or as loss of the perpendicular orientation of the nuclei in relation to the basal membrane. Often, mitoses are numerous, and atypical
mitoses also may be present.[34,35,39]

Other, less common, histologic variants of GED have been recognized as well. Foveolar-type
dysplasia, also known as hyperplastic or type II dysplasia, is usually seen in nonintestinalized
mucosa.[38] It resembles normal surface-foveolar epithelium and lacks goblet and Paneth cells. The
cells are cuboidal or low columnar and they variably have clear cytoplasm or retain eosinophilic
apical mucin. Frequent immunoreactivity for the gastric-type mucin Muc5AC, but not for the
intestinal mucin Muc2, is typical.[36] Foveolar dysplasia has been noted in some series to be more
commonly associated with poorly differentiated tubular adenocarcinoma.[38,40] A significant proportion of gastric dysplasias, about 30%, was recently reported to have a hybrid adenomatous/
foveolar phenotype, defined as having at least 10% of the alternative histologic type.[36]

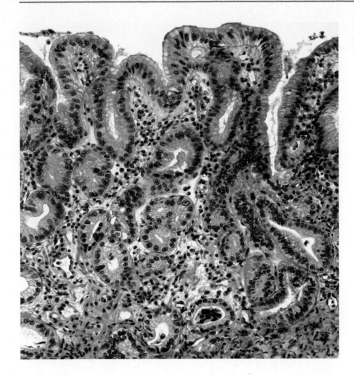

FIGURE 22-3 Low-grade foveolar dysplasia, with oval, basal nuclei, inconspicuous nucleoli, and mild stratification.

Stratification of foveolar GED into low- and high-grade categories is not well established, and the diagnosis of low-grade dysplasia can be challenging. The presence of architecturally simple gastric foveolar-type epithelium with elongated, hyperchromatic nuclei and some degree of pseudostratification is categorized as low-grade foveolar dysplasia (Fig. 22-3). High-grade foveolar dysplasia is characterized by complex glands of variable size and shape with papillary infoldings, serration, and occasional cystic dilatation. Nuclei are round to oval and vesicular with prominent nucleoli (Fig. 22-4).[36]

Finally, some dysplastic lesions show a pyloric phenotype characterized by cuboidal cells with eosinophilic cytoplasm and round nuclei and highlighted by Muc6 immunoreactivity (Fig. 22-5).[41]

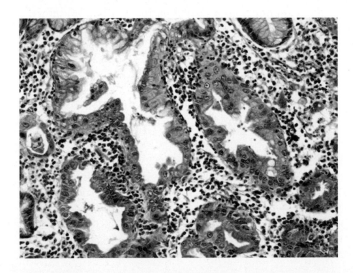

FIGURE 22-4 High-grade foveolar dysplasia. The complex glands of variable size and shape present papillary infoldings, serration, and occasional cystic dilatation. The nuclei are round to oval, with vesicular chromatin and prominent nucleoli.

FIGURE 22-5 Low-grade pyloric-type dysplasia. The lesion is composed of small cuboidal cells with eosinophilic cytoplasm and round nuclei.

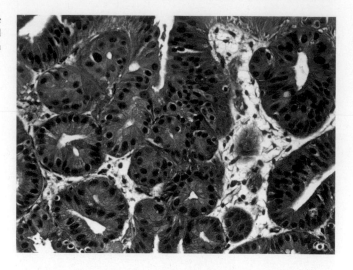

Tubule neck dysplasia is a rare type of GED that is not well defined. It usually occurs in nonmetaplastic gastric epithelium and is thought to be a precursor of diffuse-type gastric carcinoma.[42] Typical features include pale and polygonal or nondescript neoplastic cells confined to markedly elongated tubular structures occupying the midportion of the mucosa that corresponds to the mucous neck region.[42] The cells of dysplastic tubules do not show evidence of mucous, parietal, or chief cell differentiation. Transition from dysplastic tubules to overt invasive diffuse cancer can be seen in deeper parts of the mucosa, and malignant cells of invasive cancer can infiltrate between dysplastic tubules[43] (author's unpublished observations). It remains to be shown whether tubule neck dysplasia can be (a) consistently diagnosed in the absence of admixed diffuse carcinoma and (b) be reliably differentiated from atypical reactive change.[42]

Another morphologic type of precursor lesions has been described in familial hereditary diffuse gastric cancer, an autosomal dominant cancer susceptibility syndrome, characterized by signet-ring cell (diffuse) gastric cancer and lobular breast cancer.[44] It is caused by germ line E-cadherin/CDH1 gene mutations, and close to 50% of affected patients develop diffuse-type gastric cancer. In many prophylactic gastrectomies from these patients, examples of signet-ring cell carcinoma in situ have been reported. The latter corresponds to the presence of signet ring cells located within the confine of the basement membrane. From this location, the cells spread in pagetoid manner between the gastric epithelium and the basal membrane along the foveolar region[45,46] (Fig. 22-6). These lesions have been found to be multifocal, and although one study showed their predilection for the distal stomach and the body-antral transitional zone, in another study, the majority of the lesions were found in the proximal third of the stomach.[47,48] E-cadherin immunoreactivity is reduced or absent in these lesions.[49]

GED DEVELOPING IN BENIGN POLYPOID LESIONS

GED may develop in gastric hyperplastic polyps, particularly those >2 cm in size. Several studies have reported that dysplastic changes occur in 1.8% to 16.4% of hyperplastic polyps.[50,51] In sporadic fundic gland polyps, dysplasia is exceedingly rare, but it is prevalent in patients with FAP, occurring in up to 42% of patients with FAP-associated fundic gland polyps.[28,52] Gastric adenomas constitute approximately 7% to 10% of all gastric polyps[53] and occur in 2% to 50% of patients with FAP.[26,33,54] Dysplasia can also occur in gastric juvenile polyps in patients with juvenile polyposis.[55]

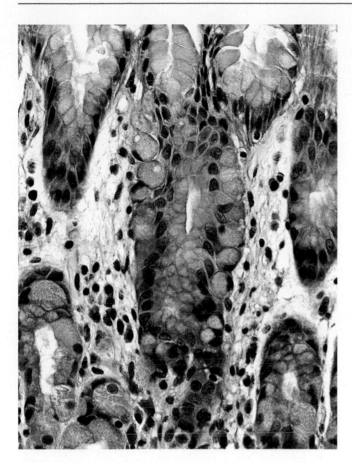

FIGURE 22-6 Signet-ring cell carcinoma in situ has been reported. Note the signet ring cells located within the confine of the basement membrane and that have spread in pagetoid manner between the gastric epithelium and the basal membrane.

DIFFERENTIATING DYSPLASIA FROM REACTIVE ATYPIA

The diagnosis of dysplasia can be challenging for multiple reasons, including orientation of the specimen, sampling, and difficulty in distinguishing it from reactive atypia. Also, while architectural and cytologic features are used in concert to reach a diagnosis, most criteria suffer from low specificity in isolation. In practice, these difficulties lead to significant interobserver diagnostic variability. Furthermore, mucosal regeneration caused by active inflammation or reactive/chemical gastropathy and reparative processes around erosions and ulcers may mimic dysplasia by demonstrating cytological atypia with severe mucin depletion, nuclear hyperchromasia, and increased mitotic activity. Clues to the reactive nature of the epithelial changes include the presence of vascular congestion and edema of lamina propria, evenly spaced nuclei without crowding or pseudostratification, gradual rather than abrupt transition between the atypical and adjacent normal cells, and maturation of the atypical cells of deeper glands as they reach the luminal surface (Fig. 22-7).[34,35]

Few markers are available to support a diagnosis of gastric dysplasia. p53 nuclear staining is reported in about one third of cases of dysplasias,[56–62] usually, but not invariably, limited to areas of high-grade dysplasia,[56,59–61,63] but others were not able to validate these findings.[64,65] Consequently, p53 immunostaining is not widely used in the diagnosis of dysplasia.

While loss of cell polarity is one of intrinsic mechanisms of malignant transformation, the biomarkers of cell polarity have not been evaluated to support a diagnosis of dysplasia. In 2009, Lisovsky et al.[66] reported the use of Lgl2, a basolateral cell polarity protein, to evaluate gastric neoplastic proliferation. They showed that Lgl2 was either entirely lost or aberrantly localized in almost all cases of GED and adenocarcinoma, while it was maintained in chronic gastritis

FIGURE 22-7 A,B: Reactive atypia in a case of chemical/reactive gastropathy. There is vascular congestion of lamina propria and evenly spaced nuclei without crowding. The mucin depletion and nuclear hyperchromasia are indicative of regeneration and should not be interpreted as dysplasia.

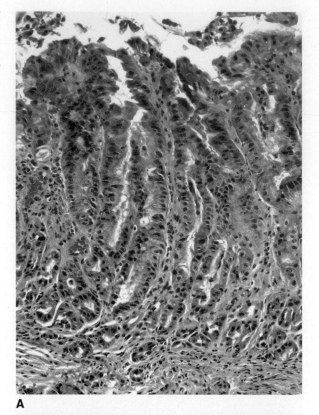

A

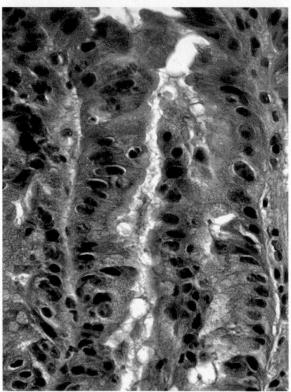

B

and reactive gastric mucosa.[66] However, since Lgl2 staining is consistently negative in intestinal metaplasia, it does not allow to differentiate dysplasia from intestinal metaplasia with reactive change. However, Lgl2 could be used to rule out dysplasia.

DIFFERENTIATION OF GASTRIC EPITHELIAL DYSPLASIA FROM INTRAMUCOSAL CARCINOMA

Intramucosal adenocarcinoma may be superficially similar to high-grade dysplastic lesions and, in the well established case, is distinguished from them on the basis of invasion through the epithelial basement membrane. At this stage, stromal desmoplasia may be absent or limited. More reliable features of intramucosal carcinoma are invasion of the lamina propria by single cells or cell clusters and fused or cribriforming glands. Another set of features of intramucosal carcinoma comprises haphazard arrangement of small and/or budding glands with effacement of the epithelial-stromal interface and occasional change in the tinctorial properties of the cytoplasm of the cells.

VIENNA AND WHO CLASSIFICATIONS OF GASTROINTESTINAL EPITHELIAL NEOPLASIA

Lack of universally accepted diagnostic criteria for each grade, and disagreement on the definition of carcinoma, in particular, between Western and Asian pathologists are well known.

For example, cytologic atypia and architectural complexity are important criteria for the diagnosis of carcinoma in Japan, while breach of the basement membrane and invasion into the lamina propria are needed for the diagnosis of cancer in the West. Noninvasive intramucosal neoplastic lesions with high-grade cellular and architectural atypia are termed intramucosal carcinoma in Japan, whereas the same lesions are diagnosed as high-grade dysplasia by most pathologists in the West. In attempt to bridge differences, a group of GI pathologists convened in Vienna, Austria, with the purpose of developing a new dysplasia classification system that would help address the limitations of the highlighted previously. Importantly, in the Vienna system, modern management strategies and implications were taken into account (Table 22-1). For example, a single diagnostic category was used for both high-grade premalignant lesions without invasion of the lamina propria and invasive adenocarcinomas confined to the lamina propria, because both are amenable to endoscopic mucosal resection.[67]

The World Health Organization (WHO) has previously recommended the terminology of low-grade and high-grade intraepithelial neoplasia for dysplasia and defines carcinoma as invasion of the lamina propria or beyond. However, in this scheme invasion of the lamina propria was not clearly defined.[68] In the upcoming version of the WHO, intraepithelial neoplasia is used to describe lesions that display cytologic and/or architectural alterations perceived to reflect

Table 22-1	Classfication and management of gastric epithelial dysplasia	
"Classic" Nomenclature	Updated Vienna Classification	Clinical Management
Indefinite for dysplasia	Indefinite for neoplasia	Repeat bx surveillance
Low-grade dysplasia	Low-grade adenoma/dysplasia	Repeat bx with or without local treatment surveillance
High-grade dysplasia	High-grade adenoma/dysplasia and Noninvasive carcinoma (carcinoma in situ)	Repeat bx EMR surveillance

underlying molecular abnormalities that may lead to invasive carcinoma and therefore, covers both lesions with morphologically identifiable and morphologically nonidentifiable alterations. At the same time, traditional dysplasia is also recognized leaving the pathologists free to use the terms with which they and the clinicians are more familiar with.

NATURAL HISTORY AND CLINICOPATHOLOGICAL SIGNIFICANCE

In a large nationwide cohort study from the Netherlands, the annual incidence of gastric cancer within 5 years of a diagnosis of atrophic gastritis and intestinal metaplasia was 0.1% and 0.25%, respectively.[4] An earlier study had reported an 11% risk of gastric cancer in patients with gastric atrophy or intestinal metaplasia over a 10-year follow-up period. However, the high incidence in this study can likely be explained by the fact that only macroscopic abnormalities were biopsied.[69]

A review of older series shows that low-grade dysplasia regresses in 38% to 75% of cases and persists in 19% to 50% of the cases. In comparison, high-grade dysplasia regresses in only 0% to 16% of cases and persists in 14% to 58% of cases.[23,29,70] Furthermore, progression to adenocarcinoma has been reported in 0% to 23% of low-grade GEDs, during an interval of 10 months to 4 years. In contrast, the rate of malignant transformation for high-grade GED has been reported in 60% to 85% of the cases over an interval of 4 to 48 months.[29–31,33,71,72] More recent studies have confirmed a low risk of progression to cancer in patients with low-grade dysplasia (0%–9%) and reiterate a more severe risk of transformation for high-grade dysplasia (6%–100%).[3,4,72]

The reasons why, on average, no more than 10% of low-grade dysplasias progress to a higher grade or adenocarcinoma are poorly understood and may be manifold. First, some cases of low-grade dysplasia could be, in fact, misinterpreted as reactive atypia. Second, it is also possible that many dysplasias are biologically nonprogressive lesions. In fact, mutations in the mutation cluster region of the exon 15 of the APC gene appear to be the marker of nonprogressive dysplasia. In a series of non-FAP Korean patients, mutations in the mutation cluster region were found in 76% of adenomas/flat dysplasias without carcinoma and only in 3% of adenomas/flat dysplasias associated with carcinoma. Importantly, gastric adenocarcinomas also had a low rate of APC mutations (4%), suggesting that dysplastic lesions with APC mutations in the cluster region of exon 15 are not part of a pathway to cancer.[73] Supporting this view is the lack of significant increase in the risk of gastric cancer in patients with FAP in the United States, albeit it is increased in Japan.[74,75] Additionally, most FAP-associated adenomas do not progress over extended periods of surveillance (7 years),[26] and rare gastric cancers in patients with FAP have been reported only from Japan where gastric cancer is highly prevalent.[26,76] Also, dysplasia in fundic gland polyps, both sporadic and FAP-associated, has frequent somatic mutations in the APC gene but almost never progresses to carcinoma.[77,78] Rarely, high-grade dysplasia and adenocarcinoma arise in fundic gland polyps associated with an attenuated form of FAP.[79–83] Notably, attenuated FAP is associated with APC mutations involving the first four exons, the alternatively spliced region of exon 9, and the 3′ half of exon 15, but not the usual mutational cluster region.[84,85] Taken together, these observations suggest that GED with APC mutations in the mutational cluster region of exon 15 is not associated with progression to adenocarcinoma. However, gastric dysplastic lesions devoid of APC mutations and with or without microsatellite instability (MSI) behave differently and likely represent the precursor lesion of tubular adenocarcinoma.[73]

While the association of adenomatous or type I dysplasia with adenocarcinoma is not disputed, the significance of foveolar dysplasia continues to be discussed.[86] One line of evidence suggests that dysplastic lesions of foveolar type are low-grade lesions that are not associated with appreciable progression to adenocarcinoma.[41,86] Another study reported that foveolar dysplasia is often high grade, and more often than adenomatous dysplasia is associated with a second dysplastic lesion and adenocarcinoma.[36] The discrepancy may be due to evaluation of biologically distinct groups of lesions. While in the studies of Abraham et al.[86] and Chen et al.[41] foveolar dysplasias were associated with fundic gland polyps and FAP or with mild *H. pylori*–negative gastritis, in the study of Park et al.,[36] 40% of the lesions were depressed or flat, 60% were associated with *H. pylori*, and none were associated with FAP or fundic gland polyps. Notably, several Japanese studies also suggested an association of gastric phenotype with high-grade dysplasia based on mucin immunophenotype.[64,87]

MOLECULAR ABNORMALITIES IN GED

Most gastric adenocarcinomas develop as a result of a combination of predisposing environmental conditions and genetic and epigenetic abnormalities. Many of the molecular alterations are observed in gastric dysplasia, albeit with a lesser frequency. Chromosomal instability, MSI, and CpG-island methylation can be observed. Importantly, there are currently no immunohistochemical or molecular assays that can help stratify the risk of progression of gastric dysplastic lesions.

Chromosomal Instability

The APC gene is mutated in 20% to 76% of gastric dysplasias.[73,88–90] However, <10% of gastric carcinomas contain APC mutations, suggesting that these are not critical in gastric carcinogenesis.[91] On the contrary, p53 mutations are detected in 22% of high-grade dysplasias[64] and in 30% to 50% of gastric carcinomas consistent with their role in cancer progression.[58]

The role of K-ras mutations in gastric adenomas is debatable. Present in atrophic gastritis,[92,93] they are not found to predict progression to premalignant lesions.[94] In addition, several studies have failed to show a significant prevalence rate of K-ras mutations in either gastric adenomas or adenocarcinomas.[73,89,95,96]

Mutations of the beta-catenin gene were not identified in gastric adenomas.[73,88,97] However, abnormal nuclear accumulation is seen in 11% to 38% of adenomas, suggesting that dysregulation of the Wnt signaling pathway may be involved in the neoplastic process.[97]

Microsatellite Instability Phenotype

Gastric carcinomas may arise through inactivation of the DNA mismatch repair pathway, due to promoter hypermethylation and loss of expression of MLH1. Accumulating genomic mutations manifest as MSI, which increases with neoplastic progression.[98,99] MSI-high phenotype (MSI-H) may be present in up to 21% of gastric adenomas, equaling its frequency in tubular adenocarcinoma ("intestinal type"),[57,60,73,96,100] whereas it is uncommon in chronic gastritis and intestinal metaplasia.[101,102] Some authors have reported an association between MSI-H and high-grade dysplasia.[100] In a recent study, MSI was reported in 20% of dysplastic precursor lesions without associated carcinoma, again suggesting that it is an early event in gastric carcinogenesis.[103]

CpG-Island Methylation Phenotype

Aberrant DNA methylation of tumor-related genes is present in chronic gastritis and intestinal metaplasia, and an increasing frequency of methylated promoters is associated with histologically progressive lesions that lead to gastric adenocarcinoma.[104–106] Genes hypermethylated in gastric adenomas include, among others, those involved in cell cycle regulation (p14, p16, COX-2),[105–107] signal transduction (APC),[106] DNA repair (hMLH1 and MGMT),[105–107] and invasion and metastasis (E-cadherin and TIMP3).[105,106] The frequency of methylation of APC, E-cadherin, MGMT, and hMLH1 is not different between precursor lesions and cancers, indicating that these are potential early events in gastric carcinogenesis.[104,106] On the other hand, methylation of p16 is present in only 7% of intestinal metaplasias and 18% of adenomas but 29% of dysplasias/adenomas associated with adenocarcinomas, and 44% of adenocarcinomas, suggesting a role in both neoplastic and malignant transformation of gastric lesions.[107] Methylation of RUNX3, a recently recognized tumor suppressor gene for gastric cancer, appears to be important at later stages of carcinogenesis, since the rates of methylation are similar in intestinal metaplasia and gastric adenoma, but increase 2.3-fold in gastric cancer.[108] Concurrent promoter methylation in three or more genes among p16, Runx3, MGMT, and DAP-kinase was recently found in 11% of GED and in 31% of early gastric carcinoma, further attesting to the role of methylation in cancer progression.[109] Silencing of tumor suppressor gene TFF1/pS2 by promoter hypermethylation also has been implicated in gastric cancer,[110] and progressively reduced expression of pS2 has been shown in intestinal metaplasia and gastric dysplasia.[111]

MOLECULAR DIFFERENCES BETWEEN DYSPLASIAS OF ADENOMATOUS AND FOVEOLAR TYPE

Very few studies have addressed molecular differences between adenomatous and foveolar dysplasia. However, one study found no significant differences between gastric adenomas of intestinal and foveolar phenotypes for the presence of APC gene alterations, high-level MSI, and K-ras mutations.[88]

STEM CELL MODEL OF GASTRIC CARCINOGENESIS, GASTRIC ATROPHY, AND SONIC HEDGEHOG

Although cancer stem cells have been identified in many solid tumors, gastric cancer stem cells remain to be demonstrated.[112] Preliminary results suggest the existence of such cells, and gastric multipotential stem cells or lineage-restricted progenitor cells appear to be plausible candidates.[113,114] According to the cancer stem cell model of carcinogenesis, gastric dysplasia can be viewed as a process driven by stem cells or progenitor cells that gradually acquire features of cancer stem cells. The exact mechanism leading to acquisition of stem cell features is unclear; however, a basis for one explanatory model is abnormality of Sonic Hedgehog, a member of the family of Hedgehog proteins that are involved in regulation of patterning and growth in development. Sonic Hedgehog is expressed in parietal cells of corpus/fundic glands, and available evidence suggests that Sonic Hedgehog has an inhibitory effect on epithelial cells, restricting mucosal hyperplasia and gland branching.[115] Loss of Sonic Hedgehog expression has been reported in *H. pylori* atrophic gastritis.[116] It is hypothesized that reduced Sonic Hedgehog levels could result in increased proliferation and accumulation of undifferentiated progenitors, which then progress along the metaplasia-dysplasia-cancer pathway in the presence of chronic inflammation.[21,117,118]

MANAGEMENT OF GED

Current recommendations include local treatment with careful topographic mapping of the entire stomach, along with additional biopsies from any endoscopically visible abnormalities.[119] *H. pylori* eradication therapy is also recommended in these patients; however, the cancer risk, albeit decreased, is not eliminated completely if either atrophy or intestinal metaplasia is present at the time of the index endoscopy.[120,121]

Given the low rate of malignant transformation of low-grade dysplasia, annual endoscopic surveillance with rebiopsy is typically performed, and surgical resection is usually not necessary.[122] It must be also emphasized that low-grade dysplasia occurring in a background of extensive intestinal metaplasia may be associated with a higher risk of malignancy.[123] In patients indefinite for dysplasia, follow-up endoscopy and targeted biopsies are performed. Since most of these lesions are flat, techniques such as chromoendoscopy may be helpful.

Patients who have high-grade dysplasia (flat or polypoid) should undergo definitive therapy. Chromoendoscopy and endoscopic ultrasound are used widely to evaluate the extent and depth of these lesions. Complete excision of mucosal-based lesions may be performed by endoscopic mucosal resection or dissection, which in most cases obviates the need for surgical resection.[124,125]

References

1. Riddell RH, Goldman H, Ransohoff DF, et al. Dysplasia in inflammatory bowel disease: standardized classification with provisional clinical applications. *Hum Pathol.* 1983;14(11):931–968.

2. Oehlert W, Keller P, Henke M, et al. Gastric mucosal dysplasia: what is its clinical significance? *Front Gastrointest Res.* 1979;4:173–182.

3. Rugge M, Cassaro M, Di Mario F, et al. The long term outcome of gastric non-invasive neoplasia. *Gut.* 2003;52(8):1111–1116.

4. de Vries AC, van Grieken NC, Looman CW, et al. Gastric cancer risk in patients with premalignant gastric lesions: a nationwide cohort study in the Netherlands. *Gastroenterology.* 2008;134(4):945–952.

5. Uemura N, Okamoto S, Yamamoto S, et al. *Helicobacter pylori* infection and the development of gastric cancer. *N Engl J Med.* 2001;345(11):784–789.

6. Shibata D, Tokunaga M, Uemura Y, et al. Association of Epstein-Barr virus with undifferentiated gastric carcinomas with intense lymphoid infiltration. Lymphoepithelioma-like carcinoma. *Am J Pathol.* 1991;139(3):469–474.

7. Spigelman AD, Williams CB, Talbot IC, et al. Upper gastrointestinal cancer in patients with familial adenomatous polyposis. *Lancet.* 1989;2(8666):783–785.

8. Shinmura K, Goto M, Tao H, et al. A novel STK11 germline mutation in two siblings with Peutz-Jeghers syndrome complicated by primary gastric cancer. *Clin Genet.* 2005;67(1):81–86.

9. Kondo K. Duodenogastric reflux and gastric stump carcinoma. *Gastric Cancer.* 2002;5(1):16–22.

10. Wood MG, Bates C, Brown RC, et al. Intramucosal carcinoma of the gastric antrum complicating Menetrier's disease. *J Clin Pathol.* 1983;36(9):1071–1075.

11. Cai X, Carlson J, Stoicov C, et al. *Helicobacter felis* eradication restores normal architecture and inhibits gastric cancer progression in C57BL/6 mice. *Gastroenterology* 2005;128(7):1937–1952.

12. Takaishi S, Okumura T, Wang TC. Gastric cancer stem cells. *J Clin Oncol.* 2008;26(17):2876–2882.

13. Weis VG, Goldenring JR. Current understanding of SPEM and its standing in the preneoplastic process. *Gastric Cancer.* 2009;12(4):189–197.

14. El-Zimaity HM, Ota H, Graham DY, et al. Patterns of gastric atrophy in intestinal type gastric carcinoma. *Cancer.* 2002;94(5):1428–1436.

15. Schmidt PH, Lee JR, Joshi V, et al. Identification of a metaplastic cell lineage associated with human gastric adenocarcinoma. *Lab Invest.* 1999;79(6):639–646.

16. Yamaguchi H, Goldenring JR, Kaminishi M, et al. Identification of spasmolytic polypeptide expressing metaplasia (SPEM) in remnant gastric cancer and surveillance postgastrectomy biopsies. *Dig Dis Sci.* 2002;47(3):573–578.

17. Halldorsdottir AM, Sigurdardottrir M, Jonasson JG, et al. Spasmolytic polypeptide-expressing metaplasia (SPEM) associated with gastric cancer in Iceland. *Dig Dis Sci.* 2003;48(3):431–441.

18. Wang TC, Goldenring JR, Dangler C, et al. Mice lacking secretory phospholipase A2 show altered apoptosis and differentiation with *Helicobacter felis* infection. *Gastroenterology.* 1998;114(4):675–689.

19. Nomura S, Baxter T, Yamaguchi H, et al. Spasmolytic polypeptide expressing metaplasia to preneoplasia in *H. felis*-infected mice. *Gastroenterology.* 2004;127(2):582–594.

20. Goldenring JR, Nomura S. Differentiation of the gastric mucosa III. Animal models of oxyntic atrophy and metaplasia. *Am J Physiol Gastrointest Liver Physiol.* 2006;291(6):G999–G1004.

21. Fox JG, Wang TC. Inflammation, atrophy, and gastric cancer. *J Clin Invest.* 2007;117(1):60–69.

22. Farinati F, Rugge M, Di Mario F, et al. Early and advanced gastric cancer in the follow-up of moderate and severe gastric dysplasia patients. A prospective study. I.G.G.E.D.—Interdisciplinary Group on Gastric Epithelial Dysplasia. *Endoscopy.* 1993;25(4):261–264.

23. Bearzi I, Brancorsini D, Santinelli A, et al. Gastric dysplasia: a ten-year follow-up study. *Pathol Res Pract.* 1994;190(1):61–68.

24. Stockbrugger RW, Menon GG, Beilby JO, et al. Gastroscopic screening in 80 patients with pernicious anaemia. *Gut.* 1983;24(12):1141–1147.

25. Ye W, Nyren O. Risk of cancers of the oesophagus and stomach by histology or subsite in patients hospitalised for pernicious anaemia. *Gut.* 2003;52(7):938–941.

26. Iida M, Yao T, Itoh H, et al. Natural history of gastric adenomas in patients with familial adenomatosis coli/Gardner's syndrome. *Cancer.* 1988;61(3):605–611.

27. Domizio P, Talbot IC, Spigelman AD, et al. Upper gastrointestinal pathology in familial adenomatous polyposis: results from a prospective study of 102 patients. *J Clin Pathol*. 1990;43(9):738–743.

28. Bertoni G, Sassatelli R, Nigrisoli E, et al. Dysplastic changes in gastric fundic gland polyps of patients with familial adenomatous polyposis. *Ital J Gastroenterol Hepatol*. 1999;31(3):192–197.

29. Lansdown M, Quirke P, Dixon MF, et al. High grade dysplasia of the gastric mucosa: a marker for gastric carcinoma. *Gut*. 1990;31(9):977–983.

30. Di Gregorio C, Morandi P, Fante R, et al. Gastric dysplasia. Gastric dysplasia. A follow-up study. *Am J Gastroenterol*. 1993;88(10):1714–1719.

31. Rugge M, Farinati F, Di Mario F, et al. Gastric epithelial dysplasia: a prospective multicenter follow-up study from the Interdisciplinary Group on Gastric Epithelial Dysplasia. *Hum Pathol*. 1991;22(10):1002–1008.

32. You WC, Blot WJ, Li JY, et al. Precancerous gastric lesions in a population at high risk of stomach cancer. *Cancer Res*. 1993;53(6):1317–1321.

33. Saraga EP, Gardiol D, Costa J. Gastric dysplasia. A histological follow-up study. *Am J Surg Pathol*. 1987;11(10):788–796.

34. Lauwers GY, Riddell RH. Gastric epithelial dysplasia. *Gut*. 1999;45(5):784–790.

35. Goldstein NS, Lewin KJ. Gastric epithelial dysplasia and adenoma: historical review and histological criteria for grading. *Hum Pathol*. 1997;28(2):127–133.

36. Park do Y, Srivastava A, Kim GH, et al. Adenomatous and foveolar gastric dysplasia: distinct patterns of mucin expression and background intestinal metaplasia. *Am J Surg Pathol*. 2008;32(4):524–533.

37. Park do Y, Srivastava A, Kim GH, et al. CDX2 expression in the intestinal-type gastric epithelial neoplasia: frequency and significance. *Mod Pathol*. 2010;23(1):54–61.

38. Jass JR. A classification of gastric dysplasia. *Histopathology*. 1983;7(2):181–193.

39. Rugge M, Correa P, Dixon MF, et al. Gastric dysplasia: the Padova international classification. *Am J Surg Pathol*. 2000;24(2):167–176.

40. Murayama H, Kikuchi M, Enjoji M, et al. Changes in gastric mucosa that antedate gastric carcinoma. *Cancer*. 1990;66(9):2017–2026.

41. Chen ZM, Scudiere JR, Abraham SC, et al. Pyloric gland adenoma: an entity distinct from gastric foveolar type adenoma. *Am J Surg Pathol*. 2009;33(2):186–193.

42. Ghandur-Mnaymneh L, Paz J, Roldan E, et al. Dysplasia of nonmetaplastic gastric mucosa. A proposal for its classification and its possible relationship to diffuse-type gastric carcinoma. *Am J Surg Pathol*. 1988;12(2):96–114.

43. Kumarasinghe MP, Lim TK, Ooi CJ, et al. Tubule neck dysplasia: precursor lesion of signet ring cell carcinoma and the immunohistochemical profile. *Pathology*. 2006;38(5):468–471.

44. Guilford P, Hopkins J, Harraway J, et al. E-cadherin germline mutations in familial gastric cancer. *Nature*. 1998;392(6674):402–405.

45. Carneiro F, Huntsman DG, Smyrk TC, et al. Model of the early development of diffuse gastric cancer in E-cadherin mutation carriers and its implications for patient screening. *J Pathol*. 2004;203(2):681–687.

46. Lynch HT, Grady W, Suriano G, Huntsman D. Gastric cancer: new genetic developments. *J Surg Oncol*. 2005;90(3):114–133; discussion 133.

47. Charlton A, Blair V, Shaw D, Parry S, et al. Hereditary diffuse gastric cancer: predominance of multiple foci of signet ring cell carcinoma in distal stomach and transitional zone. *Gut*. 2004;53(6):814–820.

48. Rogers WM, Dobo E, Norton JA, et al. Risk-reducing total gastrectomy for germline mutations in E-cadherin (CDH1): pathologic findings with clinical implications. *Am J Surg Pathol*. 2008;32(6):799–809.

49. Oliveira C, Seruca R, Carneiro F. Hereditary gastric cancer. *Best Pract Res Clin Gastroenterol*. 2009;23(2):147–157.

50. Kamiya T, Morishita T, Asakura H, et al. Histoclinical long-standing follow-up study of hyperplastic polyps of the stomach. *Am J Gastroenterol*. 1981;75(4):275–281.

51. Hattori T. Morphological range of hyperplastic polyps and carcinomas arising in hyperplastic polyps of the stomach. *J Clin Pathol*. 1985;38(6):622–630.

52. Wu TT, Kornacki S, Rashid A, et al. Dysplasia and dysregulation of proliferation in foveolar and surface epithelia of fundic gland polyps from patients with familial adenomatous polyposis. *Am J Surg Pathol*. 1998;22(3):293–298.

53. Snover DC. Benign epithelial polyps of the stomach. *Pathol Annu*. 1985;20 Pt 1:303–329.

54. Utsunomiya J, Maki T, Iwama T, et al. Gastric lesion of familial polyposis coli. *Cancer*. 1974;34(3):745–754.

55. Subramony C, Scott-Conner CE, Skelton D, et al. Familial juvenile polyposis. Study of a kindred: evolution of polyps and relationship to gastrointestinal carcinoma. *Am J Clin Pathol.* 1994;102(1):91–97.

56. Brito MJ, Williams GT, Thompson H, et al. Expression of p53 in early (T1) gastric carcinoma and precancerous adjacent mucosa. *Gut.* 1994;35(12):1697–1700.

57. Chang MS, Kim HS, Kim CW, et al. Epstein-Barr virus, p53 protein, and microsatellite instability in the adenoma-carcinoma sequence of the stomach. *Hum Pathol.* 2002;33(4):415–420.

58. Feng CW, Wang LD, Jiao LH, et al. Expression of p53, inducible nitric oxide synthase and vascular endothelial growth factor in gastric precancerous and cancerous lesions: correlation with clinical features. *BMC Cancer.* 2002;2:8.

59. Lauwers GY, Wahl SJ, Melamed J, et al. p53 expression in precancerous gastric lesions: an immunohistochemical study of PAb 1801 monoclonal antibody on adenomatous and hyperplastic gastric polyps. *Am J Gastroenterol.* 1993;88(11):1916–1919.

60. Nogueira AM, Carneiro F, Seruca R, et al. Microsatellite instability in hyperplastic and adenomatous polyps of the stomach. *Cancer.* 1999;86(9):1649–1656.

61. Rugge M, Shiao YH, Correa P, et al. Immunohistochemical evidence of p53 overexpression in gastric epithelial dysplasia. *Cancer Epidemiol Biomarkers Prev.* 1992;1(7):551–554.

62. Shiao YH, Rugge M, Correa P, et al. p53 alteration in gastric precancerous lesions. *Am J Pathol.* 1994;144(3):511–517.

63. Joypaul BV, Newman EL, Hopwood D, et al. Expression of p53 protein in normal, dysplastic, and malignant gastric mucosa: an immunohistochemical study. *J Pathol.* 1993;170(3):279–283.

64. Jin Z, Tamura G, Honda T, et al. Molecular and cellular phenotypic profiles of gastric noninvasive neoplasia. *Lab Invest.* 2002;82(12):1637–1645.

65. Anagnostopoulos GK, Stefanou D, Arkoumani E, et al. Immunohistochemical expression of cell-cycle proteins in gastric precancerous lesions. *J Gastroenterol Hepatol.* 2008;23(4):626–631.

66. Lisovsky M, Dresser K, Baker S, et al. Cell polarity protein Lgl2 is lost or aberrantly localized in gastric dysplasia and adenocarcinoma: an immunohistochemical study. *Mod Pathol.* 2009;22(7):977–984.

67. Stolte M. The new Vienna classification of epithelial neoplasia of the gastrointestinal tract: advantages and disadvantages. *Virchows Arch.* 2003;442(2):99–106.

68. Hamilton S AL, eds. *Pathology and genetics of tumors of the digestive system.* Lyon: IARC Press; 2000.

69. Whiting JL, Sigurdsson A, Rowlands DC, et al. The long term results of endoscopic surveillance of premalignant gastric lesions. *Gut.* 2002;50(3):378–381.

70. Burke AP, Sobin LH, Shekitka KM, et al. Dysplasia of the stomach and Barrett esophagus: a follow-up study. *Mod Pathol.* 1991;4(3):336–341.

71. Fertitta AM, Comin U, Terruzzi V, et al. Clinical significance of gastric dysplasia: a multicenter follow-up study. Gastrointestinal Endoscopic Pathology Study Group. *Endoscopy.* 1993;25(4):265–268.

72. Yamada H, Ikegami M, Shimoda T, et al. Long-term follow-up study of gastric adenoma/dysplasia. *Endoscopy.* 2004;36(5):390–396.

73. Lee JH, Abraham SC, Kim HS, et al. Inverse relationship between APC gene mutation in gastric adenomas and development of adenocarcinoma. *Am J Pathol.* 2002;161(2):611–618.

74. Offerhaus GJ, Giardiello FM, Krush AJ, et al. The risk of upper gastrointestinal cancer in familial adenomatous polyposis. *Gastroenterology.* 1992;102(6):1980–1982.

75. Iwama T, Mishima Y, Utsunomiya J. The impact of familial adenomatous polyposis on the tumorigenesis and mortality at the several organs. Its rational treatment. *Ann Surg.* 1993;217(2):101–108.

76. Watanabe H, Enjoji M, Yao T, et al. Gastric lesions in familial adenomatosis coli: their incidence and histologic analysis. *Hum Pathol.* 1978;9(3):269–283.

77. Abraham SC, Park SJ, Mugartegui L, et al. Sporadic fundic gland polyps with epithelial dysplasia: evidence for preferential targeting for mutations in the adenomatous polyposis coli gene. *Am J Pathol.* 2002;161(5):1735–1742.

78. Bianchi LK, Burke CA, Bennett AE, et al. Fundic gland polyp dysplasia is common in familial adenomatous polyposis. *Clin Gastroenterol Hepatol.* 2008;6(2):180–185.

79. Garrean S, Hering J, Saied A, et al. Gastric adenocarcinoma arising from fundic gland polyps in a patient with familial adenomatous polyposis syndrome. *Am Surg.* 2008;74(1):79–83.

80. Ong ES, Alassas MA, Bogner PN, et al. Total gastrectomy for gastric dysplasia in a patient with attenuated familial adenomatous polyposis syndrome. *J Clin Oncol.* 2008;26(21):3641–3642.

81. Attard TM, Giardiello FM, Argani P, et al. Fundic gland polyposis with high-grade dysplasia in a child with attenuated familial adenomatous polyposis and familial gastric cancer. *J Pediatr Gastroenterol Nutr.* 2001;32(2):215–218.

82. Hofgartner WT, Thorp M, Ramus MW, et al. Gastric adenocarcinoma associated with fundic gland polyps in a patient with attenuated familial adenomatous polyposis. *Am J Gastroenterol.* 1999;94(8): 2275–2281.

83. Zwick A, Munir M, Ryan CK, et al. Gastric adenocarcinoma and dysplasia in fundic gland polyps of a patient with attenuated adenomatous polyposis coli. *Gastroenterology.* 1997;113(2):659–663.

84. van der Luijt RB, Meera Khan P, Vasen HF, et al. Germline mutations in the 3′ part of APC exon 15 do not result in truncated proteins and are associated with attenuated adenomatous polyposis coli. *Hum Genet.* 1996;98(6):727–734.

85. Su LK, Kohlmann W, Ward PA, et al. Different familial adenomatous polyposis phenotypes resulting from deletions of the entire APC exon 15. *Hum Genet.* 2002;111(1):88–95.

86. Abraham SC, Montgomery EA, Singh VK, et al. Gastric adenomas: intestinal-type and gastric-type adenomas differ in the risk of adenocarcinoma and presence of background mucosal pathology. *Am J Surg Pathol.* 2002;26(10):1276–1285.

87. Tsukashita S, Kushima R, Bamba M, et al. MUC gene expression and histogenesis of adenocarcinoma of the stomach. *Int J Cancer.* 2001;94(2):166–170.

88. Abraham SC, Park SJ, Lee JH, et al. Genetic alterations in gastric adenomas of intestinal and foveolar phenotypes. *Mod Pathol.* 2003;16(8):786–795.

89. Maesawa C, Tamura G, Suzuki Y, et al. The sequential accumulation of genetic alterations characteristic of the colorectal adenoma-carcinoma sequence does not occur between gastric adenoma and adenocarcinoma. *J Pathol.* 1995;176(3):249–258.

90. Sanz-Ortega J, Sanz-Esponera J, Caldes T, et al. LOH at the APC/MCC gene (5Q21) in gastric cancer and preoplastic lesions. Prognostic implications. *Pathol Res Pract.* 1996.;192(12):1206–1210.

91. Endoh Y, Sakata K, Tamura G, et al. Cellular phenotypes of differentiated-type adenocarcinomas and precancerous lesions of the stomach are dependent on the genetic pathways. *J Pathol.* 2000;191(3): 257–263.

92. Gong C, Mera R, Bravo JC, et al. KRAS mutations predict progression of preneoplastic gastric lesions. *Cancer Epidemiol Biomarkers Prev.* 1999;8(2):167–171.

93. Hiyama T, Haruma K, Kitadai Y, et al. K-ras mutation in *Helicobacter pylori*-associated chronic gastritis in patients with and without gastric cancer. *Int J Cancer.* 2002;97(5):562–566.

94. Hunt JD, Mera R, Strimas A, et al. KRAS mutations are not predictive for progression of preneoplastic gastric lesions. *Cancer Epidemiol Biomarkers Prev.* 2001;10(1):79–80.

95. Koshiba M, Ogawa O, Habuchi T, et al. Infrequent ras mutation in human stomach cancers. *Jpn J Cancer Res.* 1993;84(2):163–167.

96. Isogaki J, Shinmura K, Yin W, et al. Microsatellite instability and K-ras mutations in gastric adenomas, with reference to associated gastric cancers. *Cancer Detect Prev.* 1999;23(3):204–214.

97. Kim HS, Hong EK, Park SY, et al. Expression of beta-catenin and E-cadherin in the adenoma-carcinoma sequence of the stomach. *Anticancer Res.* 2003;23(3C):2863–2868.

98. Baek MJ, Kang H, Kim SE, et al. Expression of hMLH1 is inactivated in the gastric adenomas with enhanced microsatellite instability. *Br J Cancer.* 2001;85(8):1147–1152.

99. Fleisher AS, Esteller M, Tamura G, et al. Hypermethylation of the hMLH1 gene promoter is associated with microsatellite instability in early human gastric neoplasia. *Oncogene.* 2001;20(3):329–335.

100. Kim JJ, Baek MJ, Kim L, et al. Accumulated frameshift mutations at coding nucleotide repeats during the progression of gastric carcinoma with microsatellite instability. *Lab Invest.* 1999;79(9): 1113–1120.

101. Leung WK, Kim JJ, Kim JG, et al. Microsatellite instability in gastric intestinal metaplasia in patients with and without gastric cancer. *Am J Pathol.* 2000;156(2):537–543.

102. Kashiwagi K, Watanabe M, Ezaki T, et al. Clinical usefulness of microsatellite instability for the prediction of gastric adenoma or adenocarcinoma in patients with chronic gastritis. *Br J Cancer.* 2000;82(11):1814–1818.

103. Rugge M, Bersani G, Bertorelle R, et al. Microsatellite instability and gastric non-invasive neoplasia in a high risk population in Cesena, Italy. *J Clin Pathol.* 2005;58(8):805–810.

104. To KF, Leung WK, Lee TL, et al. Promoter hypermethylation of tumor-related genes in gastric intestinal metaplasia of patients with and without gastric cancer. *Int J Cancer.* 2002;102(6):623–628.

105. Kang GH, Shim YH, Jung HY, et al. CpG island methylation in premalignant stages of gastric carcinoma. *Cancer Res.* 2001;61(7):2847–2851.

106. Kang GH, Lee S, Kim JS, et al. Profile of aberrant CpG island methylation along the multistep pathway of gastric carcinogenesis. *Lab Invest.* 2003;83(5):635–641.

107. Lee JH, Park SJ, Abraham SC, et al. Frequent CpG island methylation in precursor lesions and early gastric adenocarcinomas. *Oncogene.* 2004;23(26):4646–4654.

108. Kim TY, Lee HJ, Hwang KS, et al. Methylation of RUNX3 in various types of human cancers and premalignant stages of gastric carcinoma. *Lab Invest.* 2004;84(4):479–484.

109. Zou XP, Zhang B, Zhang XQ, et al. Promoter hypermethylation of multiple genes in early gastric adenocarcinoma and precancerous lesions. *Hum Pathol.* 2009;40(11):1534–1542.

110. Kirikoshi H, Katoh M. Expression of TFF1, TFF2 and TFF3 in gastric cancer. *Int J Oncol.* 2002;21(3): 655–659.

111. Taupin D, Pedersen J, Familari M, et al. Augmented intestinal trefoil factor (TFF3) and loss of pS2 (TFF1) expression precedes metaplastic differentiation of gastric epithelium. *Lab Invest.* 2001;81(3): 397–408.

112. Lobo NA, Shimono Y, Qian D, et al. The biology of cancer stem cells. *Annu Rev Cell Dev Biol.* 2007;23:675–699.

113. Takaishi S, Okumura T, Tu S, et al. Identification of gastric cancer stem cells using the cell surface marker CD44. *Stem Cells.* 2009;27(5):1006–1020.

114. Bjerknes M, Cheng H. Multipotential stem cells in adult mouse gastric epithelium. *Am J Physiol Gastrointest Liver Physiol.* 2002;283(3):G767–G777.

115. van den Brink GR. Hedgehog signaling in development and homeostasis of the gastrointestinal tract. *Physiol Rev.* 2007;87(4):1343–1375.

116. Shiotani A, Iishi H, Uedo N, et al. Evidence that loss of sonic hedgehog is an indicator of *Helicobacter pylori*-induced atrophic gastritis progressing to gastric cancer. *Am J Gastroenterol.* 2005;100(3): 581–587.

117. Xiao C, Ogle SA, Schumacher MA, et al. Loss of parietal cell expression of Sonic hedgehog induces hypergastrinemia and hyperproliferation of surface mucous cells. *Gastroenterology.* 2010;138(2): 550–561, 561e1–561e8.

118. Waghray M, Zavros Y, Saqui-Salces M, et al. Interleukin 1 beta promotes gastric atrophy through suppression of Sonic Hedgehog. *Gastroenterology.* 2010;138(2):562–572, 572e1–572e2.

119. Hirota WK, Zuckerman MJ, Adler DG, et al. ASGE guideline: the role of endoscopy in the surveillance of premalignant conditions of the upper GI tract. *Gastrointest Endosc.* 2006;63(4):570–580.

120. You WC, Brown LM, Zhang L, et al. Randomized double-blind factorial trial of three treatments to reduce the prevalence of precancerous gastric lesions. *J Natl Cancer Inst.* 2006;98(14):974–983.

121. Leung WK, Lin SR, Ching JY, et al. Factors predicting progression of gastric intestinal metaplasia: results of a randomised trial on *Helicobacter pylori* eradication. *Gut.* 2004;53(9):1244–1249.

122. Rugge M, Nitti D, Farinati F, et al. Non-invasive neoplasia of the stomach. *Eur J Gastroenterol Hepatol.* 2005;17(11):1191–1196.

123. Rugge M, Leandro G, Farinati F, et al. Gastric epithelial dysplasia. How clinicopathologic background relates to management. *Cancer.* 1995;76(3):376–382.

124. Jang JS, Choi SR, Qureshi W, et al. Long-term outcomes of endoscopic submucosal dissection in gastric neoplastic lesions at a single institution in South Korea. *Scand J Gastroenterol.* 2009;44(11): 1315–1322.

125. Nakajima T. Gastric cancer treatment guidelines in Japan. *Gastric Cancer.* 2002;5(1):1–5.

Index